Dynamic Consultations with Psychiatrists

Dynamic Consultations with Psychiatrists

Understanding Severely Troubled Patients

Jason Maratos

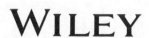

This edition first published 2022
© 2022 John Wiley & Sons Ltd

The right of Jason Maratos to be identified as the author of this work has been asserted in accordance with law.

Registered Office
John Wiley & Sons, Inc., 111 River Street, Hoboken, NJ 07030, USA
John Wiley & Sons Ltd, The Atrium, Southern Gate, Chichester, West Sussex, PO19 8SQ, UK

Editorial Office
9600 Garsington Road, Oxford, OX4 2DQ, UK

For details of our global editorial offices, customer services, and more information about Wiley products visit us at www. wiley.com.

Wiley also publishes its books in a variety of electronic formats and by print-on-demand. Some content that appears in standard print versions of this book may not be available in other formats.

Limit of Liability/Disclaimer of Warranty
The contents of this work are intended to further general scientific research, understanding, and discussion only and are not intended and should not be relied upon as recommending or promoting scientific method, diagnosis, or treatment by physicians for any particular patient. In view of ongoing research, equipment modifications, changes in governmental regulations, and the constant flow of information relating to the use of medicines, equipment, and devices, the reader is urged to review and evaluate the information provided in the package insert or instructions for each medicine, equipment, or device for, among other things, any changes in the instructions or indication of usage and for added warnings and precautions. While the publisher and authors have used their best efforts in preparing this work, they make no representations or warranties with respect to the accuracy or completeness of the contents of this work and specifically disclaim all warranties, including without limitation any implied warranties of merchantability or fitness for a particular purpose. No warranty may be created or extended by sales representatives, written sales materials or promotional statements for this work. The fact that an organization, website, or product is referred to in this work as a citation and/or potential source of further information does not mean that the publisher and authors endorse the information or services the organization, website, or product may provide or recommendations it may make. This work is sold with the understanding that the publisher is not engaged in rendering professional services. The advice and strategies contained herein may not be suitable for your situation. You should consult with a specialist where appropriate. Further, readers should be aware that websites listed in this work may have changed or disappeared between when this work was written and when it is read. Neither the publisher nor authors shall be liable for any loss of profit or any other commercial damages, including but not limited to special, incidental, consequential, or other damages.

Library of Congress Cataloging-in-Publication Data applied for

Paperback ISBN: 9781119900504

Cover Design: Wiley
Cover Images: © Ken Welsh/Alamy Stock Photo

Set in 11/13.5 pt and SabonLTStd by Straive, Pondicherry, India

Printed and bound by CPI Group (UK) Ltd, Croydon, CR0 4YY

C122098_130622

Contents

Introduction

This publication developed from a collaboration across more than 10 years between hospital psychiatrists and JM. JM's contact with these psychiatrists started with a series of *interprofessional consultations*. JM was invited to conduct an educational event in their country twice. The first was on the introduction of Group Analysis and the second was a comparison between Group and Individual analyses.

The consultation sessions were often referred to as "supervision sessions," but this was a misnomer. JM was not in a position to supervise the work of any doctor working in a different setting and, more so, in a different country. JM had no wish to intervene in the hierarchy that has to exist in a well-functioning hospital with the inevitable lines of accountability and responsibility. Furthermore, supervision would be against the ethos of arriving at a new insight via *collaboration* of professionals of varying experiences in different fields. For example, the doctors in training were more aware of the culture of their patients and often taught consultant (JM) quite bit but who was also not ignorant of their culture and history. The consultations were meant to be and were, indeed, a two-way process. JM feels that he benefited from the process at least as much as the consultees.

A local doctor took the initiative to organize this series of consultations that would be available to psychiatrists in training at their hospital. Successors in her role took up the torch with enthusiasm. In this way, consultations between hospital trainees and JM were established monthly and were conducted via video conferencing.

The hospital's ethical committee approved the project. The hospital authority insisted that extra care be taken to preserve patient confidentiality. No case was discussed without the patient's consent. Furthermore, the names of patients were fictitious, the names of doctors and of hospitals were withheld, and any reference to the country was deleted.

JM was impressed by the high standard of practice at the hospital, by the receptiveness of the trainees to analytical concepts, and by their willingness to learn from the experience. It is a credit to all participants that, over the years, only one or two consultations were canceled, and these were for good reasons. The coronavirus disease 2019 (COVID-19) pandemic was an unavoidable interruption. The trainees were not able to meet as a group because of the risk of increasing the transmission of the virus. Due to the commitment of the doctors, a Zoom account was established, and the meetings restarted with each participant engaging via their own terminal.

Dynamic Consultations with Psychiatrists: Understanding Severely Troubled Patients, First Edition. Jason Maratos.
© 2022 John Wiley & Sons Ltd. Published 2022 by John Wiley & Sons Ltd.

It was thought that many other psychiatrists, who are expected to treat traumatized and disturbed patients, could benefit from the study of the history of such cases and the consultation that followed if they had access to a transcript of these consultations.

The doctors started submitting the text of their presentations in a standardized format. We thought that a full and proper exposition (according to the Maudsley Hospital standard) would take too much space and time and should be sacrificed for the sake of a more focused, reader-friendly, and less time-consuming presentation. Each presented case is of a person with a dysfunction on the severe end of the spectrum. The aim of the consultations was not to offer or get patients to engage in psycho-analysis or other form of dynamic psychotherapy but to use analytical concepts to gain a deeper understanding of the patients' "disorder" and to adjust, through this understanding, their psychiatric management. Being aware of the possibility of development of an antagonism between approaches, JM was particularly mindful to make sure that the consultations are seen as **complementary** to the treatment provided by the hospital and the services of that country as a whole. There is no implication that one approach is "better" or more suitable than the other.

The presentation of each case, and particularly of the consultation, is meant to demonstrate the process by which insights were gained. The consultation was audio-recorded, and JM, based on this recording, dictated the content aiming to preserve the interaction that led to the gained insights. Searching for more details of this therapeutic interaction is part of this process and should not be seen as criticism of the material presented by the trainee. JM has not forgotten his days as a trainee, the stressfulness of encountering a new patient in crisis, and of having to come up with a helpful measure that would make a difference. JM is still practicing and knows that the work of a practicing clinician does not always permit perfection but always demands a helpful conclusion.

The consultation is written in plain English with deliberately avoiding terminology, especially that of psychoanalytic jargon. In the consultations, the reader may detect the presence of the psychoanalyt-ical concepts even though reference to them is descriptive and using language understood by all mental health professionals. There are several reasons for avoiding terminology; at first, jargon often leads to misunderstandings and, second, makes the flow of reading harder to those not familiar with it. If ter-minology were to be included, it would make the text incomprehensible for those who it is written. A particular effort is made to explain what is meant by the occasional inevitable use of terminology.

We are grateful that the appropriate ethical committee approved the recording of the consultations with a view to publication. Naturally, all identified features of the patients have been deleted or changed so that patients' privacy is not compromised. The author is grateful to the hospital for agree-ing to fund this series of educational events consistently over many years. We are encouraged by the fact that only few patients withheld their permission, and we, naturally, have respected their wishes and have made no mention of them in this book.

The structure of the book is not according to a diagnosis but according to "presenting problem" or to the most prominent feature. Presenting problem in this context is the first impression that the doc-tors formed on either being referred the patient or on seeing them. Presenting problem is not meant to replace "diagnosis," which is important in a different context. Indeed some cases could be allo-cated to different diagnostic groups. The philosophy of this book is to present how a doctor is faced with a patient who is suffering in their own particular way and gradually, after a painstaking process, the clinician gets to develop a deeper understanding of their predicament. The doctor will try to make sense of the patient's present state in the context of their personal history, present family situation, intimate relationships, work situation, understanding of their future, and the cultural context (histor-ical and contemporary) in which they live. The sections of this book do not correspond to any diag-nostic category, although diagnoses are inevitably in the author's mind and are occasionally mentioned in the text.

The reader of this book will gain a sense of the wide range of difficulties doctors encounter and the challenges they face both in their personal emotional well-being and in their relationships with the other professionals (seniors of the same discipline and those of other disciplines, such as psychology, nursing, and the various therapies) both within their hospital and also with other agencies.

The ordering of the sections is arbitrary and does not imply order of severity or importance. The doctors have presented some but few patients with psychosis, though they have presented patients with psychotic and borderline symptomatology. The author has not engaged in an exhaustive consideration of the "right" diagnosis nor has he entered in the extensive professional dialogue (which justifiably exists) about the epistemological standing of various diagnostic categories, such as that of Borderline Personality Disorder. Where appropriate, mention of "borderline features" has been made.

The reader may feel that some of the details in the histories is redundant. They may be right, but the histories are included that so that there is a seamless exposition, as much as possible, of how the conclusions of the consultation have been reached. The author hopes that the readers of this book will feel that they become part of the journey that the consultation process represents and may be able to use similar activities in their own work setting.

Although this work has been developed with hospital psychiatrists, other mental health professionals such as psychologists, mental health nurses, occupational therapists, and social workers may find it useful because it is and, more so, as a prompt to develop similar activities in their work setting.

Jason Maratos

Section I

Affective Presentations

1
Depression

Ms. A

Introduction

Ms. A is a 60-year-old woman, divorced housewife, and living with her daughter in her 30s, her son-in-law, and two grandsons (5 and 10 years old). Her eldest son and her youngest daughter, both in their 30s, live separately from her.

History of Present Illness

Ms. A met her ex-husband in the city; he is a distant relative, 10 years her senior, working as restaurant staff. They were married in her early 20s after a courtship of 1 year. Her first two pregnancies were planned, whereas the third pregnancy was unplanned but wanted. There were no immediate postpartum depressive episodes. She found that her ex-husband became aloof after the birth of their children; he supported the family financially but did not attend to his wife or their children, including the puerperal periods. He spent most of his time playing with birds (keeping birds as pets), gambling, and horse racing after work. There was no physical violence, but there was verbal aggression.

Ms. A's mood deteriorated from the age of 26; she had frequent crying spells. Ms. A found it hard to cope with the care of three children on her own because there was no local relative or friend to support her. She feared any stepmother might maltreat her daughters if she divorced and her husband remarried. Ms. A feared that her own experience of being brought up may have been reenacted. She had decided to leave her husband when her elder daughter reached the age of 18.

Ms. A's low mood was associated with initial and middle insomnia, fatigue, and fleeting suicidal ideas of jumping onto rail tracks but there were no suicidal attempts. Her major hope was from caring and obedient children when they were small. At times, she experienced free-floating anxiety, dyspepsia, chest tightness, and shortness of breath. She visited a general practitioner. She was prescribed a hypnotic, which was useful only for the initial period.

Dynamic Consultations with Psychiatrists: Understanding Severely Troubled Patients, First Edition. Jason Maratos.
© 2022 John Wiley & Sons Ltd. Published 2022 by John Wiley & Sons Ltd.

Early in her 40s, when her elder daughter reached the age of 18, she decided to divorce, and she was awarded custody of her younger daughter'. Ms. A could not afford raising her, and eventually, her younger daughter lived with ex-husband while the other 2 children lived apart from her and from each other (one married and one living with a partner). Ms. A rented a room on her own and worked as a server. Ms. A was expecting her mood to improve on leaving her husband, but it did not. Ms. A was feeling guilty about leaving her youngest daughter (aged 12). This was not described excessive guilt. She was unable to work after a wrist injury, which she suffered while on duty, because she could not lift loads.

Her general practitioner referred ger and she has been known to psychiatric services since she was 42 years old (in 1998). She was diagnosed with dysthymia and was prescribed Deanxit, trazodone, and promethazine. Her sleep had improved only slightly.

Ms. A lived with elder daughter's family in the last 10 years since her daughter became pregnant. She claimed that she had a good relationship with her daughter. Her mood improved when she started to look after her grandsons, but she never reached complete remission. She was later referred to the family medicine clinic in 2009. She had defaulted follow-up in 2014 because she felt that the contact was not useful.

In the past 2 years, her mood deteriorated because her daughter was annoyed by what she considered to be an overinvolvement in childcare. For example, Ms. A repeatedly asked her daughter not to punish her children. She asked her daughter to prevent the children from making mistakes rather than letting them have a try. Ms. A also blamed her daughter for failing to correct the children when they did not follow Ms. A's commands.

Ms. A's mood deteriorated again. She developed crying spells, insomnia with poor sleep, and fatigue. She lacked daytime engagement. Her memory and concentration worsened; for example, she would forget to turn off the stove at times. She would ask "Why was it not me?" when watching news on fatal car accidents. Four months before admission, Ms. A expressed her intention to return to live alone in her hometown the following year. Her daughter responded, "you can go anytime you like." She was distressed by this response and developed fleeting suicidal ideas of dying by burning charcoal. However, she did not purchase charcoal when she saw it at a supermarket.

She was referred from the "positive ageing center" to the family medicine clinic. She had tried escitalopram 5 mg nightly when she waited for psychiatric reactivation. Her sleep remained poor with frequent dreams and sleep-talking. She also complained of constipation and dry eyes. She went to the emergency department under clinical advice in view of suicidal ideas and was admitted to a psychiatric unit.

Family History

Her youngest daughter suffered from depression.

Personal History

Ms. A was born in her hometown and was the second of four siblings. Her parents sold her to another family when she was 1 year old. This was attributed to poverty. She was illiterate. The "mother" in the "owning" family often scolded her and instructed her to care for the other "siblings." There is no history of physical abuse. The "father" looked after her and allowed her to leave the family at 20 years of age. Ms. A then migrated illegally to the city. She was a nonsmoker and nondrinker. She had no history of substance abuse or a forensic record.

Past Medical History

Ms. A had no significant medical problems (menopause at 50 years old).

Premorbid Personality

Ms. A described herself as rigid with absolute beliefs about what "right and wrong" are. She adopted avoidance as a coping mechanism.

Mental State Examination

Ms. A appeared not sophisticated but was tidy and established good contact with staff. She was dysthymic with appropriate affect. Her speech was coherent and relevant, with normal tempo and soft voice. She had difficulties in articulating her worries and frustrations. She was preoccupied with her daughter's negative responses. She thought of leaving her daughter as an escape from stress. Somatic complaints were present. She had no active suicidal ideas or psychotic features. Her insight was partial: She actively sought help for mood, sleep, and memory problems.

Physical examination and investigations were unremarkable.

Impression

The impression was that Ms. A suffered from depression of moderate severity with somatic complaints, related to relationship problems with daughters, over a background of dysthymia, and prominent sleep disturbance.

Management

The treatment involved medication (mirtazapine and clonazepam for mood and insomnia); referral to psychologist for cognitive behavioral therapy (CBT) for depression and insomnia and referral to occupational therapist for daytime engagement and cognitive assessment.

Progress

Ms. A's mood improved quickly after admission. Mirtazapine was titrated to 30 mg nightly. Clonazepam 0.5 mg nightly was also given. Pregabalin was added for restless leg syndrome related to mirtazapine and clonazepam. Ms. A had a good response to mirtazapine and refused to switch to an alternative antidepressant. She enjoyed when her family visited her. Sleep improved from 3 to 5 hours per night with structured routine, good sleep hygiene, and medication.

Ms. A wanted to live in her hometown for a short while and wait there for a singleton public housing unit to become available. Ms. A felt that living separately would prevent any conflict developing with her daughter. She was encouraged to develop leisure activities and participate in social gatherings. During discussion on postdischarge life, she often claimed sleep was still suboptimal and requested further hospital stay.

After the first discharge from hospital, Ms. A had repeated admissions for suicidal thoughts when she was feeling that she was being abandoned by her family. She still had insomnia with poor sleep hygiene. She continued to lack any daytime engagement, and this was more so when grandchildren grew up and did not need much of her care.

Consultation

JM thanked the doctor for the full presentation, but in view of the limited information available for Ms. A's early life history, he asked the doctor to clarify if there were any more data about this important period in her life. The doctor responded that Ms. A was reluctant to talk about that period in her life. Ms. A remembered "repeated scolding" but denied any abuse—physical or sexual. Ms. A spent most of that time looking after the young "siblings" of that family. JM invited the doctor to give some more information about this woman's experience of living with this family, such as "what was it like being adopted?" The doctor clarified that her state was not one of adoption; she was expected to work for the family in return for meals and shelter. Later, the doctor explained that Ms. A had described her experience as a form of emotional "torture" and had explained that the "mother" treated her as a maid and not as a family member.

JM asked if this was slavery and the doctor responded that Ms. A perceived it this way. She further perceived that she lacked parental care and that her childhood was deprived. JM inquired if she was educated, and the doctor replied that she was not allowed to go to school, and the family did not spend any money on her education. JM asked about her status as a worker and if from the age of 1 she was an unpaid worker for this family and if the deprivation of education was common at that time in such villages in her home area. The doctor responded that she was an unpaid worker and the absence of education was common in many poor families at that time in similar villages.

JM asked the doctor to clarify what Ms. A's perception of growing up would be. Would she see herself as having a similar life experience as the other children in her "bought-in" family? Did the other children receive education? The doctor responded that she would see herself as disadvantaged because the other children did receive education. Ms. A. often "grumbled" that her biological siblings received better care that she did. She knew who her biological family was. JM said, so she was aware that she was not the child of the family in which she had been sold. Yes, because she was in contact with her biological siblings. JM asked about her understanding of why she was sold and not any of the other children. Ms. A. did not have a clear idea of why that was the case. She attributed the sale to poverty and to the fact that her elder biological sibling was needed to look after the other children because the parents had to work to sustain the family.

JM summarized the predicament of Ms. A as that of someone whose life was far from ideal but not unique in that cultural setting. She lived with her daughter's family (not unusual in that culture), she had been divorced (not uncommon in today's city—or elsewhere), she remained in contact with her children, and she was unable to work (5 years from retirement age). Her situation could not completely explain her depression. Not many women in her situation suffer from recurrent depressive illnesses and gain hospital admissions because of suicidal ideation. One needs to look deeper and further to gain a genuine understanding of her depression. Another important feature of her condition is that Ms. A improves rather quickly after admission to hospital. She improves before any medication has time to cause a lift in mood.

JM inquired what the doctor's understanding of why Ms. A responds in this way to her predicament. The doctor replied that she has no role in her daughter's family. She did have a role when she was bringing up her children and her grandchildren; since she lost her job, she lost not only a role but also the social contact and she felt lonelier. JM replied that she had to contend not only with the *absence* of a role and of connections but also with the *loss* of them (role and connections) and that she was becoming more isolated and without a purpose in life. JM asked if her connections were related to her "feeling useful?" The doctor said yes.

JM noted that it seems that when she lived with her daughter, she was fulfilling a number of functions; she was useful and in return she had connections and a purpose in life. With the loss of these functions and connections, she not only feels redundant and isolated, but she is without a useful role and without meaningful connections. JM asked if she has any other connections, such as with friends. She is friendly with some neighbors with whom she plays cards sometimes, but this activity "bores" her at present and so, she does not seek their company as much. JM then stated so, she does not have any friends. The doctor replied, none at all. JM then said, and is this the reason why she is dreaming of returning to her hometown? Is she hoping that she will find some connection there? The doctor agreed with this. JM noted that her predicament is depressive; she has not managed the present transition in her life in a creative way and asked if she could have stayed with her daughter if she had managed the situation there more positively. The doctor said that it is common for grandmothers to stay with one of their children's families in that culture, and it would be possible for her to do so (live with her daughter). JM asked if the aspect of Ms. A's behavior that was making their living together difficult or untenable was known. The doctor said that she wanted her daughter to follow Ms. A's style of bringing up children. JM summarized then she was not respectful of her daughter's and her son-in-law's views on how they should bring up their children. She was critical of them. She would not accept the different way that they had decided to bring up their children.

JM responded that it is not only a matter of her beliefs about upbringing of children but it is also the matter of her actions. Ms. A insisted on criticizing and on influencing her daughter's family so that their family would be brought up in Ms. A's way. He then asked if she was aware that her intervention was going to influence the relationship with her daughter negatively. The doctor said that she knew of the effect that her behavior was having, but she insisted that hers was the right way. JM noted that although Ms. A's main need was one of being connected, her behavior was putting that connection in danger and asked if she was clear that her behavior was working against her own needs and that for the sake of doing things in the way that she believed was right she was endangering her relationship with her daughter? The doctor replied that she was aware. JM then responded, so she was consciously prepared to sacrifice her relationship with her daughter for the sake of struggling to do things in the way that she thought was right.

JM inquired how the doctor made sense that Ms. A sacrificed the most important thing in her life for the sake of doing things in the way that she thought (she felt) was right and what the point of conflict with her daughter about the bringing up of grandchildren was. And more, what was the nature of the conflict between her and her daughter? Ms. A's daughter felt that her mother was overprotective. Ms. A believed that her daughter should correct her children's errors, while her daughter believed that she should allow her children to experience the consequences of their mistakes. JM asked if there was a way of helping Ms. A to maintain the connection with her daughter by changing her behavior in relation to the grandchildren and if there was a way of helping her understand that her beliefs about the values of bringing up the grandchildren are connected with her own experience as a child. Ms. A feels strongly that the children's needs should be addressed in an immediate way, whereas her daughter was prepared to hold back. Can Ms. A's current behavior toward the grandchildren be linked to her own early childhood experiences? The doctor noted that when she was a child, Ms. A was aware that her needs were not addressed and only demands were placed on her.

JM responded that her own privation as a child remained a powerful force for her current behavior toward her grandchildren. It was emotionally impossible for her to allow what she perceived to be some privation in her own grandchildren. The meaning she gave to the current situation was a replication of her own privation as a child. Analytically it is important to see how she had not overcome the trauma of her early privation and that it was these feelings that were driving her (even to her own cost) to rush to meet the grandchildren's needs immediately. In this way Ms. A was attempting to overcompensate for her own privation, and this feeling was so powerful that living with her daughter had become impossible.

In view of this understanding, if Ms. A were to be receptive to analytical therapy, what would you set as the objective of therapy? Therapy would be directed toward resolving the feelings arising from her early painful experiences. JM concurred; she needs to mourn and grieve the deprived childhood that she had. After the mourning is complete, she will be more likely to be able to separate her own childhood experiences from the present experiences of her grandchildren. For example, her relationship with her daughter will be a lot better if she allowed her daughter to bring up her children in a way that her daughter thought right, instead of seeing that as a repetition of her own privation. She will be in a better position to allow her daughter to be the authority over her own children. She will be able to see that her grandchildren, being brought up in her daughter's way, are not being deprived in the same way that she had been when she was a child.

JM asked if there any chance that she may live with her daughter again. It was clear that her daughter will welcome her back. JM responded that there is a hope that if she resolves this mourning that she will be able to live with her daughter and have a life in which her need to be connected is more likely to be satisfied than it is presently. This change will address one of the main reasons for her depression. Once she has resolved that grief, she is more likely to see the separateness of her own experience from the experience of her grandchildren and she will be able to have a more contemporary life experience with her daughter. Ms. A is likely to feel that her grandchildren, being raised in the way that her daughter and her husband wish, is not a repetition of her own deprivation and that her grandchildren are having a pretty good life. Feeling like this, will make it easier for her to take a grandparenting role, which is secondary to that of her daughter. She will be a grandmother helping her daughter instead of going against her. This will enable her to adopt the new role of "the helpful grandmother" and will remove one source of frustration and conflict in the new extended family situation.

JM noted that because her depression has a large element that is reactive to the situation, an improved life situation is likely to improve the feelings of depression. It is fortunate that the relationship with her daughter is not irrevocably broken down and it is conditional. "Mum, if you respect my way of bringing up my children, I will welcome you to live with my family." So the line of therapy could be two-pronged: one line is to help her accept, mourn, and complete the grief about her own childhood experience and the second to point to the direction that she can strengthen the connection with her daughter (instead of threatening it with antagonism) and in this way remove one of the main sources of her depression.

JM noted that another aspect of her life is her need to develop other relationships not related to her eldest daughter and her family. She needs to have her own adult and separate connections and sources of support. If she remains with the only connection of that with her daughter and her family, this is likely to create serious difficulties. There is a high risk that she will become overbearing and overdemanding. There will need to be a separate focus on why her relationships with her own peers have not gone well. Relationships with her peers are a whole new chapter. My guess is that she breaks the relationships with her peers before they have any chance of becoming genuinely supportive. It seems that she does not have the patience to negotiate the relationships with her peers so that they become mutually supportive. Ms. A's approach is good in the beginning of a relationship, but she seems to break it at the initial stage without working at developing the relationship with her peers. She misses the opportunity of advancing the superficial relationship to make it a more substantial one. The doctor agreed to work with her in moving through her previous experience and on developing new relationships with her family and with her peers.

JM then noted that it seems that her difficulty in proceeding in the mourning process is reflected in her reluctance to even contemplate her early life experience. She needs to be shown that it is possible with a professional's presence and sympathetic understanding to undertake this painful mourning process. Her chances of moving on will improve if she completes this mourning process and accepts that the past was past and is not being repeated in the present. This has been an interesting case; thanks for presenting it so well.

Scientific Literature

This case is of particular interest because it highlights the long-term impact of child selling. This is, of course, an abusive practice that was common in several countries during times of famine or other social privation. Children are also sold for sexual exploitation, prostitution, or for organ transplantation for a financial reward to, usually, the father. Most commonly the sold children are females. Surprisingly there is no scientific literature easily accessible on this issue. One can find the case of the sold child in the literature of Child Abuse and Neglect.

The other focus for this case is one of the "loss of role" and loss of connections in the later stages of life. References to "retirement" in more general terms (not only from gainful employment) are cited in relation to other cases in this work.

Mrs. Z

Introduction

Mrs. Z is a 56-year-old unemployed woman, living alone in her elder brother's public housing unit.

History of Present Illness

Mrs. Z began to complain of low mood in the last 2 to 3 years. She also realized that she was never happy throughout her life. She had on-and-off crying spells. She slept poorly. She had intense anticipatory fear when she knew that her brother would be returning to the city. She had fleeting suicidal ideation from time to time, but there were never actual attempts or related preparation. She sought help from general practitioner and was later referred to psychiatric outpatient department.

Personal History

Mrs. Z was born in the city. She has two older brothers and one younger sister, with each sibling was born 2 years after the previous one. She reported that she was treated badly by her father and elder brothers since childhood. She was often blamed and scolded by them for being "stupid," while her mother turned a blind eye toward such treatment. She had always been a submissive child to her young sister and to her father and elder brothers, hoping that she would be scolded less frequently. She tended not to express her feelings to others. She stopped studying after the first year of secondary education and started working. She recalled that she never had plans to study further or get married because her father kept telling her that she should stay at home to care for her parents. During this time, her siblings moved out of the family home one by one after having their own families; Mrs. Z continued to live with her parents.

Mrs. Z's mother died 10 years ago (2007) from breast cancer, and her father died of a heart attack 6–7 years ago (2011). Although she put much effort in taking care of her parents when they became ill during their final years, she never received any gratitude from her father until the last moments of his life. Yet, she continued to take care of her parents and never considered abandoning them.

After her parents died, her younger sister moved back to live with her because she was having marital problems and was in the process of divorcing. After several years, her younger sister remarried and her husband moved in to live with them. As it was inconvenient to live with her brother-in-law, she moved to her second elder brother's home 3 years ago. Her second elder brother's family had already emigrated, and they returned to visit the city several times a year. She described that whenever her second elder brother returned to the city that he criticized her daily for being useless and told her to go to die so that she would not be a burden to this world, although she would prepare meals for her brother's family when they were in the city. Her brother's wife and children seemed not to notice the criticism at all. Mrs. Z stopped working 5 or 6 years ago (2012).

Past Psychiatric History

Mrs. Z is new to psychiatry; she has no history of violence or suicide attempt. There is no family history of mental illness.

Past Medical History

Mrs. Z suffered from bilateral knee pain and was diagnosed with osteoarthritis. She had operations on her knees (bilateral knee replacement carried out in a private hospital in 2013), but the pain persisted, making it difficult for her to walk normally. Mrs. Z also suffers from hypertension, hyper-cholesterolemia, and allergic rhinitis; there is no known drug allergy.

Mental State Examination

Mrs. Z is an obese lady walking slowly with a stick; she is neat and tidy, wearing a surgical mask, calm and settled; she made fair eye contact and showed no psychomotor disturbances. Mrs. Z's mood was low and her affect congruent. There were no psychotic symptoms, and she denied any active suicidal ideas; she was orientated to time, place, and person. Mrs. Z. had good insight.

Diagnosis

Dysthymia, which was perpetuated by poor stress coping strategies.

Consultation

The consultation was started with the request to clarify a few points of history. Mrs. Z. started earning at the age of 14–15 years. She is obese with a body mass index (BMI) of 30. Her intelligence was considered to be slightly below average. She had undertaken semi-skilled jobs. The siblings were "well off" with one sibling running their own business and a sister being a housewife.

The therapeutic contract was not clear, but it involved the use of antidepressants (on account of low mood and anxiety); the medication was not significantly helpful but had led to some "partial improvement." The improvement had been noticed to take place 3 to 4 weeks after onset of medication. The staff noticed that she demonstrated fewer crying spells, fewer temper outbursts, less self-harming-harming, and fewer ruminations but no change in interest in activities. Her sleep was normal when brother was absent but problematic when he lived with her. Mrs. Z did not complain of anhedonia and did not demonstrate any diurnal variation of mood.

The use of antidepressants was justified based on the sleep disturbance. This was questioned because the sleep disturbance was conditional on her brother's presence. The next question was, if the presence of her brother is so unsettling, why did she continue living with him? Could she not live in a place of her own?

The provisional formulation was that this was a woman who was depressed because she was being criticized by her brother, was submissive, and had been previously criticized by parents.

Mrs. Z did not see herself as the agent of her own predicament but that she was at the mercy of other people's wishes and actions. The doctor clarified that the arrangement by which she lived was not a necessary part of the culture prevailing in the city and was unfair to her as a younger sister. The doctor added that this arrangement was not the result of Mrs. Z's generosity but an expression of her being taken advantage. There was no doubt that she was being exploited. It seemed that this woman of limited ability was in an unfortunate position in which the only resort of comfort for her was to (over)eat.

In conclusion, Mrs. Z was exploited and was not in a position to take charge of her own life. She had a serious difficulty in becoming the agent of her own predicament. Therefore, the therapeutic intervention needed was the provision of a professional (counselor or social worker) who would support her and direct her in establishing a way of living that was fairer to her and which would secure her human rights. The counselor may mediate on her behalf with key family members. Mrs. Z. could be supported to improve her physical health (she needs to lose weight because her obesity limits her ability to move and restricts her independence).

It is unlikely that analytical therapy would be appropriate for her. Mrs. Z. is more likely to respond to a continuous intervention that would have realistic (and finite) expectations for change of a pattern of a lifetime. Ambitious therapeutic objectives can only lead to failure in the patient and disappointment in the therapist. The services of occupational therapy may provide support, socialization, and a program toward some work in the final years before retirement.

One can see how her early life experience of being psychologically and emotionally abused led her to see herself as a person of lesser value and as one who is not entitled to fair treatment because she was not as able as her siblings. Mrs. Z unfortunately continued relating to her family (and possibly to others) in the same way that had been established in her family of origin from a young age.

Any change in her approach needs to be gradual and coupled with considerable amount of support and small increments of interpretations. She may be helped by comments like: "Even if you are not as able as your siblings, this does not give them the right not to respect you and certainly does not mean that exploiting you is justified." Mrs. Z could also be given opportunities to build her self-esteem by being engaged in tasks that carry a realistic chance of success, which will then be demonstrated that she (and her work) is valued. A simplistic example is she may be given a chance to carry out a job that is not too intellectually demanding and is attainable by her despite her knee disability—perhaps something like answering the phone at a center. Being useful and successful can only help to improve her self-esteem and the confirmation by colleagues and seniors may help consolidate this improvement.

Ms. B

Ms. B is a 21-year-old single unemployed woman living with her family in a public housing unit.

Presenting Condition

Ms. B was voluntarily admitted to the hospital on 21 May 2018 because of unstable emotions, following a suicidal gesture after an argument with her boyfriend.

History of Present Complaint

Ms. B has had a stormy relationship with her boyfriend ever since they started courting when they were Form 3 classmates (7 to 8 years previously). Over the years, they broke up many times and, in between, Ms. B also had many short-lived relationships. Ms. B would throw temper tantrums and employ self-harming behaviors when she expected to be abandoned by her boyfriend. In January 2018, they reunited. The couple agreed that they would not lie to each other, and there would be no personal privacy in the relationship. Her boyfriend promised that he would not do anything harmful to her. Ms. B also treated her boyfriend better as a kind of compensation.

However, later, Ms. B searched her boyfriend's smartphone and found that he had sent WhatsApp messages to two female colleagues with flirtatious content. Ms. B was so angry that her boyfriend was not totally loyal to her. Upon confrontation, instead of explaining the meaning of the suspect WhatsApp messages, her boyfriend would linger on her past maladaptive coping and unstable emotions. He labeled her mentally ill. She was dissatisfied with her boyfriend's response, implying that she was the only one who should bear the responsibility for their disharmony. She slashed her wrist to get the painful feeling and to remind herself that she did not treat her boyfriend well at the beginning. She had poor sleep when she ruminated about her boyfriend's WhatsApp messages. In the previous month, Ms. B had two episodes of drug overdosing and one episode of climbing at the edge of a high slope. She had left a suicidal note to her family. Yet, Ms. B denied a pervasive depressive mood. She still enjoyed part-time work as basketball match referee assistant. Her self-care and hygiene were satisfactory.

On the day of admission, Ms. B reported that she and her boyfriend had been arguing from morning to night. She had discovered in WhatsApp a message in which her boyfriend had asked his friends' opinion whether he should send a bunch of flowers to his former girlfriend. She calmed down a little after an afternoon nap. The couple later went out and met their shared friends. Ms. B consumed two bottles of apple cider and became emotional again. She scolded their friends as she felt that they were colluding with her boyfriend for his unfaithfulness. She cried loudly and threw an empty glass bottle on the floor. She impulsively banged her head on a lamppost and hit the gate of a street shop. She also attempted to rush into the traffic but was stopped by her boyfriend. Later, her father and maternal aunt were called for help. She hid in a restaurant's toilet and expressed negative ideas to relatives: "You will regret this. . ... you can never find me; this will be the last time that you saw me." Ms. B was subdued by father and was eventually sent to casualty.

There was satisfactory self-care and hygiene, and she was cooperative and respectful to the staff. Her mood was stable; she was not overly depressed and presented with congruent affect. Her speech was coherent and relevant, and she freely shared her feelings. She was not psychotic, suicidal, or aggressive. She had mixed feelings toward her boyfriend with grievance and guilt. She showed no psychomotor retardation.

Ms. B was physically fit. There were many old slash marks over the volar aspect of both wrists. There was a tattoo (with the boyfriend's name) on her right thumb.

Family History

Her mother and maternal grandmother had been diagnosed with depression. Her mother committed suicide by jumping from height at the age of 32. Her father is 55 years old and, together with her stepmother, owned a logistic company. He suffered from hypertension, dyslipidemia, and ischemic heart disease. Her stepmother, 32 years old, had moved to the city from the country. Ms. B has a distant relationship with her stepmother. Her stepmother was thought to be greedy and irresponsible because she kept buying luxury goods even when the logistic company had financial deficit. Father and stepmother are currently living separately. Ms. B has three younger half-siblings ages 15, 12, and 4. Ms. B has a close relationship with her second younger sister.

Personal History

Ms. B was born in the city; she felt that she was deprived of love from her parents. Her mother died when she was 2 years old, and she has no recollection of her. She felt that there was lack of emotional caring and love from her father who otherwise provided the patient with enough money and other material goods. Ms. B was brought up by her maternal grandmother. Ms. B felt that she was spoiled by her maternal grandmother and felt loved by maternal grandparents, uncle, aunt, and cousin. Ms. B described her primary school life as happy and had a good relationship with her teachers. Ms. B's academic results were below average.

When she was in higher forms in primary school, she was betrayed by one of her best friends in the class who had hacked into her internet account and spread a rumor about her relationship with some classmates. Ms. B was promoted to a local band three secondary school (not for high achievers). Ms. B felt isolated and picked on by classmates; she played truant. Her school attendance was around 80%. Ms. B maintained good relationship with her teachers.

Ms. B achieved a pass grade on four subjects in the city diploma of secondary education examination. Ms. B then stayed in abroad for 1 year with her boyfriend who studied while there. She came back to the city and worked in her father's logistic company as a clerk for 1 year. She also worked in sales in a computer company for few months. Ms. B is currently employed as part-time basketball match referee assistant. She is financially supported by her father.

Ms. B has had many short-lived courtships since Form 2. She started a relationship with the current boyfriend while in Form 3. They broke up and reconciled many times. Ms. B agreed that she was manipulative in the relationship and not loyal to her boyfriend; she initiated breakups on a few occasions. She had threatened her boyfriend with self-harm behaviors and made suicidal threats during conflicts and when she was worried that she would be abandoned.

Ms. B has no forensic record. She had made regular use of "ice" (an amphetamine) under peer influence at the age of 17. She stopped taking ice for 1 year when she lived abroad. She restarted taking ice at the age of 20 for 1 year after she came back to the city. Ms. B denies having used ice in the last year but believed that "amphetamines" gave her increased energy, euphoria, and weight loss. Ms. B experienced transient auditory hallucinations after taking ice. Ms. B made less frequent but regular use of cannabis at the age of 17; the last use of cannabis was a few days before admission. Ms. B also took slimming pills prescribed by her general practitioner from January to June 2017.

Ms. B had a personality of being "hot tempered," impulsive, outgoing, and willful. Her hobbies were outdoor activities, basketball, hiking, swimming, and badminton. Ms. B is not religious and enjoyed good past health. She is a smoker of about seven cigarettes per day and a social drinker.

Past Psychiatric History

Ms. B has been known to a private psychiatrist since 2011 when she experienced depressive symptoms after a relationship breakup (in her first relationship in Form 2). She consulted a private psychiatrist on an "as necessary" basis. In the last 2 months, Ms. B consulted a psychiatrist on three occasions. She presented with unstable emotions attributed to relationship problems Ms. B commented that "she had too much to ruminate about negative thoughts." She felt that the doctor did not understand her needs and concerns. Ms. B was not known to the public mental health service.

There is a history of a drug overdose of 20 tablets of Panadol/clonazepam (medications from maternal grandmother), which she took with alcohol in April 2018. She had then been admitted to the casualty and discharged. There is a history of overdoses with 80 tablets of hypnotics and an incident of climbing over the railing of a high slope in May 2018. Ms. B would eventually vomit the medications.

Present Treatment and Management of Case

Ms. B was given the diagnosis of Borderline Personality Disorder, adjustment disorder, and cannabis misuse with the possibility that she may have been suffering from a depressive episode. She was treated with antidepressant medication and counseling, which was focused on her relationship difficulties and her maladaptive coping techniques as well as anger management. She was offered a short stay (1 week) at the psychiatric hospital.

Ms. B settled well and was cooperative throughout the admission. She had no overt or pervasive depressive symptoms. She had no craving for substances or alcohol. She could sleep well without hypnotics. She was quite attentive and constructive when talking about relationship problems. She had no intention of giving up her boyfriend even though he appeared to be suspicious and unfaithful. She kept daily phone contact with her boyfriend. When her boyfriend visited her in the hospital (once), she mentioned that he cried in front of her. Ms. B said she missed the ward "a bit" at the time of discharge. She considered the hospital a safe and secure place. Ms. B also respected the staff and her doctor and asked to be followed-up in the public sector.

It was felt that the following factors were playing a part in her condition: a strong family history of depression; mother committed suicide; insecure attachment to parents; lack of care, love, and emotional expression from father and stepmother; lack of discipline from maternal grandmother who often satisfied her demands, irrespective of whether they were thought to be reasonable. There was a history of being betrayed by peers in primary school, which may have further intensified her feeling of insecurity. Repeated self-harm behaviors and suicidal threat as a kind of manipulation to induce the boyfriend's guilt whenever Ms. B considered the relationship unstable, which contributed to a vicious circle.

Consultation
JM thanked the doctor for the thorough presentation and for developing a good relationship with Ms. B. JM then asked the doctor to state what the treatment plan was. The doctor explained that the treatment plan had been discussed with Ms. B, her father, and her aunt, and it was jointly decided that she should have counseling psychotherapy by a private professional. The doctor explained that one of the factors determining treatment provision was the limitations of the health service. JM pointed out that an additional factor probably was the doctors need to have the experience of seeing patients through to the end of treatment. JM pointed out that Ms. B had not managed to improve her ability of dealing with her emotions in a more constructive way despite the years of therapeutic efforts.

JM then asked the doctor about his understanding of the reason why Ms. B finds it so difficult to manage her feelings in a more constructive way, without resorting to destructive actions. The doctor responded that her early life experience could provide an answer. He pointed out that Ms. B had lost her mother at the age of 2 and that her father was not available for her because he was preoccupied with the survival of his business. The doctor pointed out that Ms. B felt insecure in her childhood and that this feeling was accentuated with the betrayal that she experienced in primary school. Her upbringing led her not to feel secure in any environment. JM then asked the doctor if he could clarify in what way Ms. B did not feel secure at present because history is important, but the present is equally significant. The doctor pointed out that the main source of security for Ms. B was the relationship with her boyfriend, and unfortunately, his behavior had given her grounds to feel less secure with him.

JM then drew a distinction between the realistic insecurity and the "core" insecurity that Ms. B carries with her all the time. The realistic insecurity is appropriate in her case because her boyfriend does not give her grounds to feel that the relationship is stable and long term. Her perception is not a matter for treatment. In contrast, a matter for treatment is the insecurity that she carries with her and that she perceives in many other settings.

Ms. B enters relationships without expecting them to be secure. She does that at a level that is well beyond the understandable and expects uncertainty in any new relationship. By beginning a relationship with excessive suspiciousness combined with a tendency to act destructively, Ms. B plays a part in damaging the relationship and bringing about the thing that she fears (i.e., the breakup and the resulting insecurity). This was a description of the vicious circle through which one's feelings and behavior cause their worst fears to become reality. JM pointed out that the doctor had correctly identified that this was a pattern that she developed from early age and that she applies at present.

JM then moved on to the immediate therapeutic task of enabling Ms. B to move out of this vicious circle. The focus of therapy needs to be on making Ms. B stronger emotionally so that she can cope with difficult feelings in a more constructive way. JM redefined the question of "how can this Ms. B be made to feel secure enough so that she can handle her emotions more constructively?" JM suggested that the first secure attachment that this she could have is that with the therapist. A therapist can become a secure figure for her if they are able to provide a strictly professional and predictable relationship. The first parameter is being "strictly professional." The importance of the therapeutic alliance has been adequately researched. See studies by McCabe and Priebe (2004) and Krupnick et al. (2006). There is often the temptation to become friendly, parental, or, worse, flirtatious or amorous with a patient to respond to the patient's needs for a secure attachment. Medicolegal literature is full of cases in which therapists have not been able to maintain the professional role to the detriment of their patients and themselves.

The second dimension of the professional is that the appointments are prearranged, and the patient knows when they are going to take place, how long each session will last, and that this is not a forever relationship that has to end. In that way, the conclusion of therapy will be seen as that (conclusion of a period of treatment) and not as a further rejection. Additionally, the therapist will be able to support the patient not in the sense of colluding with her but in the sense of enabling her to reflect on her feelings and adapt them so that they correspond to reality and are not determined by the early life experiences. JM gave several examples where this process happens in a healthy and constructive way in well-functioning families and in well-functioning schools where staff help the children who get upset by various interactions to recover as well as mend relationships.

Finally, a therapist can help the patient develop a sense of perspective. This means that the patient will be more able to see their difficulties in context and to have hope that a better future lies ahead through a resolution of the present difficulties and the ability to develop better relationships in the future. These are some of the changes that psychotherapy can bring about. They are referred to in the scientific literature as transformative factors. For those interested in group analysis, see Garland (1982, 2015).

JM then decided to divert the attention to the area of Ms. B's view of herself. JM pointed out that the relationship between one's ability to have a relationship and one's view of themselves; for example, a person with a more realistic view of their self is more likely to develop a realistic relationship with others, and a person with a damaged view of their self is more likely to handle relationships in a dysfunctional way. At this point in the consultation, the doctor gave an excellent summary of the essence of the consultation so far, and it was natural then to move on to exploring Ms. B's self-psychology. JM pointed out the need for the therapist to retain credibility with Ms. B and that the main basis of credibility is that they should be realistic. A tendency to idealize or to be overly hopeful often reduces the therapist's credibility in the patient's view and therefore reduces their ability to be effective. In Ms. B's case, reality means that she has the future potential to develop appropriate and functional relationships, but she will need to do some work to reach that point.

The doctor pointed out that Ms. B does not like herself at present and that she does not see herself as loveable. This is made worse by her awareness that she has negative emotions. The doctor added that Ms. B does not like herself for her feelings or for her actions in the recent past. JM then pointed out that it seemed that Ms. B only defines herself on her negative characteristics and that she attends only to the negative responses that she receives from other people. JM pointed out that Ms. B may well be ignoring any positive feedback that may come her way. In search for positives, the doctor pointed out that Ms. B was happy when she was working as an assistant basketball referee.

The doctor pointed out that Ms. B remembered that there was little challenge to her decisions as an assistant referee and that when she was refereeing there was little argument in the game.

The doctor was finding it difficult to define further positive aspects of Ms. B's personality. JM then clarified that he was not asking the doctor as a teacher who knows what the right answer is but as a consultant raising issues with him that he could then explore together with his patient. In this way Ms. B would begin to look for the positive and realistically positive aspects of herself, so that Ms. B will develop a more balanced and realistic view of herself. This view will replace the damaged and almost totally negative view of herself that was based on her early traumatic life experiences. The doctor then added that there were times when Ms. B was attractive and charming. JM then concluded that a good professional relationship with the therapist would enable her to be more conscious of the positive attributes of her personality and, as a result, develop a more balanced view of herself.

References

Garland, C. (1982). Group analysis: Taking the non-problem seriously. *Group Analysis, 15*, 4–14.

Garland, C. (2015). Group analysis: Taking the non-problem seriously. In J. Maratos (Ed.), *Foundations of group analysis for the twenty-first century* (pp. 53–70). Karnac.

Krupnick, J. L., Sotsky, S. M., Elkin, I., Simmens, S., Moyer, J., Watkins, J., & Pilkonis, P. A. (2006). The role of the therapeutic alliance in psychotherapy and pharmacotherapy outcome: Findings in the National Institute of Mental Health Treatment of Depression Collaborative Research Program. *Focus, 4*(2), 269–277.

McCabe, R., & Priebe, S. (2004). The therapeutic relationship in the treatment of severe mental illness: A review of methods and findings. *The International Journal of Social Psychiatry, 50*(2), 115–128.

Mrs. A

Mrs. A is a 60-year-old widowed housewife living with her two grown sons.

Presenting Condition

Mrs. A presented with a depressive mood of 1 month, with negative ruminations, chest tightness, dizziness, and insomnia. She had decreased motivation and was barely able to maintain her usual interests in exercise and church activities.

History of Present Complaint

Mrs. A had two recent stressors leading to the current episode of depressive mood. The first was that her younger son, who lives with her, was having some work problems but did not elaborate the details to her. She said her son was quiet and she was afraid that he might have depression.

The second stressor was that she had a gathering with her old classmates and during that, she compared herself to her classmates. She felt herself shorter, widowed, lower financial status, and could not achieve what her friends had achieved in their careers. She felt that she was inferior to them. She ruminated about these two ideas and started to develop a pervasive low mood, chest tightness, dizziness, and insomnia.

Family History

Mrs. A had no known family history of any mental or mood disorders. She had two older sisters.

Personal History

Mrs. A was married at 21 years. She enjoyed a good marital relationship. She described her husband as tall, strong, reliable, and caring. She felt grateful for having a good husband, and her husband was not bothered by their difference in height. Her husband died in December 2015 of cancer.

Mrs. A has two sons and one daughter, all in their early 30s. Her older son divorced and is currently living with her. Her older son worked in the government in the environmental and health department. Her younger son is also living with her and is currently working as a fireman. Her younger son will be getting married early next year and will be moving out later this year to live in a flat, which he has bought with his fiancée. Her daughter lives abroad and is currently a student in nursing school. Mrs. A. has regular contact with her daughter over the phone. Her daughter has a stable boyfriend abroad and has no plans to return to the city.

Mrs. A is happy about her younger son's upcoming wedding. However, she preferred them to have a private marriage, perhaps somewhere overseas, instead of having a big banquet. She felt that it would be troublesome for her to organize a banquet, and she would have difficulty finding a suitable dress because she felt she was short and not good looking.

Personal History

Mrs. A. was born in another city. She had two older sisters, who were caring toward her during her childhood. She grew up in the country with normal upbringing, and her childhood was uneventful. She was educated in the country until secondary 2 level. She then came to the city early in her 20s and got married.

Mrs. A worked in a garment factory and in a restaurant as a food seller before. Her longest employment was for 3 years in a restaurant. After she got married, she became a housewife.

Mrs. A is a nonsmoker and nondrinker. She has no substance abuse or forensic record. She is even-tempered, a little prone to anxiety, pessimistic, and passive in her personality. She enjoys exercise every morning as a hobby. She is a Christian and goes to church weekly. Her friends are mostly her old classmates, neighbors, and "church-mates."

Past Psychiatric History

Mrs. A was first known to the mental health service in 2006. She was seen twice in the clinic at that time for generalized anxiety disorder with insomnia, but she defaulted at follow up. That episode was triggered by an event of a gas explosion in the flat below her apartment. This event was widely publicized in the city. The explosion occurred in the context of domestic conflict. There were three deaths in the incident including two residents of the flat and an old lady of a neighboring flat. The person who set the gas explosion was an elderly man who was the owner of that flat and who was later jailed. In the afternoon of that day, Mrs. A was suddenly woken up by a loud noise and some smoke. She saw her own windows and glass drawers broken. She evacuated downstairs immediately. When she arrived at the balcony, she looked up to see the fire scene and was overwhelmed with fears. It was arranged for her to stay in the community center for one night and then in a temporary housing unit for 3 months. Afterward, she suffered from a startling response and apprehension whenever she heard a loud noise or passing the floor of the incident when she returned to live at home. These symptoms lasted for about a year and then gradually subsided. She was referred by a social worker to receive a psychological intervention at that time. She recalled that the clinical psychologist taught her some relaxation techniques involving muscle relaxation and listening to relaxing music. She did not practice the techniques often and the psychologist service was terminated after 1 year when her symptoms subsided.

A few years later in 2011, Mrs. A presented to the psychiatric clinic again. This time she was troubled by menopausal symptoms. She developed low mood, poor sleep, and appetite, was feeling anxious, experienced chest tightness, dizziness, and had poor motivation. She attributed these complaints to depression because she felt her symptoms were similar to the description of depression she read in newspaper articles. She was started on fluoxetine and had regular follow up in the clinic. She achieved remission shortly after the start of antidepressants.

Two years later, in 2013, Mrs. A suffered a relapse of depression. This time it was triggered by her daughter having a road traffic accident abroad. It was a minor accident; her daughter was only mildly injured and made a good recovery. She was worried and then developed persistent low mood, poor sleep, loss of appetite, chest tightness, and dizziness. She had lack of motivation, and she did not want to see anyone at that time. She stopped her usual habit of daily exercise with her neighbors. She was added on Deanxit in the clinic. She achieved remission again shortly after adjustment of the medication.

In the next 2 to 3 years, her husband suffered from multiple physical problems, including cancer of the lung and prostate, with brain metastases, complicated by epilepsy. Her husband was physically frail in the last few years of life, and she had to take care of him. Her husband eventually died in December 2015. She had a normal grief reaction. She missed her husband, but she soon accepted the loss. She felt that his death was a good way to end her husband's long-term suffering from the illness.

Mrs. A then had a stable mental state until the current episode of depressive mood, which was triggered by younger son's change in work duty and her gathering with old classmates. She advanced her clinic appointment this time, and her antidepressant dosage was adjusted. She soon achieved remission again after around 1 month.

Present Treatment and Management of Case

The diagnosis for her was recurrent depressive disorder. Her current medications included fluoxetine 40 mg daily, Deanxit (mixed medication of flupentixol and melitracen) 1 tab daily, zopiclone 3.75 mg at bedtime when necessary, and propranolol 10 mg twice a day as necessary. She achieved remission again after 1 month after medication adjustments. She was keen on psychological intervention for relapse prevention, reducing reliance on medication, and learning relaxation techniques.

She was seen a few times and reported that her greatest concern at this stage was reliance on sleeping pills. Sleep hygiene was discussed, and she successfully cut down the use of hypnotics. She reported no other distress at this moment. Further work would be needed to focus on relapse prevention for her.

Consultation

JM congratulated the doctor for the excellent presentation. JM first focused on the timing of Mrs. A's remission after the onset of medication and whether the remission could be pharmacologically explained or if the timing was related to some other factor. The doctor believed that the timing of her improvement was earlier than what would be expected pharmacologically. JM then asked about the significance of this early remission. The doctor wondered whether this was related to a placebo effect. JM then asked about the nature of the therapeutic factor, which was called "placebo." The doctor found it difficult to respond to this question, and JM suggested that a doctor is not expected to know all the answers but when a matter like this confronts a patient and doctor, then it is worthwhile exploring it with the patient. For example, JM suggested that the doctor mentions to Mrs. A that they have noticed that her recovery occurs earlier than medication had time to have effect and whether doctor and patient could explore this and come to a shared insight. That exploration would help the patient to start thinking more psychologically and less organically. The doctor repeated that Mrs. A's understanding was that it was the medicine that was making her better, and JM pointed out to the doctor that he was aware that the build-up of serotonin in the synaptic cleft takes longer than the first 2 or 3 weeks to make a clinically significant improvement.

JM then asked now that it was established that her mental state improvement took place before the biochemical effect of medication, do we have a better understanding of the therapeutic factor? The doctor pointed out that Mrs. A had said that when she tried to speak with her son or daughter, they only offered reassurance that seemed quite facile. Mrs. A felt that her children could not understand her illness. Mrs. A explained that she felt that the professionals at the hospital had a better understanding of her condition. JM then asked, "what was the reassurance given by the healthcare professionals?" The doctor responded that Mrs. A was probably not offered reassurance, but it was the opportunity to talk with professionals at a different level to that of the discussion with her own children.

JM then asked if the doctor had any thoughts of what the qualitative difference was in the communication with the healthcare professionals and with her children. The doctor replied that Mrs. A felt that doctors could understand her illness better and that the doctors could be more effective in helping her by adjusting the medication. JM then suggested that Mrs. A was given a sense of security on a false premise. The false premise being that it was the change in medication that would get her better. JM pointed out that although the premise was false, it was nevertheless effective. The therapeutic factor was that Mrs. A had a feeling that she was in the right hands and that she would receive the right and effective treatment. The contact with the hospital gave her the security that she needed and that was the therapeutic factor.

JM then raised the issue of whether it would be appropriate to disabuse Mrs. A of this false assumption and deprive her of a sense of security or whether the doctor should leave this "false assumption" unchallenged. The decision will depend on whether the doctor's assessment is that Mrs. A can cope with the new reality. JM pointed out that for some people this is the best that one can hope for: That they live with the belief that every now and then, events will overwhelm them and they will become depressed (meaning clinically depressed) and that they will then be sorted out by adjustment in medication by specialist doctors.

Only after the doctors form the opinion that Mrs. A can cope with being disabused—of losing a system of beliefs that she had to date found helpful—can one proceed with a more psychological exploration. For example, only then could she be asked why being short and being less successful than her fellow churchgoers is something that is depressing for her. For an exploration of the relationship among religion, spirituality, and mental health, see the excellent recent review by Dein (2018).

Mrs. A could be asked to reexamine the way she evaluates herself. For example, we do know that the value of people is not measured by a tape measure. Why is Mrs. A rating herself according to height rather than as a human being? Mrs. A was depressed at the thought of appearing at her children's wedding being as short as she is. Why has Mrs. A not gained a realistic evaluation of herself despite her height? JM then repeated the issue that if the doctors felt that Mrs. A could cope with this kind of exploration, this is one issue that they could begin to look at again with her.

JM then pointed out that Mrs. A rates herself by comparing herself to her "fellow churchgoers" on the dimensions of height, wealth, and career. JM asked the doctor about other dimensions along which Mrs. A could begin to rate herself so that she develops a more realistic evaluation of herself. The doctor pointed out that Mrs. A could begin to value herself as the mother of three good children, that the children are independent, they have good jobs, and they contribute to society. JM then pointed out that Mrs. A may feel that she has not been as good a mother because none of her children are high-achieving professionals nor are they great earners. JM asked how the doctors could anticipate this depressive slant that Mrs. A is likely to give to her achievements. The doctor responded that the value of a job is not measured by the amount of money they earn but on the worth of the contribution to society. JM confirmed this as a useful line to follow with Mrs. A. JM then added that this was an excellent idea because the doctors could apply the same evaluation to how she values herself. For example, bringing up three children who are useful members of the society is of enormous value even though it brought no income to her. The doctor also added that the children's emotional development was also largely positive in the sense that they had not presented with any psychiatric conditions although they were reserved. It could be pointed out that with her husband, they raised three children who have not become a burden to society, who have not become dysfunctional, and who are dealing with the stages in their lives (like developing a career and personal relationships) constructively. Mrs. A has a good reason to feel proud of this achievement.

JM then asked the doctor if Mrs. A had good reason to feel proud in her role as a wife. The doctor pointed out that Mrs. A could feel proud of the dedication that she showed to her husband, especially through the last difficult years of his illnesses. JM then summarized that Mrs. A could value herself as a good mother and as a good wife and that she has contributed to society in that way.

JM pointed out that once Mrs. A felt secure in the relationship with a therapist, the therapist can invite her to reexamine the dimensions that she values herself and think not only of the limitations of her achievements but also of the positive contributions. This would enable her to have a more global, balanced, and realistic view and evaluation of herself and not judge herself only by comparing herself negatively. JM then summarized that contact with the professionals enables her to have a more realistic view of herself and also to develop a shared "understanding."

JM then expanded a little on the notion of understanding by pointing out that people feel understood only if the other person shares the same belief or the same view as they do. JM pointed out that young people particularly often accuse their parents of not understanding when their parents see the same events in a different perspective. The security of the relationship with a professional enables patients to reexplore their understanding of and their own interpretations of events or of themselves. In Mrs. A's case, the shared understanding that was based on a false premise was helpful in treating the individual episodes but was not helpful in preventing a relapse. Challenging the original shared understanding would lead to an improved evaluation of herself and an increased personal strength and resilience to face challenges and threats to her self-esteem. Put more simply, only if she values herself more as a person will she be able to face the reception of her children's wedding with the height and a dress that suits her and that she can afford. Only with an improved sense of self-worth will she be able to accept, for example, a reception that is appropriate to their financial status.

JM then suggested, as simple techniques, to use extreme examples of either intellectual brilliance or exorbitant wealth. JM pointed out that he sometimes challenges patients who present with such difficulties by pointing out that most people are not professors at universities and most people are not exorbitantly rich. This comparison often stimulates people to value what they can contribute rather than rating themselves negatively according to what they cannot. The doctor concluded that this was a line of approach that he had already initiated and that Mrs. A was already showing signs of improving.

References

Dein, S. (2018). Against the stream: Religion and mental health—the case for the inclusion of religion and spirituality into psychiatric care. *British Journal of Psychological Bulletein*, 42(3), 127–129.

Bob

Presenting Condition

Bob presented with depressed mood, suicidal ideation, preoccupation, and anxiety.

History of Presenting Complaint

Bob is a 30-year-old married primary school teacher living with his wife. Bob is new to the mental health services. In early April 2018, he downloaded a new software called "FOX" on his computer, which would automatically download web pages and videos after entering a few keywords. He had entered words related to explicit sexual intercourse. He had difficulty engaging in sexual intercourse with his wife. He claimed that he did not know what videos he had downloaded.

He was reported to be mentally well until April 26, 2018 at around 5:00 a.m., when police arrived at his home and arrested him for "possession of child pornography." He claimed that he was misled by police to confess that his computer was only used by him, although in fact it could be accessed by others (including his younger brother, wife, his wife's younger brother, and colleagues). He was brought to the police station, interrogated alone, and finally admitted the charge "under coercion." The case was opened for investigation, and he was concerned regarding possible legal consequences including imprisonment. Since then, he had pervasive depressed mood with weeping episodes. His volition was low. He developed psychomotor retardation, was slow in actions and thoughts, with memory and attention deficits. He was socially withdrawn and preoccupied. He had increased anxiety, and described constantly being "on the verge," with associated shortness of breath, chest discomfort, numbness of his fingers, and hand tremors. He had increased negative cognitions of worthlessness, helplessness, and hopelessness. He was admitted to the emergency ward of a medical center from April 29 to May 1, 2018, where he was seen by the visiting psychiatrist. He was given fluoxetine, diazepam, and lorazepam and was discharged. He sought help from legal advice on May 1, 2018, and the possible legal consequences were explained to him. He first attended the out-patient department on May 31, 2018, where a voluntary admission to a hospital was arranged. Since he was charged, he was suspended from duty as a primary school teacher and is on sick leave.

Family History

His father has depression with follow-up. His mother has a delusional disorder, with past admissions to psychiatric hospitals; she presented with a belief that there were ghosts following her since her paternal grandmother died. His elder brother (33 years old) has severe-grade mental retardation, attention deficit hyperactivity disorder (ADHD), and autism, with hospital follow-up. Bob is the second of three sons.

Personal History

Bob was born in the city. His father was a shop assistant, described to be hot-tempered, and often scolded and hit with bare hands, a bamboo cane, with hangers, or keys. His mother was a housewife, described to be even-tempered, but also used corporal punishment.

Bob was described to have normal development milestones but had poor social interaction with his classmates. He was reported to have poor eye contact, often felt scared to see people, and refused to talk to others. He had interest in memorizing bus and train lines. He enjoyed watching TV advertisements with jingles and often sang these jingles in the wrong social context. He reported that he had been speaking only English since 2001 because he believed that he was an English teacher and that he "should not" speak the local language. He recalled watching the news in English and tried to imitate a British accent. Since then, he had been speaking in English obsessively, even when it was socially inappropriate for him to do so. For example, he insisted on speaking English to his students' parents even though they could not understand. He was told by his school principal and his colleagues that he shouldn't be rigid, but he ignored the advice. At school, he was described as socially awkward and weird. He had no friends. Growing up, he was bullied throughout primary and secondary school for being "weird." He had no confiding relationships. He reported various episodes of intense anxiety during his school years prior to school examinations or being asked to do public speaking. He described his baseline anxiety to be high, and trivial events were enough to cause a surge of intense anxiety.

Other than corporal punishment and physical abuse by his parents, he reported an episode of sexual abuse/harassment when he was 12. He was at home watching cartoons with his two brothers and the phone rang. A man claiming to be a policeman asked him how many people were at home and then asked him to do as he was told or else the police would come and arrest him. He was asked to take out his penis and to measure the size. He was then asked to masturbate and then measure the size again. He was then asked to do the same to his two brothers. He was then asked to stimulate his elder brother's penis with his mouth, but he found it disgusting so he sucked his own fingers instead. His mother then came home and asked what had happened. She told them to hang the phone up. Since this occurrence, Bob believed that some adult men were dirty, especially those who smoked and spoke foul language.

Bob met his wife at university. It was his first relationship. The couple started dating while they were still at university. His wife found Bob to be socially awkward at times but admired his ability to speak in fluent English. His wife was also a primary school teacher. The couple married in August 2016. However, they found it difficult to have sexual intercourse because Bob did not know what position he should be at. When he tried to penetrate her, he claimed his wife would experience pain, and he would stop to avoid hurting her. As a result, Bob and his wife developed a fear of sexual intercourse. As the couple wanted children, they downloaded pornography online to watch together and hoped that by imitating the actors, they would be able to have successful sexual intercourse. They tried for 2 years already without making any progress.

Past Psychiatric History

There is no history of other psychiatric episodes or of suicide or violence.

Present Treatment

His symptoms on presentation satisfied the diagnostic criteria for severe depressive episode without psychotic symptoms He also has predominant anxiety symptoms His rigidity/stubbornness, insistence to speak English even when it was socially inappropriate, lack of social reciprocity, poor social communication, and poor social interaction, all of which starting from childhood, satisfied the diagnostic criteria for childhood autism.

Pharmacologically, he was prescribed venlafaxine and quetiapine for mood regulation. He took lorazepam as needed to help with his anxiety. He was seen by the clinical psychologist for social skills training as well as for coping with stress.

The doctor concluded by clarifying that he wished to form an opinion whether this patient was likely to respond to psychological interventions.

Consultation

JM thanked the doctor for the comprehensive presentation. He also praised the doctor for managing to establish a good relationship with Bob because he is someone who has difficulties in interpersonal relationships. JM then proceeded asking the doctor to clarify if there was a diagnosis of severe depression as well as a diagnosis of autistic spectrum disorder. Regarding the sexual dysfunction, the doctor stated that he saw this as part of the autistic disorder. As such, he did not feel that it merited special diagnostic classification. The case of him suffering from pedophilia (a disorder of sexual preference) had not been established yet. And the difficulty in consummating the marriage was again seen as part of the autistic disturbance.

The doctor added that he knew that the couple had some help from a fertility clinic, which found that there was no physiological reason for them not to be able to have children. To JM's question, the doctor responded that the couple do not have sexual intercourse. JM then queried the logic of going to a fertility clinic when they don't have sexual intercourse, though this is not a rare phenomenon. The doctor stated that Bob had told him that he "was not sure" whether they have had intercourse. JM questioned the veracity of this statement and suggested that because one cannot be not sure whether they have had intercourse that Bob is avoiding answering this question meaningfully. The doctor added that Bob had expressed fear of penetrating his wife. What became clear was that embarrassment inhibits Bob from giving a full history of his sexual life, and a full history is essential for a proper diagnosis of his difficulties. The doctor then expanded on Bob's sexual development. The onset of secondary sexual characteristics seemed to have proceeded naturally. Bob began masturbating at the age of 11. The doctor added that Bob had told him that he thinks he is heterosexual. In recounting the images that were associated with his masturbation Bob made some vague mention of boys but subsequently he made it clear that he was only interested in women. The doctor remained unsure whether Bob was interested in boys or not. Bob did mention to the doctor that once he had been attracted to a 12-year-old boy.

JM then raised the issue of confidentiality and the law regarding pedophilia. JM pointed out that in the UK if a doctor is treating a patient who is a threat or a danger to anyone else, they have a duty to take whatever action is necessary to protect the public. This is much more so when the welfare of children is concerned. The legal situation will need to be clarified with Bob even before the psychiatric or the therapeutic consultations are initiated. The doctors need to be aware that according to UK law, a court can subpoena the records of a doctor if there is an issue of possible harm to children.

In view of the prevailing legal situation, it is important for Bob to know that if he has been found to be downloading pornographic pedophile material, that he accepts this as his own personal problem so that he can proceed to explore it openly within the therapeutic sessions and reach a level where he can receive the appropriate therapy and work toward overcoming this dysfunctional situation. It is not only that he may be attracted to boys aged 12 and that he feels trapped in a 12-year-old body, but it is also the global sexual dysfunction that he has and his attitude about tenderness, warmth, sexual foreplay, and the other aspects of heterosexual interaction.

JM then reflected on the management of pedophiles especially because this is a condition that is particularly resistant to therapeutic interventions. He should certainly avoid working in environments where he would be coming into contact with children and that means that he should change his job as a primary school teacher. In any case, if this case goes to court and he is found guilty, then presumably his name will be put on a register, and would have to disclose this with any application for job that he makes. JM pointed out the predilection of pedophiles for jobs that bring them into contact with children and that one finds frequently pedophiles among the professions of teachers, gymnastic coaches, foster parents, care workers, priests, and even doctors who deal with children such as pediatricians and psychiatrists for children. JM pointed out that many of these unfortunate people choose a profession that will give them access to children. JM referred to the numerous cases of historical sexual abuse that have come to the surface and have shaken many institutions including the Catholic Church.

JM then referred to psychotherapy of pedophilia. This is a highly specialized branch that requires trained professionals who have experience in the field. General psychotherapeutic interventions have not been shown to be therapeutically effective. For practical purposes pedophilia should be considered a condition with guarded prognosis that needs to be managed as well as treated.

JM made a comment about the doctor's record and where he refers to *facts*, information that is only an allegation against Bob. More specifically, Bob's attribution of his confession to pressure from the police must be clearly stated that this is what Bob felt not that this was a fact, although such interrogations are almost never without a personal sense of threat and pressure.

It is of interest that Bob seems to want to shift the responsibility for the downloaded images to the other people who had access to his computer. This is a matter for the police investigation and the psychiatrist needs to keep an open mind until a judgment is passed. JM pointed out that for the police to be involved, this must have been an activity that he was engaged in for some time and for which he probably paid money. He must have accessed these sites in a naïve way because currently, sophisticated pedophiles use the "dark web" and make themselves undetectable. The psychiatric approach needs to be informed by the details of this activity and by the methods Bob used to record this in his hard drive.

JM then pointed out that the event that Bob described when he was telephoned (aged 12) and ordered to carry out certain sexual acts may have been defining and traumatic for him, taking to account the overall personal structure of his psychology that was that of somebody who is suffering from an autistic spectrum disorder. JM pointed out that Bob does have some abilities that mainline autistic people do not have such as the ability to communicate and the well-developed language.

JM then questioned the diagnosis of a depressive illness. He pointed out that the present emotional state could be a reaction to an enormous stress and threat that he must be under. The present detection and interrogation by the police has implications on Bob losing his job, going through court, his private difficulties becoming public, having to register as a pedophile, having to declare this on every job that he seeks an appointment, and challenging the relationships with his wife and with his family. It would be surprising if somebody facing this enormous constellation of changes and losses was not in some emotional turmoil. JM then asked if the doctor knew if there was a service that was oriented therapeutically toward the treatment of people with sexual dysfunction of Bob's type. The doctor was not sure, although he had the impression that the forensic department does treat some cases with antiandrogens. JM's view was that prescription of antiandrogens was not a highly effective way of helping people with this condition.

JM then began his conclusion by saying that the role of a general psychiatrist would be to get Bob to accept that he has a complex problem for which he needs treatment. Denying its existence is not a good foundation for any kind of treatment.

JM then pointed out that Bob may not think that viewing child pornography is harmful. That is pure ignorance because he denies the process by which children are made to take part in acts that are then filmed and put on the internet. The process of developing the pornographic images is itself enormously damaging to children, and by viewing them, he is funding this crime. If he saw the viewing of this activity as innocuous, he simply needs to be informed why viewing these images is criminal.

References on Autism and Pedophilia
A good introduction to the subject of paraphilia is the chapter by (Fedoroff, 2009) in the *New Oxford Textbook of Psychiatry*. It is general and does not address adequately the issue of autism and these

disorders. The same limitation applies to the volume on *DSM-V*. Several studies establish a link between autism spectrum disorder and the paraphilias (Fernandes et al., 2016; Schottle et al., 2017). Of special interest is the study of Kolta and Rossie (2018), which describes a case with both these conditions.

Obviously, the fields of paraphilias and of autistic spectrum disorders are vast. Those interested in the psychoanalytic aspect of paraphilias could study the works of Socarides and Loeb (2004) and of Woods and Williams (2014).

References

Fedoroff, J. P. (2009). The paraphilias. In M. G. Gelder, N. C. Andereasren, J. J. Lopez-Ibor, Jr., & J. R. Geddes (Eds.), *New Oxford textbook of psychiatry* (Vol. 1, pp. 832–842). Oxford University Press.

Fernandes, L. C., Gillberg, C. I., Cederlund, M., Hagberg, B., Gillberg, C., & Billstedt, E. (2016). Aspects of sexuality in adolescents and adults diagnosed with autism spectrum disorders in childhood. *Journal of Autism and Developmental Disorders, 46*(9), 3155–3165.

Kolta, B., & Rossi, G. (2018). Paraphilic disorder in a male patient with autism spectrum disorder: Incidence or coincidence. *Cureus, 10*(5), e2639.

Schottle, D., Briken, P., Tuscher, O., & Turner, D. (2017). Sexuality in autism: Hypersexual and paraphilic behavior in women and men with high-functioning autism spectrum disorder. *Dialogues in Clinical Neuroscience, 19*(4), 381–393.

Socarides, C. W., & Loeb, R. (2004). *The mind of the paedophile: Psychoanalytic perspectives.* Karnac.

Woods, J., & Williams, A. (Ed.) (2014). *Forensic group psychotherapy.* Karnac.

Mrs. C

Mrs. C is a 68-year-old woman, widowed, and living alone in a public housing unit. Mrs. C walks with the aid of a walker (a Zimmer Frame) outdoors and with a walking stick indoors because of arthritis in both knees. Mrs. C functions on activities of daily living, level I (can look after herself).

Presenting Condition

Mrs. C was referred to the psycho-geriatric day hospital from a psycho-geriatric center due to low mood, poor social support, and daytime engagement.

History of Present Illness

Mrs. C reported having fleeting suicidal ideas but no concrete plans or actions. She was diagnosed with a recurrent depressive episode, the current episode being severe, without psychotic symptoms. Upon receiving psychiatric attention since 2015, her mood had shown some improvement, but she still often maintained that she had fulfilled her duties to her family and had no reason for living any more. Mrs. C continued having a sense of worthlessness and hopelessness. She reported having an early death wish and that she wished for a quick natural painless death. Mrs. C had no actual suicidal plans because she was afraid that she would be a burden to her family if the suicide was not successful. She was dysthymic and tearful when husband was mentioned. There was no abnormality of speech. There were no psychotic symptoms. She was not suicidal or aggressive.

Personal History

Mrs. C was born in the city and was the third of four siblings. Her eldest brother died when he was an infant after a fever and before Mrs. C was born. Her eldest sister remained in the country under the care of her maternal grandparents when her parents immigrated to the city. Mrs. C and her younger brother were born in the city. Mrs. C has a distant relationship with her eldest sister because they have lived apart all their lives.

Mrs. C reported having a good relationship with her younger brother and her parents; she claimed that her parents loved both her and her brother dearly because they did not have many children. Mrs. C felt that she had led a happy childhood despite being poor and living in a wooden hut. From a young age, she knew the importance of bringing money home. Mrs. C claimed that her mother died in her arms in her 80s and that her mother had waited for her to come to the hospital to see her final moment. Her father moved in with her, after her younger sister-in-law died, and stayed with her until his death. Mrs. C has no family history of mental illness.

Mrs. C studied until Form 2 at night school and then worked as a factory worker until she was about 50 years old. When her husband had a stroke, when she was around 60 years old, she attended a course to learn how to care for the debilitated and became a helper at an old age home after attending the course. She later studied at the open university (in 2009–2010) because she wanted to have a better work-life balance. Mrs. C was keen on learning.

Mrs. C married after dating for 2 years. She had a good relationship with her husband. Mrs. C commented that her husband was outgoing and liked small gambling but was never in debt. Her husband would take her to trips or buy her good food when he won on betting. When her husband suffered the stroke in 2000, she claimed there was not much support or education given to her at the time. She was told by the doctor that her husband may have recurrent strokes and told her to be careful, but she claimed that she did not know what was meant by this. Mrs. C felt that the doctors were not helpful in advising her how to look after her husband, and as a result, Mrs. C felt helpless. He had stayed in the intensive care unit with a Ryle's (nasogastric) tube at the time, and he was bedbound. Since his discharge from hospital, she had a transient thought of pushing him out the window and jumping from the height with him, but she later changed her mind after thinking that her husband's father was still alive. She later took him to see practitioners of traditional Chinese medicine (each appointment costing the equivalent of about US$50) and hired a maid to help care for him. She claimed she had spent her life savings and sold their minibus to pay for his medical bills. Her husband used to work as a minibus driver. When he entered hospital, she was mocked by relatives for placing him there. Mrs. C claimed that her husband's father was unsupportive, and he claimed that her husband deserved the stroke because he smoked. There was no further support from family members. He eventually had some improvement and was able to walk with a stick but then suddenly developed an infection and died within 3 days. She was disappointed that after she had achieved such an improvement in him, he would die so suddenly.

Mrs. C has two daughters and one son. Her son emigrated when he was in his 20s; her eldest daughter studied in Australia and later worked in the country. Her younger daughter works on a nearby city, she visits her weekly and gives her the equivalent of about US$300 a month. She reported having a quite distant relationship with her children because they work abroad and have their own lives.

Premorbid Personality

Mrs. C is a responsible and independent person who tends to bottle up her feelings. She feels that she is a good listener, a helper, and a giver instead of a recipient of help. Her present limitations (as in mobility) force her to a situation of dependency in which she feels uncomfortable. Mrs. C feels that everyone has their own set of problems and understands that others do not have the time to listen to her difficulties. She is a Buddhist.

Past Psychiatric and Medical History

Mrs. C presented to the hospital in July 2015 with low mood that had persisted since her husband's death in May 2015. Her husband had suffered a stroke in 2000, and Mrs. C had cared for him since that time. Her husband had entered a sub rented old age home in 2004, and Mrs. C used to visit him daily. Her relatives were critical of her because they implied that she should have looked after him at home with the help of the maid whom they had employed. Mrs. C's husband died suddenly within 3 days after admission to hospital where he developed fever and vomiting. After her husband's death, Mrs. C reported to have lost her reason for living. She felt she had done everything she wanted to do in this world already and her responsibilities had been fulfilled. She developed low mood and a loss of energy and interest. She had early morning waking and poor appetite.

After her husband's death, Mrs. C reported to have seen her husband's ghost twice at night but did not feel distressed because she felt it was her husband visiting her.

She felt helpless and had thoughts of pushing her husband out of a window and jumping out of the window after him. Her sister-in-law had also died around that time. Mrs. C was known to the mental health services for more than 15 years. Her sister-in-law had died around that time, leaving her 8-year-old nephew behind. Mrs. C claims that she only attended a psychiatric clinic once and was given antidepressants that made her drowsy and for this reason she did not continue with follow-up. Since attending the hospital, she had tried various antidepressants, which she felt had doubtful therapeutic effect and considerable unwanted effects.

Mrs. C was limping and walking slowly supported by a walker. Mrs. C continued being worried about her progressive bilateral osteoarthritis of her knees, with varus knee, and back pain affecting her mobility. Mrs. C has suffered from dyspepsia, hypertension, hyperlipidemia, empty sella syndrome (which was thought to be nonsignificant at follow-up), spinal stenosis with left foot drop, and obesity.

Mrs. C had been on a waiting list for total knee replacement since 2015 but claimed that she had been advised that she needed to wait until 2018 for it to be done. Last year, Mrs. C also developed hypertension and felt more concerned about her failing health. Her knee pain and poor mobility had limited her from pursuing her interests, such as hiking and doing volunteer work. However, old case notes reported she had previous plans of hanging herself in the mountain, but Mrs. C denied it during current psychiatric clerking. She claimed that since her husband's stroke, she had already completed the bank account rearrangements and written her final notes in case something was to happen to her.

Present Treatment and Management of Case

Mrs. C had been advised to accept inpatient admission, but she strongly refused. She was referred to a clinical psychologist for grief therapy and to a community psychiatric nurse for community supervision; she was started on fluoxetine 30 mg daily. She was referred to PGDH for daytime engagement and support. Mrs. C is sensitive to the side effects of antidepressants and she often complained of fatigue.

Mrs. C had started attending PGDH in July 2017 with the aid of transportation service. She had been reluctant to attend at first, but after joining, she started to enjoy the activities (including physiotherapy and occupational therapy) and liked chatting with other patients. Mrs. C claimed that she had made friends and liked listening to other's problems She is receiving meals on wheels at home and would also do volunteer work at the city society for the aged around once a week whenever her knee and hip pain is better. She had continued receiving cognitive behavioral therapy (CBT) from a clinical psychologist and felt that she had ruminated less about her husband and had resolved some of her anger regarding his death. Mrs. C was not keen to have further psychiatric medication because she was concerned about their side effects. Mrs. C felt that her primary difficulty was her mobility. She had also been referred to the district elderly community center for further support. She also applied for medical fee waivers because she is financially dependent on her daughter only and old aged allowance.

Consultation
The doctor expressed the feeling that, as a clinician, she felt helpless; as a psychiatrist she was in no position to improve Mrs. C's mobility (could not hasten the knee replacement operations) or address the other physical problems and medical treatment, which was within her field of expertise (antidepressants).

JM summarized the case as a case of a woman of 68 who had led an active and creative life, who became married, supported her husband, developed a good relationship with her husband, and had three children who they raised. The children have now moved and live in different countries and so, she had no role in caring for them; this was a major loss for her. The death of her husband is an additional major loss; the other enormous loss was that of her physical fitness. Mrs. C relied on her fitness to be helpful to others and also to be able to enjoy her life (as, for example, in hiking). Mrs. C has not readjusted her ideas and feelings to fit with her present life situation as an elderly, widow, and a woman whose children do not need her anymore and who can contribute little to the wider community.

JM then added that although doctors and therapists pay considerable attention to feelings of sadness and loss, we do not pay as much attention to unpleasant feelings of anger. JM acknowledged that the anger toward doctors had been addressed somehow because she had expressed anger because they did not save her husband's life and because they had not given her adequate advice on how to help him and telling her to be careful was not good enough. The doctor added that she had acknowledged her anger at not being told on how she could prevent further strokes taking place—something that was likely to happen. The doctor added that Mrs. C had also expressed anger that the doctors did not save her husband from what was a febrile illness. JM raised the issue of anger toward her husband who inflicted part of the illness on himself by smoking. The doctor added that her husband's father had made that comment that he had brought the stroke on himself. The doctor added that she felt that her husband did not deserve to have a stroke despite his smoking because there are many people who smoke and do not suffer strokes. The doctor added that Mrs. C was forgiving toward her husband. JM added that it seemed to him that Mrs. C was idealizing her husband whom she loved.

JM referred to Mrs. C's hallucinations of widowhood (Dewi Rees, 1971; Olson et al., 1985). This was referring to Mrs. C imagining that she had been visited by her husband after his death. The doctor pointed out that she was aware of the various forms of pathological grief. JM pointed out that widowhood is, at that age, one of the most stressful events that could happen to a person (regarding mortality of widowhood, see Parkes & Fitzgerald [1969]). JM added that the only life event that could be more stressful than widowhood is the death of a child. JM then pointed out that the couple had had a good life together. They brought up their children together and they brought them up well; she was tolerant of her husband's little faults, like his gambling, which was measured (not excessive). Before the husband became ill, they had managed to have savings and some small property; they had been a well-functioning couple and it was difficult for her to readjust her thinking so that she could look forward to a future. The doctor added that having spent all their savings Mrs. C was now left with few resources and she was dependent on her daughter from whom she receives the equivalent of

US300 a month which is a small sum—a sum barely adequate to cover her needs. JM pointed out the predicament of having to live alone, aged, with difficulties and with little support from family. JM asked if Mrs. C receives any support from the Buddhist community of the city. The doctor pointed out that although she does have several friends, her mobility restricts her from visiting them. The doctor also pointed out that a visit to a Buddhist temple was not mentioned. The doctor added that it was not only her physical disability but also some reluctance to go out and meet people; she was concerned how she would appear to her peers walking with a walker. The doctor added that it would also be difficult for her to invite people to her home because the living space is limited.

JM repeated that the task for Mrs. C was to readjust her thinking on how to live the rest of her life as an elderly, physically compromised, lonely woman. JM invited the doctor to imagine what prospect could this woman have for her life in the following, say, 20 years. The doctor replied that if she were in that position, she would place most of her hopes on a knee operation taking place in the immediate future because if her mobility improved she would be able to go out a bit more and engage more in the activities that will improve her emotional state. Maybe she will be able to do some hiking again—something that she enjoyed in the past; she may be able to do some voluntary work or meet up with some of her friends. JM questioned how realistic the prospect of hiking would be for Mrs. C and asked if Mrs. C was also overweight. This was confirmed by the doctor. JM pointed out the vicious circle of arthritis limiting movement, and limitation of movement leading to increased weight, which in turn limits movement even further.

JM, having questioned the realistic level of the expectation of hiking, then moved on to invite the doctors to consider what would be a realistic prospect and asked the doctor if Mrs. C's hopelessness had become her own hopelessness as well. JM then introduced the psychoanalytic concept of *countertransference* (Heimann, 1950; Kernberg, 1965; Winnicott, 1960). JM made a summary of the concept as follows: Countertransference refers to the feelings that the therapist develops that arise not from the therapist's own experience or the result of an independent assessment, but they represent the adoption of the patient's feelings, which are seen by the therapist as their own. JM pointed out that in the case of Mrs. C, her own hopelessness became the doctor's hopelessness. JM asked the doctors whether the appropriate thinking and action for Mrs. C was to end her life because there was no realistic future for her. As this was not the case, JM started pointing out the positive elements of Mrs. C's predicament. For example, she still had her mind (she was not dementing) and still had a desire to be independent, caring, and giving. JM pointed out that Mrs. C based her relationships on her ability to offer. JM invited the doctors to consider how people who retire from active life adjust to this new pattern (Wu et al., 2016). Generally, older people are less able to offer and less able to earn. The first element on which they can rely is their history. They have a memory of a full life. This lady can have a memory of surviving adversity, coping with numerous changes, enjoying a good relationship with her husband, and fulfilling herself by bringing three children up. Mrs. C can rely on this history to feel that her life has not, to date, been wasted. That is a thought that is not depressing and is realistic.

One can be sympathetic to this woman who has lost her ability to function because of widowhood, disability, and poverty. It is going to be difficult for her to make this adjustment, but it is not impossible to use the residual resources that she has, which are her intellectual ability and her personality. Once she develops a more realistic approach to her future, she is more likely to accept help to engage in interaction with other people such as the interaction arranged at the psychiatric day hospital. Some other organizations, not related with provision of care, could perhaps be approached for her to participate as an equal member and not as a recipient of service. Mrs. C needs to value that she can be useful as a presence not only as somebody who does a job for others or somebody who offers a service. Any expectations of her offering work would be frustrated and, therefore, unrealistic. She could value the realistic expectation of offering herself for who she is and not for what she can do for other people. She could make some people happier by just spending time with them. This, in return, could make her feel happier and more useful. This would increase her own sense of self-worth. The doctor confirmed that Mrs. C feels better when she is with other people at the day hospital. JM asked if the local Buddhist community has any programs to engage isolated members of the Buddhist community. The doctor undertook to explore this avenue. JM also pointed out that a physical objective within her reach could be some reduction in her body weight. JM suggested that she could be put in touch with a dietician and perhaps an exercise program appropriate to her disability could be devised.

JM concluded that the central focus of a treatment would be for the treating doctor and all the staff to resolve the feeling of hopelessness and replace it with one of realistic expectations for Mrs. C. The doctor concluded that Mrs. C does enjoy interaction with other people and that she is able to come forward with ideas that make other people feel better. JM added that this experience, that she has a positive effect on other people, could be pointed out to her and encourage her that she is still useful to others, and she should not write herself off because she is appreciated by others as a person and not as a job.

References

Dewi Rees, W. (1971). The hallucinations of widowhood. *British Medical Journal*, 4(5778), 37–41.

Heimann, P. (1950). On countertransference. *The International Journal of Psycho-Analysis*, 31, 81–84.

Kernberg, O. F. (1965). Notes on countertransference. *Journal of American Psychoanalysis Assessment*, 13, 38–56.

Olson, P. R., Suddeth, J. A., Peterson, P. J., & Egelhoff, C. (1985). Hallucinations of widowhood. *Journal of the American Geriatrics Society*, 33(8), 543–547.

Parkes, C. M., Benjamin, B., & Fitzgerald, R. G. (1969). Broken heart: A statistical study of increased mortality among widowers. *British Medical Journal*, 1, 740–743.

Winnicott, D. W. (1960). Countertransference. *The British Journal of Medical Psychology*, 33, 17–21.

Wu, C., Odden, M. C., Fisher, G. G., & Stawski, R. S. (2016). Association of retirement age with mortality: A population-based longitudinal study among older adults in the USA. *Journal of Epidemiology and Community Health*, 70(9), 917–923.

2
Postnatal Depression

Margaret

Presenting condition

Margaret is a 28-year-old married housewife, mother of two (a boy aged 3.5 years and a girl aged 2 months), who lives with her husband and children in a rented subdivided room. Her infant daughter is mainly breastfed. She was referred by Maternal and Child Health Centre with an Edinburgh Postnatal Depression Scale score of 27 out of 30 in January 2018.

History of present complaint

Margaret presented with low mood with suicidal ideas. She was new to the mental health service. She delivered a baby girl on November 19, 2017, via vaginal delivery with no complications. She had multiple stressors from before her daughter's birth. These included her husband indulged in gambling and, recently, even online gambling; he would disappear for a few days a month in the past 3 years. The debt had increased to the point that the debt was paid using credit cards, and the debt now totals about US$30,000. The second source of stress was her son's problematic behavior since she became pregnant. The third source of stress is the crowded living environment. She had decided to live in the city because this would enable her son to attend kindergarten year 1 from January 2018. Margaret has limited support from her family of origin.

Margaret developed low mood, with a sense of worthlessness and helplessness. She would look at her children and become worried about their future; she felt that they were poor. Since giving birth, her mood further deteriorated, with her experiencing reduced energy and poor concentration at work. Her sleep was also disturbed by childcare. Margaret experienced appetite loss and lost 1–2 kg. She does not enjoy activities, feels the lack of money, and has no time for any entertainment; they do not even have a television set at home. Previously, she had fleeting suicidal ideas of jumping from heights, but these became less frequent since she moved to the city. In the city, her husband tended to stay at home most of the time. Margaret denied having a concrete suicide plan, had not acted on any

Dynamic Consultations with Psychiatrists: Understanding Severely Troubled Patients, First Edition. Jason Maratos.

suicidal impulses, was remorseful, and still cared about and worried for her children. Margaret denied alcohol or substance use and denied the existence of any psychotic symptoms. Occasionally, she would hit her son with bare hands or with a hanger; however, she would feel remorse afterward. There were no previous hypo-manic or manic episodes.

Family history

There is no family history of mental illness or suicide.

Personal history

Margaret was born in the country. She is the eldest of four siblings (two sisters who are 2 years younger and one brother). Margaret graduated from secondary school. She came to the city when she was 17 years old. She had a fair relationship with her family of origin. Her mother works in the market and her father works as a casual worker.

Margaret had an unhappy childhood; her father would hit her with a belt and a hanger until she developed skin lacerations; her mother would kick her over trivial matters. Her family was patriarchal. She was physically punished by her parents until she reached high school. Her parents disliked her studying and wanted her to work and earn for the family. Margaret insisted on working part-time and supporting her studies. She felt that she was an "extra" in her family. She had a better relationship with her younger sisters and brother.

Margaret was married at 24 years of age and moved back to the country; she would travel daily to work as a saleslady in a part of the city, which is near the country; she was the main breadwinner of the family. Her family of origin was not supportive of her marriage; they disliked her marrying and moving back to the mainland. Margaret does not "dare" to express her feelings to her family of origin and does not feel that she can ask them for support. She gave up her job in January 2018 to allocate her time to childcare. Margaret is currently unemployed and has been working as a housewife since moving to the city.

Her husband is 28 years old and from the country; he is without a city identity card. He previously worked as a waiter but became unemployed recently to take care of their son while Margaret worked and was the breadwinner. Her husband is currently waiting for his identity card and so he can find work. Husband and family depend on Margaret's savings. Margaret is a nonsmoker and nondrinker; she has no history of substance or alcohol misuse.

Past psychiatric history

Margaret is new to the mental health service.

Present treatment and management

On the first consultation in February, Margaret was found to have low mood and to be calm and settled, even though she was weeping. She presented within the normal range. Her speech was coherent and relevant and was of normal tone and tempo. She claimed that she had been troubled by fewer suicidal ideas. No psychotic features were detected. She had no violent ideas or any harmful ideas toward her children.

The overall impression was that Margaret was suffering from a moderate depressive episode whose onset was well before the birth of her last child and which was related to multiple stressors. Margaret felt initially relieved to live away from her family of origin but found that since moving to the city she was facing more problems, such as financial stress and stress in relation to the care of the children, with limited social support.

Treatment options were discussed with Margaret who was then started on Sertraline 25 mg and was referred to a medical social worker and to the community psychiatric nurse service. The issue of the use of benzodiazepines while breastfeeding was also considered.

Consultation

JM acknowledged that this was a thorough and thoughtful presentation. JM addressed the question of why Margaret developed depression after the second child and not after the first. The doctor responded that Margaret had to change her living environment on this occasion so that her son could attend the nursery in the city. This move brought greater financial stress on the family. It was clarified that Margaret had lived in the country with her first child and her husband. It was therefore made clear that the family is under stress because of the opinion that the children would have a better education in the city than in the country. The doctor pointed out that Margaret was familiar with the city where she lived from her early teenage years. Furthermore, Margaret had been working in the city while living in the country for quite a few years. The doctor pointed out that quite a few families do this as a matter of course. The doctor also pointed out that many people who live in the country believe that the city offers better education, better social care, and better health care.

JM pointed out the disappointment that Margaret must have felt when she was expecting the move to the city to represent an improvement in her family life and living conditions and found quite the opposite. The doctor pointed out that the family had taken steps to make their stay in the city permanent, such as applying for an identity card for her husband and expecting their son to continue making improvement and a good adjustment at the nursery. They expect that after the identity card is obtained, the husband will be able to work and, therefore, contribute to the family finances. The doctor added that this was a realistic plan, but also noted that employment in the city is difficult to obtain.

JM then inquired about the debt. The doctor clarified that the debt had accumulated because of the husband's gambling. The doctor added that husband was gambling his own and his wife's savings. JM inquired further about husband's gambling, and the doctor added that there is an indication that husband is still gambling online from home. The doctor further added that husband is likely to be given an identity card in a few months' time.

JM then asked, because there probably was a group of county people who worked without an identity card in the cash economy, in the black market, or simply manual jobs for lesser money but cash in the city, why the husband wasn't doing something of the sort. JM pointed out that the family situation is not an adequate explanation for husband's staying at home and gambling instead of going out to earn a living to support the family. JM then inquired further about the husband's role in the family and, in particular, whether he was supportive of his wife in other ways.

JM summarized that the basis of Margaret's depression is her view of her own future as without hope of something getting better. JM inquired whether her feeling of hopelessness was based on the absence of any active steps that her husband could be taking to improve their situation. In this sense, her view of the future was realistic; that is, that things are not going to get better if the husband continues to behave the way that he has been.

JM then shifted the focus to Margaret's psychopathology. As the eldest child, she was brought up to feel that she was responsible for supporting the family. She may have carried the same expectation—the expectation that her parents had for her—as her expectation of herself now and, as such, had low expectations of receiving help from her husband. In other words, she expected that everything was her responsibility, and that if things were not going well, she had only herself to blame. Therefore, one of the early therapeutic objectives would be to alter Margaret's expectations of herself and of her husband. In other words, they should share more balanced expectations, but at the moment, she has to give priority to the care of a 3-month-old child. And, instead of wasting family resources by gambling, her husband, who has much more free time, should go out and earn money for his family.

JM then shifted the focus to Margaret's perception of the future. Although under the present dynamics, it did not look optimistic, they were not inevitable or unalterable. It was not inevitable that the husband would not pull his weight and that their finances would not improve. These may change if the correct support and direction was given to this family by the involved professionals. By professionals, I mean not only the clinical psychologist but also the social worker who would give them more directive advice. The likelihood is that her husband will get an identity card and, therefore, will be able to obtain legal employment. This would give the family a better living standard to which they can improve their predicament. They could be helped to have a more long-term perspective and accept that, although in the immediate future finances will be tight, they do not have to be so in the long term. Margaret could be helped to see herself in a few years; time, when both children are at school, when both parents are employed, when the debt will have been repaid, and they will be able to pour the fruits of their labor into making a better family life for themselves and their children. The reality is that they are both healthy and young, and they can make a good life for their family in the city. They also have the alternative of possibly settling in the country and working in the city like so many people do. The point is to give Margaret the ability to have a more realistic perspective of the future rather than the present perspective, which is one of hopelessness.

JM summarized that these were the two dimensions of therapy; the first dimension is her internal dynamic and the expectations that she has of herself (as shaped by the abusive parenting of which she was subjected) and others, and the second dynamic is to develop a more realistic and more long-term perspective of her future. For further study on effect of physical abuse on parenting see (Buist, 1998a; Buist, 1998b; Lang et al., 2010).

The doctor then added the dimension of parenting skills. Margaret sometimes hits her children physically and then feels remorseful about this. She feels unhappy that she is repeating the pattern with which she was brought up and is keen to give her children a different family experience. The doctor pointed out that although she wants to give her children a different family experience, when she is distressed and angry, she acts impulsively and hits them. JM responded to the doctor's added dimension by inviting her to focus on the reasons why her son was misbehaving. The doctor suggested that her son may be feeling jealous that much more attention was being given to his infant sister. JM suggested that it would be helpful to find out more about how her 3-year-old son developed the troubling behavior that he has and what is the feeling that drives this behavior. More particularly, the exploration needs to be directed to whether these parents give direction and proper attention to their son or whether they are neglectful of him because they are absorbed in other activities, some of them necessary, such as the care of their infant daughter, and some unnecessary, like the husband's online gambling. JM invited the doctor to explore the role of the father with his son and, in particular, whether the father actually spends a reasonable amount of time in some enjoyable or creative activity with him.

JM suggested that the possibility that the boy is misbehaving because he is neglected by his parents and, particularly, by his father should be explored more fully. JM pointed out that the overall impression is one of a mother who is overinvolved with her own sense that she should be responsible for the welfare of everyone and a father who is underinvolved and rather self-indulgent in gambling and perhaps not carrying his share of weight for the family. This family dynamic needs to be more balanced if the children are to be more content and exhibit less disturbing behavior.

JM concluded the session by repeating that Margaret and her husband are two young people who are physically healthy and have the potential to work and provide for their family and shape a better future for themselves. This is the baseline from which they can both be given some realistic hope for their future and such hope would motivate them to channel their energies in a more creative way.

References

Buist, A. (1998a). Childhood abuse, parenting and postpartum depression. *The Australian and New Zealand Journal of Psychiatry, 32*(4), 479–487.

Buist, A. (1998b). Childhood abuse, postpartum depression and parenting difficulties: A literature review of associations. *The Australian and New Zealand Journal of Psychiatry, 32*(3), 370–378.

Lang, A. J., Gartstein, M. A., Rodgers, C. S., & Lebeck, M. M. (2010). The impact of maternal childhood abuse on parenting and infant temperament. *Journal of Child and Adolescent Psychiatric Nursing, 23*(2), 100–110.

3
Bipolar Affective Disorder

Miss C

Introduction

Miss C, is a 21-year-old woman suffering from Bipolar Affective Disorder.

History of present illness

Miss C was noted since July 2017 to be showing increasingly irritable and labile mood when she was taking her evening school examinations. She scolded her mother and sister on trivial matters. She had recently joined an insurance course and planned on taking the qualifying exam. She spent about US$1,000 this month on clothes and handbags and was spending more on dining. She mentioned that she needed to be someone "with class." She mentioned that she will get rich and be the breadwinner of the family. She tended to lock herself in a room at night and listen to music, experiencing decreased sleep as well. She absconded from home 2 weeks before admission and stayed at her classmate's home for 5 days. She enjoyed her time there, chatting with the family, but they found her unmanageable and asked her aunt to take her home. She had an outburst of anger t a week before admission when she was nagging to have a portion of her sisters' food and her mother confronted her. She handed a glass bottle to her mother and asked her mother to kill her. Her mother smashed the bottle and pointed it to herself said she would kill herself instead. Miss C eventually locked herself in the toilet and splashed water on her face. She was seen at the outpatient department in August 2017 and a compulsory admission was arranged by F123 of the Mental Health Act due to manic relapse.

Personal history

Miss C is an evening school Form 6 student and part-time waitress; she lives with mother and elder sister in a private flat.

Dynamic Consultations with Psychiatrists: Understanding Severely Troubled Patients, First Edition. Jason Maratos.
© 2022 John Wiley & Sons Ltd. Published 2022 by John Wiley & Sons Ltd.

Miss C was born in the city. Her birth and developmental history were unremarkable. She was raised by her parents and maternal grandparents. She is quite fond of her maternal grandfather who is gentle with her. Her maternal grandmother was deaf and had frequent conflicts with patient.

Her father came from a family associated with a criminal society. However, her father was not involved in any criminal activity, and he ran a cigarette and alcohol business. Her father was an alcoholic who tended to drink after 3 p.m.; he would scold her but would not hit her. Her mother and her mother's younger sister employed frequent physical punishment when Miss C was rebellious and would hit her with sticks.

Miss C's parents divorced when she was 9 years old and she was raised by her mother since that time. After her parents divorced, her mother worked as a waitress to support them. Her parents got back together later but never remarried. Miss C enjoyed a good relationship with both her parents. She respects her mother for the hardship that she endured in sustaining the family. She has good memories with father about their shared interest in movies and food.

Miss C had good academic results before Form 2 when her father died. She was always in the advanced class of the year. She described herself as "a shy kid" but enjoyed a good relationship with her classmates; she has five close and supportive friends with whom she's still in contact.

She has had one courtship from Primary 6 to Form 2 (ages 10–13), which she described as "puppy love." When she was in Form 3, she was bullied by a classmate. That classmate would throw a basketball at her and would also threaten to beat her. Miss C gave up day school in Form 4 because of repeated hospital admissions as well as sedation resulting from psychiatric medication. She stayed at home and played computer games most of the time after quitting day school but later joined evening school. She worked as waitress on a short-term basis to earn money.

Her maternal grandfather died in 2014 from pneumonia, and she was discharged from the hospital just in time to see him before he passed. She resents psychiatrists for depriving her time to accompany her maternal grandfather in his last days and for delaying her academic progression. She plans to get a university degree and work in an office. She said that her dream job would be in movie production but that would be after she holds a stable job that can sustain her to pursue her dream.

Past psychiatric history

The onset of her mental illness was shortly after her father's death in January 2010; her father died of a chest infection. Miss C was then in Form 2. She experienced low mood and weeping spells for 1 to 2 months after that. Her mental condition deteriorated in June 2011, when she was in Form 3; she presented with social withdrawal, frequently blaming her family for not offering her good food. She attempted suicide in September 2011 by burning charcoal in her room; she had even written a final note. Miss C was saved by her mother 1 hour later and was sent to the hospital accident and emergency department. She was stabilized and seen by a psychiatrist who diagnosed depression and discharged her on fluoxetine. A child psychiatric outpatient clinic followed up with Miss C. She could not tolerate fluoxetine; as her mood continued being labile, her medication was changed to venlafaxine 225 mg daily. Miss C showed partial improvement in December 2011.

Miss C had a manic relapse in February 2012 again with irritable mood, pressure of speech, and social withdrawal. She blamed her family for giving her poor food and would go out to buy snacks at night. She was overspending (in excess of US$2,000) for accessories and stamps for collections. She had grandiose ideas, including that she looked like a celebrity and that she might have been some prominent figure in her past life, such as Jesus, Buddha, or President Mao. She was finally admitted to hospital in March 2012 because of violent behavior against her aunt and because she was breaking objects at home. She was first tried on risperidone 6 mg nightly + sodium valproate CR 400 mg, and clonazepam 2 mg daily with suboptimal control. She developed a depressive swing during her inpatient stay with crying spells, rumination about her deceased father, paranoid ideation toward others, fleeting suicidal ideas, with persistent thoughts racing and multiple plans. Her medication was changed to olanzapine 20 mg N, sodium valproate 600 mg, and Clonazepam. Her depressive symptoms improved but manic symptoms persisted; she developed akathisia, which was partly controlled by benzodiazepines, Artane, and propranolol. Lithium was started, and manic symptoms significantly improved. Miss C discharged herself against medical advice in July 2012 and was readmitted 1 week later with manic symptoms. She was stabilized and discharged on lithium, sodium valproate, and venlafaxine.

The Child Psychiatric Clinic had followed up with Miss C and doubted drug compliance. Mirtazapine was used briefly in October 2013 for depressive symptoms and lithium was tailed off in June 2013 because "she did not like" that medication.

She was admitted to hospital in October 2014 and stayed until December 2014 for manic relapse with irritable mood, grandiose delusions, poor sleep with increase energy, and (over)spending US$100 to buy stamps. She was stabilized and discharged on lithium 800 mg, sodium valproate CR 400 mg, and Quetiapine 600 mg.

Miss C was then followed up in general adult psychiatric outpatient clinic. Escitalopram was started in October 2016 for low mood. Quetiapine was tailed off gradually due to sedation. Buspirone was added in February 2017 for anxiety. Patient was last seen in the outpatient clinic and was stable on quetiapine 150 mg nightly, lithium 600 mg nightly, sodium valproate CR 400 mg nightly, and buspirone 10 mg twice a day. A clinical psychiatric nurse and a clinical psychologist have followed up with her since March 2017 as requested.

Premorbid personality

Miss C was shy and introverted as a child. She was competitive and appears to be strong. Miss C is expressive of her emotions.

Mental state examination   Miss C appeared with dyed hair, wearing spectacles, and no makeup. She was tearful at the beginning of the session when she was talking about being admitted compulsorily. Miss C was overly friendly in the beginning, asking the case doctor to buy her snacks, trying to seek common ground with case doctor by expressing her religious and political inclination. She became more irritable when her request was turned down, and when they inquired about her manic symptoms, Miss C had a challenging attitude and questioned the case doctor's personal background information. Her speech was coherent and relevant but demonstrated pressure of speech. Her mood was labile but congruent. She did not admit to any hallucinations. Miss C had a grandiose idea about herself coming from a prominent family. There was no risk of suicide or of violent behavior. She had no insight about her manic relapse and her need for inpatient treatment.

Treatment progress

In view of oversedation, which was attributed to quetiapine, this was tailed off, and aripiprazole was added to the drug regimen and sodium valproate was titrated up. Miss C's mood stabilized, and she settled in the ward with less challenging attitude. Her sleep and appetite were maintained.

Psychodynamic observations   Miss C employed a number of pathological defense mechanisms such as *denial* of her condition and of the risk of a manic relapse. Miss C claimed that she could get a private psychiatrist to certify that she was "normal." She thought that her temperament was more expressive and irritable and that this was not related to a disease.

Splitting: Ms. C thought that a previous doctor, who was a Christian and who had bought her snacks, was a great person and she thought that other doctors were evil to force her to stay in hospital. She thought that her community psychiatric nurse, who had been her friend previously, was evil because she betrayed her and got her admitted. Miss C expressed hatred toward the psychiatrist who deprived her of the opportunity to accompany her maternal grandfather in his last days.

Miss C expressed grief on account of her delay in her career progress in comparison with her peers (who are now professionals like lawyers and dentists) because of her illness.

The doctors felt that there was a possibility of unresolved oral stage of development because there was a history of blaming her family of not serving good food during manic relapse. Her mother did not visit her in the first week of admission due to stress. Miss C repeatedly nagged the ward doctor to buy her snacks. Her mother visited her on the second week with lots of snacks, and Miss C was thrilled and offered some to the ward doctor.

Consultation   This was a comprehensive assessment of a difficult patient. Let me say at first that we are in the field of combining pure psychiatric treatment (with medication) with psychotherapy. I have no doubt, and you gave a convincing history, that this is a person suffering from a bipolar disorder and am surprised that there is not any family history of this.

The problem is that without insight, she has low compliance and low compliance leads to relapse. There are medicines that can help; pharmacology has advanced and this is something that, if you compliance can be assured, a better response can be expected. An important aspect of treatment would be that as Miss C has limited insight about the need for medication for her own welfare, somebody needs to supervise her taking medicines. Somebody in her environment needs to do that; otherwise she experiences a period of euphoria and her self-confidence increases and it veers toward grandiosity and overconfidence. She then begins to think, "I don't need all that rubbish; doctors do it for their own sake and I am going to stop taking medicines and I am going to spend lots of money to get accessories and clothes and look great." So that's when somebody else needs to take authority over her and ensure compliance or will need to arrange a prompt psychiatric appointment when they see that she is heading that way.

The other limited comment is about the developmental theory of psychoanalysis. Freud developed the developmental theory based on examining adults who gave a historical recollection of their past. Freud did not systematically examine children growing up.

Developmental psychology has done exactly that and the proposal of oral, anal, phallic, latency, preadolescent, and adolescent genital stages has been seriously challenged (Rutter, 1970, pp. 274–276). Freud's formulation is historical and interesting from a historical point of view of psychoanalysis, but it's not something considered useful by many contemporary psychoanalysts.

The second point is that such a formulation confuses normal development with pathological development. By definition, pathological development does not occur at any stage of normal maturation. So if pathological development is not appropriate, attribute it to an age. For example, Miss C is blaming her family for not serving good food, which is not something that is appropriate (consistently) at any stage of normal development as a pattern. If a 2-year-old child is served food they don't like, they will get cross and will try to weave their behavior into a pattern that is often described as representing an oral stage of development, but this is not founded on any scientific basis. So, the easiest thing would be to forget this aspect of the psychoanalytic theory because it is not a useful part of psychoanalysis.

JM pointed out that the doctor was already doing what one can expect to achieve with a patient who is suffering from a bipolar illness. The main foundation of treatment would be medication and the would be ensuring compliance. Without these, any talking aimed at changing feelings and thoughts would be wasted.

Someone who is manic and thinks they are descendants of President Mao cannot be expected to start a dialogue. The emotional conviction is so strong they will think that you don't understand who you are talking to because "I am a descendent of Jesus or I am a descendent of whomever" or "I am as beautiful and gorgeous as Naomi Campbell,"; "you just don't understand." So the approach that may be most useful in this phase is supportive and supervisory.

When Miss C becomes more receptive, then you can concentrate on building her self-esteem, building her resilience, and helping her to develop a realistic approach about her potential; she needs to be helped to value and use her "well" phases to build a realistic future for herself. But during her "ill" phases, all that can be done is concentrate on supporting and supervising her, ensuring that she is safe and that her environment understands her condition. Also, when the first signs of a relapse are seen, she should be taken for immediate psychiatric treatment because she may need hospitalization or restoration of medication because the likelihood is that she will not comply. This is the main problem with people who are manic depressive; the moment that they go toward the extreme of emotions, either toward hypomania or toward depression, they drop their medicines. When they are depressed, they think there is no point, and when they are hypomanic, they think they don't need them.

It is at this point, that someone in her life, who is not mentally ill to say: "She is going up or down too much and this is the beginning of something is going on. Let's see a psychiatrist." The psychiatrist will then institute the appropriate treatment. When Miss C is accessible, then it can be planned how she manages a genuine and serious illness. Miss C has a major risk of suicide. Her previous attempt (carbon monoxide and having left a note!) supports this view.

We have drawn an agreement between her and her mother that she needs to ensure that she takes her medication before 11:30 p.m. and are hopeful that will work.

This is exactly the right thing. And from the doctor's point of view, I think you should not have the expectation of a transformation. This is a serious illness that unfortunately has a guarded prognosis. What I am saying is that you should not be demoralized if she is not cured. Doctors who have high expectations of their patients are carrying the risk of making themselves vulnerable to disappointment and eventual burnout (Maratos, 1996). The issue of burnout among healthcare workers is of enormous significance. I attached references from the extensive bibliography that the reader may find useful (Maslach et al., 2001; Maslach & Leiter, 2016; Pines & Maslach, 1978).

References

Maratos, J. (1996). Professional burnout. In G. Manthoul, M. Manthoul, E. Besevegis, & A. Kokkevi (Eds.), *Contemporary psychology in Europe. Theory, research and applications* (pp. 301–311). Hogrefe & Huber Publishers.

Maslach, C., & Leiter, M. P. (2016). Understanding the burnout experience: Recent research and its implications for psychiatry. *World Psychiatry*, 15(2), 103–111.

Maslach, C., Schaufeli, W. B., & Leiter, M. P. (2001). Job burnout. *Annual Review of Psychology*, 52, 397–422.

Pines, A., & Maslach, C. (1978). Characteristics of staff burnout in mental health settings. *Hospital & Community Psychiatry*, 29(4), 233–237.

Rutter, M. (1970). Normal psychosexual development. *Journal of Child Psychology and Psychiatry*, 11(4), 259–283.

4
Suicidal

Iris

This is a case that demonstrates the long-term effects of child sexual abuse on how a victim approaches forming adult relationships, including some cultural contributing factors. It also demonstrates the presence of pseudo-hallucinations in depressive episodes, which is sometimes misattributed to schizophrenia.

Presenting condition

Iris is a 29-year-old single woman who is currently unemployed. She was voluntarily admitted for low mood following a suicidal gesture.

History of present complaint

Iris had deteriorated in mood after the new year in 2018. She had arguments with her boyfriend's sister after she ransacked Iris's toys and clothes. She felt that her privacy had been infringed. The incidents brought to mind her previous experiences of being sexually assaulted during childhood. She experienced fluctuations of mood and had crying spells. She had interrupted sleep. She also complained of hearing her own inner voice once every few days asking her to die and give up.

Iris had negative cognitions and was blaming herself for having depression. She had fleeting suicidal ideas. Her boyfriend brought her to see a private psychiatrist, who made the diagnosis of schizophrenia and prescribed tricyclic antidepressants. She felt dizzy and had a "hangover" feeling after taking the medication. She felt that her memory had deteriorated. There was no improvement in mood. Her boyfriend broke up with her because he could not stand her emotional fluctuations. Her appetite and low mood deteriorated further. A few days before admission, she claimed that she felt angry toward herself after she forgot to buy some things and became impulsive. She had one gesture of a jump from height a few days before admission by crossing the bench in a corridor of a building; her mother quickly pulled her back with slight effort. Iris claimed to have only a vague memory of

Dynamic Consultations with Psychiatrists: Understanding Severely Troubled Patients, First Edition. Jason Maratos.
© 2022 John Wiley & Sons Ltd. Published 2022 by John Wiley & Sons Ltd.

this incident because she was affected by drugs prescribed by her psychiatrist. There were no genuine suicidal ideas and no final act.

In March 2018, Iris took a drug overdose on impulse; she attributed this to her poor sleep. She wished to sleep better so she took 8–10 tablets of Stilnox and 20 tablets of a painkiller. She was sent to the accident and emergency department, and her mother agreed to the admission.

Family history

Her mother is reported to be suffering from schizophrenia.

Personal history

Iris was born in the city and has one older sister. She described her childhood as unhappy with an insecure attachment. Iris was in foster care by different relatives and parents' friends from the time she entered kindergarten until she was in class Primary 6 "as parents had to work." Iris described her relationship with her mother as fair, but she also felt that she was a burden and that she was loved by her parents.

Iris gave an account of four episodes of being sexually assaulted or molested. One episode was by the parents' friend who took care of her, another by a colleague at work, and yet another by a Taoism master who claimed having sexual intercourse with him would improve her fate.

Iris studied up to Form 5 and had a fair academic performance. Iris's parents divorced when she was a teenager. She has worked as a nail beautician and part-time model but is currently unemployed. Iris had been troubled by repeated ruminations and negative thoughts, a fear of abandonment, and was sensitive to unfairness; she had high expectations of herself.

Past psychiatric history

Iris has been known to the mental health service since December 2015 when she presented following a drug overdose with her mother's 10 hypnotic tablets and a self-harm gesture of wrist slashing. She was referred to a psychiatric outpatient clinic. The diagnosis, at that time, was depression. A clinical psychologist thought she had a borderline personality trait. Iris presented with two more episodes of drug overdose in 2017, which had followed relationship difficulties; she had then attended the emergency department. No psychiatric admission had been arranged. Iris was regularly followed up at the psychiatric clinic; she was last seen in March 2018, where mood fluctuations were documented following an argument with her boyfriend's sister. Antidepressant medication was titrated up.

Present treatment and management of case   Antidepressant medication was adjusted after admission. She tolerated the current dose of citalopram. Iris thought again about her relationship with her mother. She agreed that her relationship with her mother improved following her admission because she sensed her mother's love.

Methods of coping with stress were discussed. She reflected that her past trauma may affect her depressive episode. She was led to think about how her upbringing may affect her setting boundaries throughout her life. Her issue with setting boundaries was highlighted to enhance her insight on how her experience may affect her interpersonal functioning.

Iris's emotional reactivity in connection with her trauma in which people violate her privacy and rights were highlighted for her. Iris understood that she tended to overreact at times and that she could be quite impulsive. She agreed to continue to see psychologist for trauma work after discharge.

Consultation   JM thanked the doctor for the comprehensive presentation. JM then asked further questions about Iris's experience of being sexually assaulted. The doctor stated that her first sexual assault took place when she was in kindergarten. It was her parents' friend who was looking after her at the time. This was one episode of penetration. She told her parents, but her parents did not believe her at that time. Her parents did believe her when the matter was raised again with them during her teenage years. The parents did not take any measures to protect her. The doctor pointed out that there had been other episodes of sexual assault later as well. The most recent sexual assault took place 2 years previously. This was perpetrated by a fortune teller. She had been convinced by the fortune teller that her fate would be improved if she had intercourse with him. The doctor pointed out that this is not an entirely unusual practice because some fortune tellers convince their clients that they can improve their future by having intercourse with them. It is only after some time that Iris realized that she had been tricked into having intercourse with him. It was at that time that Iris reported the incident to the police. The police responded sympathetically but could not take any action because of the lack of evidence. She was told that her case had been weakened because she consented to the intercourse. JM clarified that the nature of the abuse was through deception rather than through a violent act such as rape. The doctor clarified that there had been no threats to secure secrecy.

JM asked about the effect that the abuse had on her at that time when she was 5 years old. The doctor clarified that at that time Iris felt abandoned and unwanted. The fact that her parents did not support her made her feel that she could not rely on them for protection. JM then asked if that experience had influenced her self-esteem and more specifically whether this experience had influenced her self-image and her sense of self-worth. The doctor reported that she believed that this was the case and that Iris felt unwanted by her parents. The doctor added that Iris felt that she was quite vulnerable and lost faith in relation to abuse by men. Iris also felt that she was attracting this kind of attention. JM asked if the experiences of abuse had affected Iris's view of herself and mentioned that quite a few abused people see themselves as dirty or worthless and that their only use in life is to be sexual objects. The doctor pointed out that she had explored that area and that Iris did not hold any of those feelings about herself. She only felt a target of inappropriate interest and that she was vulnerable to being abused. JM then asked about how the abuse came to an end. The doctor pointed out that four different people perpetrated all four incidents.

There were two episodes of abuse when she was an adolescent. The doctor explained that one episode was perpetrated by a colleague of hers at work and that on that occasion she put an end to it by telling the colleague that if he did that again she would report him to the police. Iris later resigned from her work. So the result was that Iris managed to protect herself when she was a teenager even though this was at a cost of losing her job. Regarding the abuse by the fortune teller, it was clarified by the doctor that a significant but small number of women in the city do believe that such action would improve their fortune and their fate. It is difficult for one to find any studies referring to this important phenomenon that is part of current culture in the city.

JM then asked the basis on which the other psychiatrist made the diagnosis of schizophrenia. The doctor pointed out that during periods of low mood, Iris sometimes hears voices. These are negative comments about herself and that she has no ability in controlling her own emotions. The doctor clarified that it was her own "inner voice" and that these hallucinations took place once every 2 or 3 days. JM pointed out that these were the characteristics of hallucinations of depression and not necessarily of schizophrenia. JM asked about Iris's insight into these experiences. The doctor reported that Iris was aware that these voices were unreal as a result; JM clarified that these were not true hallucinations but pseudo-hallucinations. JM pointed out that these experiences could not form the basis for a diagnosis of schizophrenia (Toh et al., 2015). JM then asked about the basis of the diagnosis of mother's schizophrenia. This had remained uncertain. JM then wondered if the belief that mother suffered from schizophrenia had influenced the other doctor's decision to form the opinion that Iris herself suffered from the same condition. JM wondered if the basis of diagnosing schizophrenia in the mother was just as unreliable as it was for the diagnosis of schizophrenia in Iris and whether the thought by the previous psychiatrist that Iris's mother suffers from schizophrenia made him more likely to diagnose the same condition in Iris. JM pointed out that we have reasons to doubt that diagnosis because the mother was reported to be quite functional for several years and that she worked.

The consultation then moved on to explore one of the precipitating factors of Iris's present condition, which was the breakup of the relationship with her boyfriend. The breakup took place on March 11—1 week before admission. The doctor added that she was of the impression that the boyfriend cared for Iris because he had accompanied her on quite a few of her outpatient appointments. The relationship had been going on for 1 or 2 years, and they had been living together for some of that time. Throughout that time Iris had fears of abandonment and was quite emotional at times. JM suggested that Iris's anxiety about the relationship was well founded because she had been quite difficult during the relationship. The doctor clarified that this was not exactly the case. The doctor added that Iris was aware that her emotionality may have affected the relationship and may have contributed to the breakup. JM asked about the content of these emotional fluctuations, and the doctor responded that her boyfriend saw them as overreactions. Particularly, when the boyfriend's sister disturbed her toys and Iris reacted, the boyfriend thought that her reactions were excessive. JM suggested that as it was the boyfriend's sister who had disturbed Iris's property, and Iris had a right to be not only upset but also angry.

JM pointed out that the injured party was Iris, and when such an incident takes place, it is right for the injured party to expect the offending person to own up to the error, to apologize for having caused the damage, and to make up for it. JM pointed out that just words are not enough to correct the offensive behavior and to reestablish a good relationship. JM pointed out that Iris did not expect her boyfriend's sister to own up, apologize, and correct the damage but, instead, she internalized the frustration, became depressed, and complained to her boyfriend who then, instead of correcting the harm, told her or showed her that he thought that she was overreacting. The doctor pointed out that the boyfriend urged his sister to own up and apologize but did not proceed to correct the damage. JM pointed out that without corrective action, the previous steps of owning up and apologizing amount to meaningless words. It is the action that validates the words expressed. In summary, the situation is that Iris was hurt, the boyfriend and his sister did not act to correct the damage, and their conclusion was that there was something wrong with Iris's reaction, which was considered to be excessive and probably the result of her "condition." JM then pointed out that it was difficult to correct the damage done through the earlier sexual abuse, but that compared to that abuse, the correction of the recent damage would have been easy. (For impact of sexual abuse on children, see Kendall-Trackett et al. [1993], although literature on this subject is extensive.)

JM summarized that Iris's early experiences had taught her that when she is violated or injured, she can only respond by being upset, hurt, and depressed. Her early experiences did not lead her to believe that she had the right to protect herself and the equal right to demand compensation, psychological and practical. Also, Iris has not learned that she has a right to be angry when she is injured.

JM then pointed out that although it is dysfunctional to internalize the depression and anger following an injury, it may be appropriate for Iris to see the level at which her own actions affect the relationship with her boyfriend. It was clarified that the boyfriend had been caring, but he probably changed his attitude after Iris was admitted to hospital. He used to accompany her to the outpatient appointments but has not visited her in hospital. It was clarified that the breakup seemed final and that Iris attributed the breakup to her own unreasonable behavior. Having established that Iris attributed the breakup to her own emotionality, JM then invited the doctor to explore where Iris attributed her emotionality. The doctor responded that during therapy, Iris was able to connect her behavior to the previous traumata that she suffered—referring to the incidents of abuse. JM then tried to explore the nature of the emotional reactions following interactions with her boyfriend. The doctor gave an example of when Iris was upset when she noticed some messages on her boyfriend's telephone that were directed toward another woman. The boyfriend dismissed her upset, insisting that the relationship was a purely friendly one and could not interfere with their own relationship. JM then summarized that Iris seemed to be entering a relationship with some increased uncertainty about the fidelity of her prospective partner. This sensitivity led her to be more vigilant for signs of possible unfaithfulness. The next step was to interpret potentially innocent events as signs of the boyfriend's infidelity and lead to behavior that resulted in the end of their relationship. The next step, instead of the functionally useful step of confronting the boyfriend and sorting it out, she became more upset, internalized all these feelings and became excessively emotional, in this way aggravating not only her mental state but also the relationship.

The insight that Iris could gain is that although it is understandable that somebody who had been traumatized, as she had been, would be sensitive about the fidelity of her boyfriend, she should develop the ability to judge each situation for what it is, rather than see it as a repetition of the past.

References

Kendall-Tackett, K. A., Williams, L. M., & Finkelhor, D. (1993). Impact of sexual abuse on children: A review and synthesis of recent empirical studies. *Psychological Bulletin*, *113*(1), 164–180.

Toh, W. L., Thomas, N., & Rossell, S. L. (2015). Auditory verbal hallucinations in bipolar disorder (BD) and major depressive disorder (MDD): A systematic review. *Journal of Affective Disorders*, *184*, 18–28.

Mrs. Mak

Presenting condition

Mrs. Mak is a 68-year-old woman, retired university lecturer, widowed, and living with her daughter in a private flat. This was an informal admission to the hospital via the psychogeriatric clinic for suicidal ideation.

History of present complaint

Mrs. Mak attended psychiatric follow-up one date after the original scheduled date. During her last follow-up 2 weeks previously, she had already reported low mood and an expressed wish to die but felt her daughter would not be able to cope with her suicide. A community psychiatric nurse was already involved. On the date of follow-up, Mrs. Mak claimed she had defaulted on follow-up the previous day because she wished to die. She reported that her mood deteriorated over the past 2 weeks because she had found out her daughter had moved in with her boyfriend, and Mrs. Mak claimed that she could not accept cohabitation because she was a Christian. Mrs. Mak reported that her daughter's boyfriend was of the same race, and she was afraid that her daughter would be cheated and hurt. She felt her daughter had frequently lied about why she did not sleep at home, and she had only found out accidentally she was dating someone about 2 weeks previous. She reported to have been taking Stilnox 20 mg (double the recommended dose) after lunch and 20 mg after dinner during the last 2 to 3 weeks. She claimed she wished to sleep to avoid the pain or facing reality.

Mrs. Mak claimed to have self-titrated down her antidepressant by half for about 2 months before resuming the usual dose after last follow-up. She had feelings of hopelessness, worthlessness, and suicidal ideas and plans to take a drug overdose using her psychiatric medications. She claimed she had previously thought about jumping from a height but did not wish for her body to be disfigured at death. She claimed she thought about an overdose away from the city so it wouldn't be so publicized. She had mentioned her idea of a drug overdose to her university friend, but her friend (a pathologist) told her that if she overdosed, she would require referral to the coroner and could not contribute her body to medical research as she had initially intended. She claimed, after she heard her friend's advice, that she considered donating her other organs (i.e., eyes, kidneys, etc.) instead. She denied having made a previous suicidal attempt. She claimed she did not wish to tell her daughter about her suicidal ideas in fear that her daughter would think she was threatening her with death. However, at the end of the conversation, she claimed she felt she would not actually commit suicide because she wouldn't want a lasting impact on her daughter and to have her family stigmatized. She agreed for psychiatric admission to titrate medications and for further management.

Family history of mental illness

Mrs. Mak's daughter suffered from mild depressive disorder and one of her sisters suffered from depression (her sister previously had told her if she was to die to not die in the city because it would affect their family).

Personal history

Mrs. Mak is the youngest of 11 siblings and claimed her parents favored her despite that other relatives tended to favor the boys more and the girls were stigmatized. She did well in school, which was why she was favored and was the only daughter entering university. She reported that her family was well off and that her father was a businessman and an ex-chairman of a bank who did not have much time for his family. She reported that her father was often righteous but mean. Mrs. Mak mentioned that her mother had been an alcoholic since her middle age. Since her birth, her mother would drink increasing amounts. When her mother was drunk, she could not fulfill the duty of a mother, and for this reason, Mrs. Mak was raised by a domestic maid who would often hit her. She claimed that her mother often lost control of her emotions and argued with her father. She reported her home atmosphere was full of tension and arguments. Her mother would physically burn money in front of others.

Mrs. Mak was married at age 27, which she felt was late for her age. She had courtship for 3 years before marriage. She felt her husband treated friends well but ignored her most of the time. She claimed her husband would verbally and emotionally abuse her when they were alone, and they would put a front in the presence of others. She claimed that her husband was narcissistic, critical, and judgmental man and not romantic. She gave her husband 30 out of 100 marks in the role of a husband. Her husband was a biochemist and had a PhD working at the university. She claimed to have thought to divorce him and tried moving out for a week. They had gone for marital counseling previously. Her husband had prostate cancer in 2005 and died in 2012. Mrs. Mak coped well with grief because she felt that her husband went to heaven and was given God's grace for surviving quite a few years after his diagnosis.

Mrs. Mak had one daughter. Her daughter has hearing loss in one ear since birth; this gave her some guilty feelings about her daughter. She reported that her daughter was quite rebellious. Her daughter studied fine arts and obtained a bachelor's degree; she was academically excellent. When studying before, she had tried skipping school for 2 weeks. Her daughter was back from abroad to the city in 2008 and had an affair with a divorced man who was 20 years her senior; both she and her husband did not support their relationship. She claimed her daughter previously had mild depression and taken antidepressants for 6 months. She was critical of her daughter, claiming that she was not earning considering her qualifications. Also Mrs. Mak claimed that her daughter had not sent a card to her all the time she was studying abroad.

Mrs. Mak is now undergoing family therapy, using support from the Cancer Fund with her daughter (she had been introduced to the Cancer Fund when her husband was diagnosed with cancer).

Mrs. Mak was an assistant lecturer in 1972. In 1979 she was promoted to senior lecturer and, in 1991, promoted to primary lecturer. She had interrupted her PhD study between 1992 and 1996 abroad, and when she returned as a lecturer to the university in 1996, she claimed that her seniority was lost as she studied abroad. She formally retired in 2008.

Past psychiatric history

Mrs. Mak had been known to the public mental health service in the city since December 2007 with low mood. In fact, she reported that her first onset of depression was while she was studying in the city university and reported that during exam time she was both anxious and had insomnia. She did not receive medical attention at that time. In 2002, she reported low mood precipitated by dealing with forms to help her daughter apply to study abroad. She started having poor sleep, worsened concentration and energy level, and would sleep during the day. She attended a private psychiatrist who diagnosed her with depression with bipolar trait and put her on medication. Her daughter reported that her mother had episodes of being quite talkative with increased energy and irritability in the past and that was suggestive of bipolar traits. Mrs. Mak was also undergoing family therapy under Cancer Fund with her daughter. Mrs. Mak reported a history of suicidal ideas in 2002, 2004, and 2008. She had wanted to jump from a height in 2002 and 2004 due to emotional distress. In 2008, she lost US$170,000 in the Lehman Brothers' collapse and could not cope with teaching. Had suicidal ideas was of going to a general practitioner to get hypnotics and adding alcohol. She had thoughts of checking into a hotel to die, but she canceled the plan because she had some events unfinished. Medication was titrated, and she gradually improved.

She is known to have diabetes, hypertension, hyperlipidemia, and hypothyroidism. She was diagnosed with an adjustment disorder on a background of depression.

Treatment and management   Mrs. Mak's mood improved shortly after admission with titration of lamotrigine and quetiapine. She felt that she was able to calm herself down and that she was able to engage better with her daughter. Stress coping and support were discussed. She was referred to occupational therapy, and she enjoyed setting an activity log scheduling for daytime engagements. She was referred to a clinical psychologist for psychological intervention. The psychologist had interviewed Mrs. Mak and her daughter separately and together to facilitate their communication and will continue to follow them up as outpatients. This admission was for risk assessment and to tie Mrs. Mak over the crisis and facilitate her coping with family dynamics; this aim was achieved.

Mrs. Mak had no more suicidal ideas and a long-term risk management plan for relapse prevention was discussed. A community psychiatric nurse will also continue to follow-up Mrs. Mak after discharge.

Consultation   JM thanked the doctor for the thorough presentation. JM started the consultation by inviting the doctor to look at the future from Mrs. Mak's perspective and asked what reason did she have to live. The doctor responded that in the past she had quite high educational and social status. JM interrupted by pointing out that the educational status did not apply to her future because she was retired. The doctor added that Mrs. Mak is quite functional despite her depression and also pointed out that Mrs. Mak's aspirations for the future were mostly directed toward and related to her daughter. Mrs. Mak expected her daughter to live up to her own standards. Returning to Mrs. Mak's reason for living, the doctor added that Mrs. Mak was active in the volunteer sector and was important in the community. The doctor added that Mrs. Mak also had several friends. When Mrs. Mak was in hospital, many people visited her. Mrs. Mak has many friends who are highly educated, look out for her, and seek her company. The doctor added that Mrs. Mak was still highly functional, she had no sign of dementia despite her age, and was able to manage living on her own. Mrs. Mak was the chairman of a volunteer organization; therefore, Mrs. Mak was still important to a wide range of people. She was important as a friend and as a worker and was not someone who had nothing to live for.

Mrs. Mak tended to live through her daughter. This is a situation that has been described as enmeshment between her and her daughter. Mrs. Mak sees herself as one with her daughter and not as the mother of a grown woman who will follow her own trajectory in life and will make her own life choices. JM then asked if this enmeshment was addressed in the family's therapy sessions. The doctor added that these issues had been considered at family therapy, which sometimes both mother and daughter attended but only once. The next question was whether Mrs. Mak made any shift in her attitude toward her daughter as a result of these sessions. The doctor pointed out that Mrs. Mak had some difficulty in accepting that her daughter would make her own life choices. The doctor added that Mrs. Mak used to "make" her daughter supervise her medication by coming to her flat every night; this indicated that Mrs. Mak still had a plan to keep her daughter at home.

JM pointed out that this was dysfunctional aspect of their relationship that could only lead to problems, probably for both mother and daughter. Somebody who can chair an organization, who does have an active mind, and who is important to many other people does not really need their child to come home and supervise their medication. This is something that is cognitively well within Mrs. Mak's reach and emotionally signifies a motive that is dysfunctional, to keep control of her daughter.

It is this dysfunctionality that explains to a large extent Mrs. Mak's unhappiness. She is bound to be disappointed because her objective cannot be properly achieved. It is not possible for a mother to make a daughter become like her mother.

JM pointed out that Mrs. Mak has two separate views of herself. On the one hand, she saw herself as a competent person who could take on and chair an organization and, at the same time, somebody who cannot manage without her daughter, for example, counting the pills that she must take every night.

JM then moved on to give some outline of the objectives of therapy for Mrs. Mak. The first stage would be to encourage Mrs. Mak to see herself as the competent capable person that she is. The second stage would be to accept that Mrs. Mak does have needs for personal support but that expecting her daughter to meet those needs is not likely to be acceptable. She needs to try to have her legitimate needs met through age-appropriate means, which are through linking up with other people such as her friends and coworkers in the volunteer sector but obviously not only those people.

JM then pointed out that there is legitimate, reasonable, and understandable dependency, which is separate from dysfunctional dependency (which is so because it is unlikely to ever be fulfilled). JM then gave the example of the mature adult dependency that exists between him as a consultant and the junior doctors as consultees. This is functional dependency because both parties gain something from this interaction and because both parties are free to put an end to it if it no longer serves a purpose, if the relationship became dysfunctional, if the objectives of the consultant or of the consultees were not consistent, and if the task that they agreed to carry through, which is to reach a deeper understanding of severely ill patients, was not met.

JM then pointed out that it is more appropriate in therapy to concentrate on the functionality of the interaction—the sense of what works and what does not work rather than impose any values of judgment, morality, or religion. All these higher values are important, but they confuse the issue if they are introduced in psychotherapy. Based on this, Mrs. Mak can be encouraged and given the direction to which she should employ her considerable abilities.

If Mrs. Mak were able to find a partner, a lover, or a husband, then that would be a way of having her legitimate needs appropriately met. She would be able to reciprocate and meet the equivalent and legitimate needs of the other person. There are many people, even at the advanced age of 69, who are quite able to form new relationships to people of similar age and in a similar predicament to choose that form of action. This possibility could be explored with Mrs. Mak.

JM asked if Mrs. Mak had perhaps "written herself off" as a potential partner and that it may be helpful to her if she was asked to reexamine that aspect of herself. She sounds as if she is someone who has indeed a lot to give to another person in a relationship and she may not be aware of that. The doctor then mentioned that Mrs. Mak's self-esteem may have been damaged. The doctor was pointing to the need to have some therapeutic work focused on Mrs. Mak's image of herself and that a lot of her self-esteem relied on her work, and this was removed when she retired. The doctor also pointed out that Mrs. Mak thought less of herself because she needed to rely on medication and because she was suffering from what she saw as a mental illness. JM pointed out that Mrs. Mak could be helped to have a more balanced view of herself as somebody who has talents and abilities and also who has a difficulty with her emotions and a tendency to become depressed. If she sees herself as a whole rather than as somebody who is defined only by her depression, she will be more able to seek a "real" and not an idealized relationship.

JM then suggested that Mrs. Mak's intelligence could be turned to her advantage. It could be pointed out to her that instead of directing her thinking onto how she could envelop her daughter, she could channel her energies into developing age-appropriate relationships. This can be seen as an encouragement that needs to be validated by the qualities mentioned that are real and not just words repeated by the therapist to make her feel better. The doctor added that Mrs. Mak had used her intelligence to manipulate people. JM suggested that this is a rather dysfunctional use of a powerful intellect and may indicate the despair that she experiences.

Ms. Amy

Presenting condition

Ms. Amy is a 28-year-old single woman and part-time manager of a fast-food outlet who lives with her adoptive mother, adoptive mother's older daughter, and her family. She was admitted voluntarily from the psychiatric center for low mood and suicidal ideation.

History of present complaint

Ms. Amy experienced anxiety, including symptoms of palpitations, tremors, and subjective shortness of breath. She had difficulty initiating sleep. Her appetite fluctuated with episodes of binge-eating "to cope with stress." Her volition, concentration, and energy level were fairly maintained. She was still able to go to work.

Ms. Amy attended the psychiatric center for follow-up on the day of admission. Her mood had worsened after a conflict with her adoptive brother-in-law 2 weeks previously. Her adoptive brother-in-law threatened to throw a knife at her if she made a noise again at night. She harbored more suicidal ideas in the previous week but made no plans or attempts. She had repeated impulsive ideas to harm her adoptive mother's family. She thought of taking a knife, but no actual attempts were made. She wished for psychiatric admission to titrate her medications and to stabilize her mood. A voluntary admission was arranged.

On admission, she was found to be of low mood and was observed to be tearful. Her speech was coherent and relevant; there were no psychotic features; and she was not suicidal or violent. The overall impression was that she suffered from a moderate depressive episode and an underlying Borderline Personality Disorder.

Past psychiatric history

Ms. Amy had been known to the mental health service since October 2018. She was referred by a private family doctor for anxiety and depressive symptoms. She then complained of pervasive low mood with crying spells, which occurred since March 2018; this was after she discovered that her biological mother had been trying to include her name in an application for a public housing unit over the past 10 years. Her biological mother did that to shorten the waiting time for a flat and possibly to get a bigger flat, without a genuine intention that Ms. Amy should live with her.

On her birthday in March 2018, her biological mother invited her for a birthday celebration, but it turned out she wanted her to sign some documents for her application for a public housing unit. Her biological mother again asked Ms. Amy to sign housing documents (biological mother used to ask Ms. Amy to sign many housing documents, lying to her that those were for applying for schooling allowances). Later, Ms. Amy found out that those were housing documents and that her mother included Ms. Amy's name in the tenantship of her flat so that she could have a bigger one; her biological mother needed Ms. Amy's signature on many housing documents. Ms. Amy was living with her adoptive mother.

Ms. Amy gave back her biological mother the form without signing it. Her biological mother repeated her calls to Ms. Amy's home and to the second older sister to disturb them. The second older sister then asked the biological mother to visit Ms. Amy at home at an hour that Ms. Amy was at home alone. Ms. Amy called the second older sister, and she asked Ms. Amy to sign the form. Ms. Amy felt betrayed. Although she did not have face-to-face frequent communication with her sister, they sometimes had "WhatsApp" calls and asked about each other. She recalled that years ago, when she was unhappy and slashed her arm, it was her second older sister who stopped her and comforted her. She felt disappointed that her sister put pressure on her to do something she did not want to do. Ms. Amy felt used ("Biological mother was using me," "She delivered me just to make use of me"). She also felt betrayed; she said, "elder sister pushed me to do something that I did not want to do, despite knowing my view and stance."

Ms. Amy impulsively attempted suicide by overdosing with hypnotics in April 2018. There was no prior planning, and there were no preparatory acts. She could not recall the number of hypnotics she took. She vomited out the drugs and did not seek medical attention or inform anyone about the attempt. She attempted to jump from height in May 2018 when she felt that her mood became suddenly low; she abandoned the idea after talking to her boyfriend. No psychotic symptoms were reported. She was diagnosed with an adjustment disorder and was given a possible diagnosis of depression. Ms. Amy was prescribed sertraline 50 mg nightly, propranolol 10 mg three times a day as needed, and clonazepam 0.5 mg nightly as needed.

Ms. Amy is of good past health, has no known drug allergy, is a nonsmoker and nondrinker, and has no history of substance abuse or a forensic record. There is no family history of mental illness.

Personal history

Ms. Amy was born abroad. Her biological mother lied to the adoptive family that another woman bore her. Her biological mother asked the adoptive family to take care of Ms. Amy. For the initial few months, she paid for their care, but then she stopped paying. She asked the adoptive family to send Ms. Amy to the orphanage. However, the adoptive father decided to keep Ms. Amy in their family. Her adoptive father died when Ms. Amy was in Form Primary 2. At present Ms. Amy lives with her adoptive mother; her second elder sister (10+ years older), her husband, and their children; and her eldest sister (20+ years older). The older sister moved out; the brothers (20+ years and 10+ years older) also moved out.

Ms. Amy described her adoptive father as loving and caring. Ms. Amy said that her first older sister was the one who took care of her. Her second older sister started to distance herself from her after the adoptive father died because her adoptive mother often talked negatively about Ms. Amy; the adoptive mother was critical; and the second older brother often beat Ms. Amy when she was young. This was while the family lived abroad. Both biological and adoptive families belonged to the migrant community while abroad.

Ms. Amy knew that she was adopted since kindergarten. Her adoptive father wanted Ms. Amy to change her surname, but her paternal grandmother opposed this. Ms. Amy then learned that she had come from a biologically different family. At home, Ms. Amy felt that it was her own home but sometimes she felt that she was not part of the family. She felt that she could not talk to her adoptive mother about her feelings. She felt unhappy after being criticized by her adoptive mother and could not vent about her emotions. Ms. Amy enjoyed school as she had friends at school, and she could cope well with schoolwork. She felt a sense of inadequacy, of worthlessness, of being unloved, and of not belonging. ("I am born to be manipulated and used by others," "I do not feel like I have a home; I feel like an outsider," "adoptive mother would help me when I was in need, but she is not very close or loving to me now"). She used to feel loved by adoptive father who died. She used to be close to her second older sister, who comforted her and asked about her but has become distant. Ms. Amy felt that she was coping by crying, undertaking physical exercise and by smoking, which she did since she was 20 years old. She used to have some expectation from her biological mother, hoping that she would give her a home, love, and care. However, she was repeatedly disappointed (e.g., biological mother did not appear when she asked Ms. Amy to visit her paternal grandmother together; biological mother invited Ms. Amy to attend biological father's first year celebration, but she wanted to ask Ms. Amy to sign housing documents). Ms. Amy wanted to have a place of her own and have the autonomy to live the life she wanted.

Ms. Amy studied up to degree level BBA (distance learning). Her family moved to the city in 2013. Soon after arriving at the city, she resumed contact with her biological mother.

Ms. Amy worked in various jobs. She held a part-time job in a fast-food outlet. She had a good relationship with colleagues. She had also worked as a sales assistant and later as an insurance agent for 3 years. Ms. Amy did not enjoy sales work or jobs that required a lot of socialization. She is currently only sustaining the fast-food outlet job. Her longest employment was as an insurance agent for 3 years until early 2018.

Ms. Amy has an ambivalent relationship with her family but has some good friends. She is interested in basketball and volleyball; she is usually plays with work colleagues. She is introverted, sensitive to criticism, and emotionally dependent especially on her boyfriend; she has low self-esteem (e.g., not courageous enough to proactively talk to others, even when she yearns for belongingness); she tends to underestimate her ability even when she does well, and others believe she could do well.

Ms. Amy has had two courtships; the first lasted 3 years and the second is with the current boyfriend. This relationship has lasted for 2 years, and she describes her boyfriend as supportive.

Present treatment   Ms. Amy was prescribed Zoloft 125 mg nightly and was referred to a clinical psychologist for psychological intervention; she was also referred to occupational therapy for vocational assessment.

Ms. Amy was visited by her oldest sister. She suggested that Ms. Amy change her surname to feel more part of and less alienated from the family. She also told Ms. Amy that her second older sister would visit Ms. Amy that weekend. Ms. Amy felt that she was cared for by her family. She was less angry at her second older sister and could now accept her point of view better. Ms. Amy decided to remove her name from the tenantship of her biological mother's flat and to sever any connection with her biological mother. She decided to focus on sustaining a stable clerical job. She would like to acquire her own place (a flat) in the future.

The treatment team expects that Ms. Amy can develop her ability to cope with negative emotions (such as she experiences after adoptive mother scolds her). She previously tried to cope by physically exercising, but she developed injuries as a result of excessive exercise and felt that the emotions were not relieved afterward; she currently attempts to cope by smoking.

Consultation   JM thanked the doctor for the thorough presentation and congratulated him for not only his good assessment but also for setting the foundations for this young woman to have a realistically positive life. JM pointed out that this woman is young, healthy, and has some abilities (she gained a high degree, and at work, she rose to a supervisor position), and at 28 years of age she no longer needs to depend on family for pocket money or other sources of survival. She is also able to have a good relationship with a boyfriend. Ms. Amy has the potential of developing a good life with her boyfriend. Presumably they can both apply for a flat. Ms. Amy seems to have realistic reasons to be hopeful about her future.

JM then pointed out that there are two sources of counterproductive factors (i) historical and (ii) contemporary factors. Referring to the historical factors, JM proposed that the impression that this case history gives is that the biological family has not only been rejecting from the start but that it is also currently mistreating her. For example, inducing her or pressuring her to sign papers illegally is abusive. During the presentation, it was clarified that it was not only Ms. Amy's *feeling* that she was being pressured to lie, to break the law, and that she was taken advantage of but that it was an *established fact*. Her feelings, in respect of this situation, were appropriate and not a symptom. Ms. Amy deserves to be protected by the intervention of outside agents (perhaps by her adoptive family), but if this is not possible, then she needs to develop her own sense of entitlement and self-respect so that she does not permit other people to take advantage or abuse her. She could be helped to develop a sense that she is entitled to be treated with respect.

For further study of the effects of abuse on children see the web pages of the Royal College of Psychiatrists (RCPsych 2015) and the publications of National Association for People Abused in Childhood (Kelly and Bird 2014), as well as the study by Duarte et al. (2007). One needs to take into account that the abusive relationship is not only something that happened in the past, but it is also currently being exercised through pressure to engage in something illegal.

Thinking of the historical factors, one can understand why the experience of being rejected became part of her feeling a reject and an alien who does not belong. Her experience led her to believe that she would only receive some care "out of the kindness of strangers" (to use Tennessee Williams's phrase from *A Street Car Named Desire* [1947]). The first objective of psychotherapy would be for her to develop a sense that she is somebody worthwhile who deserves to be recognized as an individual and who deserves consideration and respect. As a secondary benefit would be that she will feel that she has a right to be angry when she is abused or treated disrespectfully. In this sense, depression and frustration are not symptoms but an understandable response to anyone who is being treated abusively.

JM then addressed the issue of Ms. Amy's identity. He pointed out that there is a paradox in the concept of identity because on the one hand it is thought of as the quality that sets one apart from all the others but, on the other hand, the identity is always linked with a group to whom one feels connected or belonging to. The choice of name, in Ms. Amy's case, is an example. She wants to change her name so that she can develop an identity as part of the new and adoptive family. She wants the name to distance her from the biological family to which she does not want to belong. In general, markers of identity are those that show that we are connected with a family, a nation, a culture, or perhaps a profession, an age group, and so on.

JM pointed out that it is likely that the psychiatric service has helped Ms. Amy to resolve the confusion that she had about her own identity. He assumed that the doctor supported her in her wish to adopt the name of her adoptive family.

Ms. Amy may need to hear explicitly that the reason why she has developed feelings of not belonging and of not being entitled is understandable in view of her experience but that at the same time to continue feeling like that in the present is not justified. She does not always have to feel like that because she has developed abilities as an adult, and as an adult, she has a greater freedom to decide with which people she is going to attach to and associate. As an adult, she has a greater freedom to choose with whom she is going to develop a relationship and has greater ability to negotiate a relationship of equality and mutual dependence. She is no longer a child who is at the mercy of adults who will make decisions for her.

Perhaps Ms. Amy needs to be reminded that she has a lot of potential in the sense that she is young, that she has been found to be attractive at least by two men who wanted to be in a relationship with her, that she is valued at work because she's been given a promotion into a supervisory role, that there are some members of her family who care for her and think of her in positive terms, and that she is intellectually able because she has got a higher degree. All these characteristics amount to a significant factual and realistic evidence that she can base a solid sense of who she is and what is her worth. Once she developed a healthier and more realistic self-esteem, she will be more able to act in a way that shows others that she is entitled to be treated with respect. JM pointed out that even people without these qualities are entitled to be treated with respect. It is just in Ms. Amy's case that she may need these reminders so that she can build a sense of self-worth and is able to develop the sense of self entitlement. Such qualities give her a solid basis to have a sense of pride and of hope for her own future. Ms. Amy can take an active role in shaping of her future in a good and satisfactory way.

References

Duarte Giles, M., Nelson, A. L., Shizgal, F., Stern, E. M., Fourt, A., Woods, P., Langmuir, J. I., & Classen, C. C. (2007). A multi-modal treatment program for childhood trauma recovery: Women Recovering from Abuse Program (WRAP). *Journal of Trauma & Dissociation*, 8(4), 7–24.

Kelly, S., & Bird, J. (2014). Recovering from childhood abuse. National Association for People Abused in Childhood (NAPAC). https://napac.org.uk/wp-content/uploads/2016/06/Recovering_from_childhood_abuse.pdf

RCPsych (2015). Child abuse and neglect—the emotional impact on children and adolescents for parents and carers. Royal College of Psychiatrists. www.rcpsych.ac.uk/mental-health/parents-and-young-people/information-for-parents-and-carers/child-abuse-and-neglect---the-emotional-impact-on-children-and-adolescents-for-parents-and-carers

Williams, T. (1947). *A streetcar named desire*. New Directions Books.

Dorothy

Dorothy is a 68-year-old divorced woman, living in a home for the elderly the city.

Presenting condition

Dorothy presented with low mood and suicidal ideas.

History of present complaint

Dorothy had long history of hypnotic use and had been consuming different hypnotics, both long- and short-acting, obtained from both the public and the private sector. She was currently on many antidepressants and hypnotics and insisted on taking both sets of medications. She also insisted on visiting a particular private psychiatrist and claimed that he would prescribe as she wished. She refused to cut down the number of hypnotics she used, claiming that she felt discomfort with a sense of restlessness, internal craving, and poor sleep when she was on lower doses. She had difficulty in adjusting to life in a home for the elderly and complained about the loss of freedom; she also had arguments with the staff over her complicated drug regime. She was noted to have more unsteady gait once she was allowed to go home for a holiday. The staff of the home suspected that this was due to her resuming taking diazepam during the holiday—a drug that was not given to her weekdays. In the previous year, both of her sons signed off the responsibility for financially supporting her, so to allow her application of social welfare. This had been discussed and agreed by Dorothy and her sons, but she then started complaining about the sons cutting down the pocket money that she was given. Dorothy also complained about her sons visiting her less frequently. She felt left out and abandoned.

Dorothy repeatedly made suicidal threats to her sons. In the last 2 months, she made repeated suicide gestures and even verbally threatened to harm her grandchildren (4- and 6-year-olds). Two weeks before admission, she was found attempting to strangle herself with an electric cable at night in front of her younger son, when the couple was awake. On the night before admission, Dorothy told her social worker that she wrote a suicide note on a newspaper; the home staff reported that she had not verbalized any suicidal wishes recently and that there was no actual self-harm. She was then sent to the accident and emergency department.

Dorothy has no significant cognitive decline. She still enjoys watching TV and playing with her grandsons; she had no pervasive negative thinking; she maintained her appetite but complained of poor sleep quality despite being observed to be sleeping well in the home for the elderly.

On admission she was found to be with short hair, to look younger than her age, and to have a tattooed eyebrow and eye line. She was alert and conscious, fully oriented without a major cognitive problem; her mood was not depressed or elated. She was calm and settled and tended to be passive-aggressive when complaining about her sons. Her affect was reactive and congruent; her speech was coherent and relevant. There was no psychomotor retardation. She denied any genuine suicidal ideas. She was not psychotic or aggressive.

The diagnosis was hypnotic dependence, moderate depressive episode and the differential diagnosis was borderline, histrionic personality disorder.

Family history

There was no family history of mental illness. Her mother died of lung tuberculosis when she was 3 years old. Dorothy could not recall her face and had no memory of her mother. Her father had worked as a school janitor. Dorothy had a distant relationship with him and said, "he failed to be a father." Dorothy felt that he disliked her and that she was abandoned by her father whenever his girlfriends came to see him. Her father died many years ago following a physical illness.

Dorothy felt her elder half-sister displaced all her personal anger onto her and complained of being hit by her. She felt that her older sister did not care about her and was not welcoming her to stay with her after she left boarding school. Dorothy complained that her brother-in-law raped her when she was a teenager.

All her siblings (who were at least 10 years older than her) had died several years previously, and their deaths were caused by physical illnesses, such as cancer.

Dorothy complained that her ex-husband used to force her to have sexual intercourse and enact scenes viewed in pornographic movies. She claimed that he was a gambler and that she suffered domestic violence. For example, he dragged her on the ground. She felt her sons and daughter-in-law were not respectful to her, and she felt being "the extra one." She has a good relationship with her grandsons and enjoys playing with them.

Personal history

Dorothy was born in the country; she has an older sister and an older brother; and she also has an older half-sister. She had illegally migrated to the city at the age of 3. Her mother died, and she was raised by different relatives. She stayed 2 years in a boarding school for primary education. She then stayed with her elder sister. She had many courtships with stormy relationships; she had more than one boyfriend at a time and claimed she sometimes enjoyed seeing her boyfriends fighting for a date with her. She married in 1972 to a driver. She divorced him after he stole money from her and left. The marriage lasted a few years. She had no other courtships afterward. She had been working in textile factories and became a housewife after her marriage. She was a nondrinker and nonsmoker and has never used any slimming agents. She has had no previous features of an eating disorder.

Past psychiatric history

Dorothy had been known to the mental health service since 2001; she attended for low mood and a history of many suicide attempts. The working diagnosis, before admission, was that of mixed anxiety and depressive disorder, in partial remission with a background of dysthymia. She had been seeing psychiatrists from both the public and private sector and received multiple antidepressants and hypnotics. Dorothy chronically suffered from low mood, which was precipitated by difficulties in the relationship with her two sons and daughter-in-law; Dorothy felt that they were not respectful toward her and felt that they were trying to abandon her. She based such feelings on her impression that, for instance, they hinted that they were planning to have family activities without her. She also had chronic feelings of being the extra one in the family. She felt empty and was longing for more care from her son. She had periods of depressive mood with multiple suicidal ideas and suicidal gestures as threats to her family, including gestures of wrist slashing, jumping from heights, and banging her head against a wall. The family had become desensitized to her suicidal gestures.

Dorothy had been admitted to a mental hospital after she expressed suicidal thoughts. She felt that those were precipitated by her ex-husband's gambling and debt problems. She was then diagnosed as suffering from a depressive episode of moderate severity, with somatic symptoms. She was then followed up at the hospital outpatient clinic but had poor compliance. Dorothy complained that her case doctor at that time was "not good looking" and was not "caring enough" for her. She then sought help from a private psychiatrist, to obtain hypnotics. She was thought to be "doctor shopping" in outpatient consultation notes. She was followed up at the hospital cluster in 2016 when her diagnosis was revised to depression, in partial remission with a background of dysthymia.

Her condition was also complicated by frequent falls with head injuries since 2016. She had requested admission to a home for the elderly in response to the suggestion from her son and daughter-in-law that she should move out of the flat.

Dorothy suffered from type 2 diabetes mellitus, gastroesophageal reflux disease, hemorrhoids, migraine, mild obstructive sleep apnea (which is corrected by lateral sleeping), and some attacks of syncope. She suffered a head injury in May 2013, April 2014, and September 2014. She sustained a total abdominal hysterectomy and bilateral salpingo-oophorectomy in September 2014. She was started on hormone replacement therapy (HRT) at age of 55.

Present treatment　Before admission, Dorothy was on many medications (polypharmacy) prescribed both by the public and the private sector. The drugs were diazepam 6 mg twice daily as needed (avoided by home for the elderly); lorazepam 2 mg at bedtime; chlordiazepoxide 10 mg three times daily, triazolam 0.5 mg nightly, pregabalin 75 mg nightly, propranolol 40 mg three times daily, duloxetine delayed release 60 mg bedtime, escitalopram 10 mg twice daily, and nortriptyline 50 mg nightly.

After admission, medication was slowly simplified and the use of benzodiazepine was reduced. She was referred to a clinical psychologist.

Consultation　JM thanked the doctor for the thorough presentation. JM then asked the doctor if it was appropriate, in the city's culture, for a woman of 68 to be in a home for the elderly. The doctor felt that 68 is a relatively young age for a woman to be in a home for the elderly and that this would be rather unusual in the city, especially because Dorothy had no cognitive problems and was relatively healthy. JM then asked why Dorothy had been placed in a home when this is not the usual practice. The doctor explained that Dorothy herself had accepted it on the advice of the doctor to reduce the use of medication and the second reason was that her son was going to get married, and as the couple were to live in that home, there would not be adequate space for all. JM then asked if the placement in a home was realistic evidence on which Dorothy based the feeling of abandonment. The doctor pointed out that she did not feel that her son intends to abandon her because she experienced the son to be a rather caring person toward his mother. When JM then asked for clarification that the son asked his mother to move out so that his wife could move in, the doctor responded that it was not the son who requested that but Dorothy herself. The doctor clarified that Dorothy could live with her son and daughter-in-law if she wished to, but it was her choice to move out.

JM then asked for clarification on Dorothy's statement that she had no recollection of her mother. The doctor added that her mother died when Dorothy was 3 years old and that the mother died of pulmonary tuberculosis. This was information Dorothy gleaned from her siblings. Indeed, Dorothy was transferred to the city at the time her mother died. The doctor added that in the city, Dorothy was first looked after by a series of relatives and then, when she reached primary school age, she was placed at a boarding school where she remained for 2 years. The doctor added that Dorothy is the youngest child in her family.

JM then asked about the history of sexual abuse. The doctor responded that after Dorothy returned home from the boarding school, she stayed with her sister and it was her sister's husband, her brother-in-law, went into her room, tried to touch her sexually but did not have penetrative sex with her. Dorothy was 14 years old. This was a single episode.

Dorothy's marriage lasted "a few years" but was not able to give an exact number. The marriage was when Dorothy was in her 30s. Dorothy has not married again.

Dorothy is slightly overweight but not obese.

JM then asked the doctor to confirm that in her mental stage she was found to be not depressed and not suicidal. JM then continued to question why Dorothy was an inpatient in a psychiatric hospital. The doctor responded that this was because of the suicidal gesture.

Since admission, Dorothy explained that she had no serious suicidal intent. JM then asked whether the hospital had reconsidered the diagnosis in view of the absence of any symptoms of psychiatric illness. The doctor explained that her main complaint was the craving for hypnotics.

The doctor mentioned that Dorothy was upset that her son had not visited her on admission to hospital. The doctor felt that the son's not visiting was justified because his own son had been ill with a temperature of 40°C. JM then asked if, in view of this illness, her son was not able to leave the house to look after him and if, for example, her son had not gone to work because of this. The doctor did not have information on this matter. JM suggested that obtaining detailed information on this matter would throw light onto whether Dorothy's perception of being neglected by her son was inaccurate or whether it reflects her son's attitude toward her. JM suggested that every symptom that Dorothy is suffering from may not be attributable to her own individual pathology but maybe an understandable response to the way she had been treated. It is possible that Dorothy had been treated with neglect in her early life and that it needed to be clarified if her present perception is influenced by her early experiences or whether it accurately reflects the current way in which she is being treated. She is inappropriately placed in a home for the elderly when she could be living in a flat with her son and his family. The understanding is that it is not unusual in the city's culture for three generations of the same family to share the same flat.

JM then asked about the issue of money. The doctor repeated that Dorothy's son used to give her pocket money but that Dorothy used to spend it on luxuries and unnecessary materials. The doctor explained that Dorothy used to live in a flat with her ex-husband. That flat belonged to him, and since the marriage ended, she was left homeless and then she moved in to the flat that belonged to her son. It was not clear what independent resources Dorothy may have had. The doctor added that it is only recently that her finances have been clarified and that she did have, during the last year, some welfare financial support. It was not clear why Dorothy had not accessed the welfare resources that were available to older people in the city before. The doctor added that there was concern that Dorothy was spending her money on getting medication from the private psychiatrist. The doctor clarified that although there is a good psychiatric service, Dorothy felt that she could only access hypnotics through the private psychiatrist. In a way, Dorothy was using her money to feed her addiction to hypnotics.

JM then asked what was Dorothy's understanding of what is wrong with her. The doctor responded that Dorothy does not think there is anything wrong with her. In other words, Dorothy has no insight on her addiction to hypnotics. JM then asked if Dorothy had expressed what conditions needed to be met so that she could be content with her life. The doctor responded that she would be content if she had enough money to buy hypnotics and cosmetics. JM then asked the doctor what she felt would enable Dorothy to have a reasonable life. The doctor responded that she did not think that Dorothy needs the place at a home for the elderly; Dorothy could live independently and was justified in feeling that by entering the home she had lost some of her freedom. For example, Dorothy was not allowed to leave the home during weekdays but only at weekends. It was felt that the home for the elderly was providing some safeguard against her excessive use of hypnotics. The doctor added that Dorothy could live independently, but she should be best placed near her son.

JM then raised the issue of Dorothy's safety because she had a history of falling and hurting herself. The doctor associated these falls with excessive use of sedatives and suggested that if the intake of sedatives was controlled, then the likelihood of Dorothy falling and hurting herself would be minimized. The doctor clarified that Dorothy has had no falls when the intake of hypnotics was better controlled.

JM suggested that among the many factors that contribute to this lady's poor state is her dependency on hypnotics. JM asked to be clarified if one main target in Dorothy's psychiatric treatment was to wean her off the excessive use of hypnotics. This was confirmed. The doctor claimed that Dorothy had only been in hospital for 2 days and that the hospital was already making progress in reducing the overall amount of medication that she was taking. The doctor pointed out that the medication had already been drastically reduced. JM pointed out that Dorothy was still on at least four different medications. The doctor clarified that the intention was to discharge her only on a dose of antidepressants and no other medication.

JM asked if Dorothy would be able to sleep without hypnotics. The doctor responded that the staff of the home had observed that Dorothy sleeps well but complains that she is not. The doctor continued that part of the treatment plan is to establish a better sleep hygiene for Dorothy.

JM then asked the doctor if she felt that a random person in Dorothy's situation would be content with their life. The doctor stated that she would be unhappy because the sons are visiting infrequently, because she has lost a lot of her freedom, and because other people need to control her medication. JM pointed out that Dorothy is a vulnerable woman at her age, and she is not in a position to take full and constructive control of her life. The doctor clarified that Dorothy seems to be at least of average ability. JM then suggested that Dorothy had many things to sort out before her life became reasonable for her. Dorothy does not seem to exercise her ability to manage her life and allows other people to control matters for her. When this happens, she complains about the decisions other people make for her. One example was that although she was entitled to some pension for the last 3 years, she did not activate this to have some independent means of managing her life. Dorothy did not take the initiative to seek a public housing unit and some independent pension for herself. Dorothy did not take any steps to avail herself of the resources that are available for her in the city. It seems that her only way of coping with her distressed state is to dose herself with hypnotics. It was difficult to justify prescribing antidepressants to somebody who is not depressed (as she had been found not to be depressed on admission) but who is justifiably frustrated with her life situation. She is particularly frustrated with dependence on her son for money and for a roof over her head. It was suggested that Dorothy had a justifiable reason to be dissatisfied with her life because she was without support (as she would have had if she lived with her husband) and having to depend on her son for pocket money.

One objective of therapy would be to break this vicious circle because she does have realistic problems and her actions to address them only made matters worse for her. For example, the dependence on her son plays a part in creating further distance between them. If she were living independently and supporting herself independently, then she would have been able to have a more free and healthy relationship with her son. Dorothy's problems are not only intrapsychic but also external.

JM then suggested that the private psychiatrist who offers hypnotics to her should be contacted and they should be made aware that they are part of an unhelpful process through which, by feeding Dorothy's dependency on hypnotics, they contributes to continuing her problems. JM raised the concern that for a doctor to feed a patient's addiction is not first-class medical care. If this is controlled, Dorothy could use some of her money for her own benefit rather than the destructive dependence on hypnotics and on the finance of private psychiatric care. The doctor informed JM that Dorothy could afford one or two private consultations per month on the amount of money given to her by welfare.

JM then asked about the other sources of support that Dorothy can access. The doctor pointed out that Dorothy does have a small circle of friends but that she felt inhibited to invite them to her house either in the son's flat or in the home for the elderly; she, therefore, resorted to meeting them in tea houses, although this was obviously limited.

JM then questioned the wisdom of restricting a woman from leaving the home for 5 days a week when she is perfectly capable of going out, finding her way back, especially when going out would be a positive experience for her and a way of accessing appropriate support. JM suggested that the nursing home could be spoken to so that they could relax these rules for her.

JM repeated that it would have been useful if it was acknowledged to Dorothy that she has a right to be dissatisfied about several things in her life and that her dissatisfaction is not all the result only of intrapsychic elaboration. It would be genuinely supportive to her if she was told that it is accepted and appreciated that she has genuine reasons for being dissatisfied, even though her way of addressing her difficulties is making matters worse. This would be going some way toward reverting the vicious circle of dependency on people (who are not able or who are ambivalent about meeting her dependency needs) and the addiction to hypnotics that are making matters worse for her. The reversal of this vicious circle would be through enabling her to access healthy support and negotiate relationships with important people in her life, like that of her son in a more constructive adult-to-adult and independent way. If she negotiates her relationships in more satisfactory and effective ways she will have less of a need to resort to hypnotics.

The therapeutic team ought not to have an ambitious therapeutic objective for her and to accept that, at her age, it will be difficult to break a pattern that has been established for so many years. She will need an intervention that will be low key and long term. Dorothy, who started life with multiple carers who provided inadequate care for her, ran the risk of repeating this pattern in her adult life on a long-term basis.

Mr. Y

Presenting condition

Mr. Y is a 42-year-old married man who was voluntarily admitted from a general hospital following a suicide attempt.

History of presenting illness

Mr. Y had been known to the mental health service since 2009. At that time, he suffered from pervasive low mood with poor sleep and loss of appetite, which he attributed to work stress. He consulted a private psychiatrist and was treated with a selective serotonin reuptake inhibitor. There was improvement in mood, and he stopped medication after 5 weeks of treatment; he subsequently defaulted on follow-up. Since then, there was no major fluctuation of mood until 2018. In May 2018, Mr. Y had his first promotion after working for 22 years in the prison service. Since then, he started to experience increased stress in work as he was adjusting to the role of the new post and was coping with the new colleagues. Since then, he experienced pervasive low mood, lost his usual interest in jogging, and felt loss of energy. He also suffered from poor sleep with difficulty in initiating sleep and early morning waking (5 a.m.). Additionally, he experienced loss of concentration and attention. He also harbored feelings of worthlessness. In addition, he felt anxious with shortness of breath and chest discomfort.

Since November 2018, his work stress continued to escalate as he needed to write a report about an incident of inmates fighting. Although his supervisor was satisfied with the quality of the report, he began to ruminate that there was room for improvement, and he was disappointed with himself; his mood and sleep deteriorated. He also started thinking of self-harming. On November 20, 2018, after knowing that he would be required to compile another report, he felt he could not finish this job. For this reason, he felt like harming himself. He first used electric wires at home to tie a knot on a metal bar which was 9 feet from the ground to hang himself, but this attempt failed because the metal bar was bent by his weight. Subsequently, he used a fruit knife, which was 10 cm long, to stab himself. He failed because the knife had a blunted blade, and he was left with bruises on his abdomen without any penetrating wound. He then gave up on the suicidal act. There was no death note written, and he expected that these acts would kill him. After his wife returned from work, she found out that there were bruises on his abdomen; she took Mr. Y to seek medical advice and he revealed his act to the doctor. He was later referred to the accident and emergency department and a voluntary admission to the hospital was arranged.

Family history

There is no family history of mental illness.

Personal history

Mr. Y was born in the city. He had normal developmental milestones and unremarkable antenatal and postnatal history. He has an elder brother, and he enjoys good family relationships. He studied until secondary school. After graduation, he worked in a prison and maintained the same job. He received a promotion recently, which is his first ever promotion. He had two marriages. His first marriage took place 10 years ago, and they divorced 5 years ago due to "personality incompatibility." He met his current wife 2 years ago, and they married 2 years ago. They enjoyed a good marital relationship. They do not have any children. Mr. Y described himself as an introvert who tends to bottle up his feelings. He always had high expectations about himself.

Present treatment   Mr. Y was diagnosed with a major depressive episode and was treated with citalopram. He showed good response on 40 mg daily. He tolerated the medication well. He was referred to occupational therapy for vocational rehabilitation. Moreover, an interview with family was arranged to discuss his condition. His wife had a good understanding of the diagnosis, and she agreed to supervise his mental state and medication; she attended follow-up with him. Extensive psychoeducation was provided, and he had improved insight of his mental illness; he was able to appreciate the effect of medication on his mental illness.

Consultation   JM congratulated the doctor for the thorough assessment and expressed his agreement with the diagnosis of depression and the need for pharmacological treatment to take place at the initial stage of contact.

JM then commented on the timing of onset of psychotherapy. He expressed the view that when a patient is in such a vulnerable state as Mr. Y, he would find it extremely difficult to cope with the exploratory aspect of psychotherapy and that, therefore, at this stage, he requires more support rather than energetic treatment. JM repeated that Mr. Y's attempts at his life were serious and determined and should be considered as such. JM agreed that the psychologist's approach of trying to establish a relationship and to make him feel that he is in good hands has priority over any other therapeutic goal.

JM inquired about Mr. Y's exam results. He had received zero grades. JM felt that to obtain zero marks was quite extraordinary. JM pointed out that any student, even those who cannot get high marks, would get at least the lowest possible marks. The doctor agreed that Mr. Y could obtain more than zero grade at his exams. The doctor responded that he had asked Mr. Y about this matter, and Mr. Y had explained that he had not carried out the preparatory work required for these exams and that he spent a lot of his time relaxing and enjoying himself. Furthermore, Mr. Y had already decided to join the prison service, which did not require any exam results, so he had never taken these exams seriously. JM then asked why Mr. Y, if he had decided that the exam results were not relevant, did he take the exams. Furthermore, when he decided to take the exam, why did he not make even the slightest effort with the exam papers? As a result of this discussion, the reason Mr. Y failed with zero grade was a combination of limited ability and lack of interest in or avoidance of the result.

JM queried how was it possible for his wife not to have noticed that he was so depressed. He was not sleeping well, he was not eating well, and he must have appeared depressed to her; how come she did not notice? The doctor said that he was given one explanation: that Mr. Y was keeping his feelings secret from his wife. JM persisted that if somebody is severely depressed, they would find it extremely hard to conceal their mental state from the person they live with. The doctor suggested that the wife's limited intellectual ability (as reflected in her low achievement in education) may have been a contributory factor. At the end of the discussion, it seemed clear that both Mr. Y and his wife were people of below-average intellectual ability.

The relevance of their ability is directly related to the fact that Mr. Y became depressed after his promotion. JM suggested that Mr. Y was promoted to a level above his ability. The kind of work that he was required to do was strange to him, and he found it difficult to learn the new skills required.

JM pointed out that this is a common phenomenon for people who are promoted beyond their level of ability. They find it shaming to be faced with failure, and they cannot revert to the previous lower job for this reason but, unfortunately, neither can they perform adequately at the job to which they have been recently promoted. JM gave an example of a patient from his own experience where a senior person in a bank was promoted to beyond their level of ability and found themself in the predicament of being unable to return to their previous job and at the same time being unable to perform in the present one. Being unable to find or to think of a creative solution they, sadly, ended their life.

Another one of Mr. Y's characteristics is that when he comes face to face with a difficulty, he tends to give up rather than search for a way forward. He gave up with his examinations, and he gave up again in dealing with the new tasks of his new job. Mr. Y does not seem to have the maturity or the flexibility to make the most of a new life situation.

JM then suggested that when medication and the support from the hospital environment enables him to get to a better mental state, then the task would be to help him address his difficulties rather than panic and give up. Psychotherapy and support could lead him into adopting a problem-solving approach to his difficulties instead of abandoning hope and all efforts. JM then suggested that one target of therapy would be to help Mr. Y accept the return to his original job without a feeling of shame and without any additional damage to his sense of self-worth. Of course, a person from the health authority will need to intervene on his behalf with his employer because he is unlikely to have the negotiating skills required for this task.

JM then gave the example of a person in the same predicament but with a different approach to difficulties. Such a person would say to themselves, "I have been doing the last job for 20 years, I have gained the respect of my seniors; they have confidence that I can do the senior job. I have some difficulties in doing this job and I will ask for some help to address these difficulties. It is worth my while to persevere here because there is an increased reward in me doing this job." This example aims to illustrate that a person of the same cognitive ability but with a more mature personality would address the task in a more constructive way.

JM suggested that the return to his old job would need to be presented to his colleagues and to himself as being the result of him finding that the new job did not suit him and not that it was a job that he was unable to carry out. In this way, the return to the old job would not be an insult to his self-esteem. The doctor pointed out that the service may not be able to offer him the option of returning to his old job. JM then suggested that a service as the prison service may have available for him a job that has similar expectations as his previous one.

JM then asked if there was any realistic hope of him being helped to cope with the job to which he had been recently promoted; there is a possibility that he may have panicked at the thought of carrying out the new job when the job was within his capacity. JM repeated that supporting him to find solutions to his difficulties may be a good learning experience for him. Mr. Y tended to give up and feel that there was no hope and that was the motive behind his attempt at his own life.

There may be staff at the psychiatric service who could help him not only address the current difficulties but also to adopt an approach in his life that is more constructive when he is faced with difficulties, an approach which will lead him to say, "Ah, there is a problem therefore I will get the right help so that I can solve it." This would be more useful to him not only in his work situation but also in his life in general.

JM then suggested that it may be helpful to him if he begun to value the job that he was doing, menial though it may appear. Even the most menial and low-skill jobs have their function and their usefulness, JM often uses the example of refuse collectors, who, although they do a low-status and low-skill job, perform an enormously important function for our society. JM, without being knowledgeable about the present situation in the prison system, stated that many harmful interactions could be taking place in the space that Mr. Y was supervising; for example, a lot of bullying and a lot of drug exchange can take place in the washrooms that he was supervising. It was also possible that Mr. Y was protecting more vulnerable prisoners, simply by his presence, from being abused in various forms. Making him aware of the value of his job may help, in some way, at restoring his own sense of self-worth.

The constellation of symptoms (of depression upon promotion) have been described by Peter and Hull (1969).

Reference

Peter, L. J., & Hull, R. (1969). *The Peter principle*. Souvenir Press.

Mrs. CB

Presenting condition

Mrs. CB is a 69-year-old married woman, living with her son; she presented with depressive symptoms after her husband suffered a stroke.

History of present complaint

Mrs. CB was referred by her general practitioner to the psychiatric clinic in November 2018. Her mood had worsened for around 3 months prior to that. The low mood had been triggered by her husband suddenly suffering a stroke. Her husband was admitted to hospital, became bed-bound, and had limited improvement despite treatment and rehabilitation. The doctors at the hospital told her to arrange an old-age home placement for her husband. She visited him daily and felt stressed about the situation. Mrs. CB felt the hospital had limited manpower and had offered suboptimal care to her husband, such as often delaying the time of his changing diapers; when she wanted to ask for help from the staff, she was scolded and told to change his diaper by herself, which she could not do because her husband was of heavy built. She felt she could not accept her husband's sudden deterioration in mobility and health. She felt guilty about needing to send her husband to an old-age home because she thought all staff in old-age homes would abuse elderly residents. However, she had no choice because she did not have the ability to care for her husband at home.

As a result, her mood deteriorated, and she had frequent crying spells. She had poor sleep at night despite taking diazepam and had poor appetite with weight loss of 9 pounds in 3 months. She became busy caring for her husband and gave up her hobbies of meeting, with friends and playing cards. She felt tired and lacked energy. She had a fleeting death wish, but there was no definite idea of suicide. She did not have any hallucinations or delusions.

She was diagnosed with a moderate depressive episode. Medication was adjusted with the addition of sertraline and zopiclone. However, despite adjustments to the medication, her mood remained the same. She experienced more anxiety when the hospital put pressure on her to find an old-age home placement quicker so that her husband could be discharged from hospital. She had palpitations, tremors, and ruminations about her worries. She had severe tinnitus, leading to even poorer sleep. She felt that the stress was unbearable and decided to be admitted to a psychiatric ward for management. However, after 2 days, she requested an immediate discharge. She felt that the noises from other dementia patients in the ward made her sleep even poorer and was feeling even more distressed. She also felt guiltier about not visiting her husband in those 2 days she was in hospital. She was worried about her husband's condition. Because her family also wanted her to be discharged, she was allowed to leave and arranged for her to be followed-up in our clinic.

We continued to adjust medication for her, switching from sertraline to mirtazapine. She reported better sleep and less intense anxiety symptoms after taking mirtazapine. Her husband was discharged from hospital to an old-age home in March 2019. She felt less stressed than the time when husband was in hospital, but she continued visiting her husband daily in the old-age home to care for him because she was still worried that her husband would be abused there, she would bring her husband home for few days in a week with the help of her son. She would still feel distressed when she saw her husband in poor condition, and she felt stressed about caring for him. She also reported the ongoing symptom of tinnitus, which affected her sleep from time to time.

With some advice on her lifestyle from our clinic, she gradually reengaged with some social activities including occasionally playing cards with friends. She felt a short period of relief on the carer stress, but she also felt guilty at times about going for those social activities instead of caring for her husband. She was also referred to the clinical psychologist for psychological management.

Family history

Mrs. CB's daughter was seeing a psychiatrist for an adjustment disorder and was being treated with regular medication. Her aunt, nephew, and cousin had some mood or anxiety problems with psychiatric follow-up. She also suspected her mother and her son to have some mood problems, mostly with labile mood and temper outbursts, but they did not have any medical attention.

Personal history

Mrs. CB was born in the city and was the eldest of six siblings. She reported hardship in her childhood, with her mother being authoritarian and throwing temper tantrums most of the time. She reported that as the eldest child she was scolded most frequently and that her mother would hit her from time to time. She felt unhappy growing up in this family. She got married with her current husband late in her teenage years. She reported that she did not have significant feelings for this man, but that she resorted to an early marriage to escape from her home. She did not have a close relationship with her husband and until after her husband's stroke half a year ago, and she felt a lot of guilt about not caring enough for him.

She did not have any formal education. She worked as a handcrafting worker mostly on button work before, and then after her marriage, she worked in her husband's factory. She had two sons and one daughter. Her daughter was living overseas coming back to visit her occasionally. She is currently living with one of her sons, with whom she had a fair relationship. She described her premorbid personality as anxious prone, pessimistic, introverted, with some obsessions with cleanliness; she was responsible and hardworking.

She is a nonsmoker and nondrinker and has no history of substance abuse. Medically, she suffered from glaucoma and tinnitus.

Past psychiatric history

Mrs. CB described herself as being anxiety prone and pessimistic; she tended to be anxious or depressed over various trivial matters. However, there were no previous prolonged episodes of mood disturbance. She had chronic insomnia from around 5 years ago. She consulted a general practitioner who prescribed diazepam for sleep. She had partial improvement in sleep afterward.

Present treatment and management of the case   Mrs. CB was treated with mirtazapine to which she had a partial improvement in her mood. She was also referred to the clinical psychologist for psychological intervention. She is to be followed-up in our clinic monthly for the time being. It was hoped that in the long term, through psychological input, she could develop a more realistic appraisal of caring for her husband, with fewer guilty feelings and with an increased ability to give more credit to herself.

Consultation   JM thanked the doctor for the thorough presentation. JM then clarified that the present consultation was to consider matters in addition to the general psychiatric practice and that it would not stray into the fields of diagnostic categorization or psychopharmacology. The consultation would focus on understanding Mrs. CB and through this way aim to enable the psychiatrists to be more effective in her treatment. JM also clarified that he was not claiming that this case could be held by psychotherapy at the exclusion of other interventions.

JM then considered Mrs. CB's present predicament. She had lost a great part of the support of her husband and had gained numerous additional concerns and tasks. It is therefore normal and inevitable that she would experience some sadness for the loss and some stress for the additional demands on her. What a psychiatrist can do is address the responses that are pathological, that is responses that are beyond what one would expect from this unfortunate situation.

Along these lines, JM mentioned that one source of pathological response had already been cited previously—that of her sense of guilt. The sense of guilt needs to be understood in the context of Mrs. CB, having been a faithful wife, a woman who looked after her husband and brought up her children, and a person who contributed to the running and the well-being of the family. Her track record is not one in which she has harmed anyone through actions or inactions. Neither has she harmed her husband, nor has she neglected him. Furthermore, in the present, Mrs. CB has been doing everything that is expected of her for her family and her husband. The doctor responded that Mrs. CB had expressed guilt in connection with the fact that she was married to a man whom she was not in love with. Mrs. CB then had added that, because of this, she felt that she had not cared enough for him. JM repeated the issue of guilt being based on acts of commission or acts of omission and asked if Mrs. CB had committed any acts of commission against her husband. The doctor's response was "no."

JM asked if Mrs. CB felt she had carried out any acts of omission to which the answer was equally negative. The doctor clarified that Mrs. CB felt that she had failed because she did not have feelings of love for her husband. It was made clear that the sense of guilt was not based on any feelings of action or inaction but on the nature of the relationship of the two spouses. JM then suggested that Mrs. CB viewed emotions with a sense of duty and not a personal experience that emerges from a relationship. Mrs. CB felt that she "should" love (or should have loved) her husband. Mrs. CB was not thinking of love in the context of a relationship in which both parties play a part. JM repeated that love, as an emotion, cannot be ordered either toward other people or even toward oneself. It cannot be felt or be expressed out of a sense of duty.

JM then asked if the doctor had any information about how Mrs. CB looked after her husband and children. Although there was no comprehensive information about this, Mrs. CB had diligently carried out her duties as a wife and mother. As a result, her therapist could point out that she managed to carry out her duties despite the lack of love and that she had been able to carry out what she thought was essential even though many times she did not feel like doing it. This could be a source of pride for her. Such a new insight would go some way toward restoring her sense of self-worth.

Sometimes patients name their distressing feeling as guilt when they mean shame. Being in a marital relationship without love may well have been a source of shame for Mrs. CB.

JM then asked the doctor if he knew the content of her mood. JM clarified that he was referring to the thoughts that Mrs. CB had when she was in a low mood. The doctor referred to the sudden illness of Mrs. CB's husband. JM responded that of course such an event would cause sadness but what we were called to address was not the normal sad feeling that one experiences when they encounter a loss but on the pathological sadness that may be on top of the natural one (Freud, 1917). The doctor responded that Mrs. CB had expressed feelings of helplessness and uselessness. JM focused on her sense of being useless and asked in what sense did Mrs. CB feel that she could have been useful because uselessness or usefulness is always in relation to a task. The doctor pointed out that Mrs. CB expected to be able to look after her husband at home. This is despite that the medical team had recommended that he be transferred in a care home, implying that it would not be suitable for him to be cared for at home. The doctor added that Mrs. CB felt that she lacked the ability to care for her husband.

JM then added that it seemed that her feeling of failing her husband is not based on contemporary reality (as she had done and was doing what is reasonably expected of her) but on something different, and therefore, tracing the origin of such feelings to her early history should be reviewed. JM suggested that her background is explored to discover if the sense of responsibility and the sense of uselessness had been implanted in her mind from her early childhood experiences. Was there anything in her background that would make her feel that most things depended on her, that she was responsible for everything, and that she was expected to make everything right? The doctor added that Mrs. CB was the first of six children of strict and demanding parents. The doctor added that the parents would often use physical punishment against her and added that as the oldest child, she was often held responsible for the behavior and the needs of the younger siblings. JM responded that it seemed that the history, so sensitively obtained by the doctor, demonstrated how her sense of being responsible for everything and her sense of failing was implanted when she was a child. It seemed that the present sense of seeing herself as responsible for everything and seeing herself as failing is a repetition of views of herself from a young child.

JM then pointed out that by expecting that everything depended on her and expecting herself to be able to help with every problem, she overestimated her own abilities and overestimated the expectations that she had of herself. In other words, she had harsh and inhumane expectations of herself.

JM pointed out that there are two avenues that her therapy could follow. The first is to reduce the sense of guilt or shame because her actions have been always caring and appropriate and the second avenue would be to help her develop realistic expectations of herself so that she does not set herself up to fail and feel like a failure. Mrs. CB needs to be shown how she can look at her achievements and her contribution with contemporary adult eyes and not as a repetition of her early family experience.

The doctor added that these insights would be useful to him when he meets Mrs. CB as an outpatient. The doctor added that he had developed a rapport with Mrs. CB. In this context, Mrs. CB was receptive to the doctor's advice. JM then added, as a second thought, that Mrs. CB had never complained about herself and never spoke about her own rights as a woman. Mrs. CB had never stated any sense of being disappointed or being let down and of not being supported enough. It must have been a new and positive experience for her to have a doctor who is listening to her and is prepared to consider her needs. Part of the therapy could be the facilitation of sense of entitlement to Mrs. CB that at the age of 69 she is entitled for some help from other agencies including her children. JM then pointed out that this is the norm in many families in the city.

JM's final advice was that progress needs to be made at a slow pace, that it should not be challenging, and it should not resemble the current interprofessional consultation in any way. In a consultation, views are exchanged in a rapid and often black-and-white terms; this would be totally inappropriate for a face-to-face encounter with a patient. Mrs. CB has lived with these feelings for nearly 7 decades, and she should not be expected to change them overnight. Any overambitious therapist is likely to generate further feelings of failure and inadequacy.

Reference

Freud, S. (1917). Mourning and melancholia. In *The Standard Edition of the Complete Psychological Works of Sigmund Freud* (Vol. 14, pp. 243–258). Hogarth Press.

Mr. CK

Presenting complaint

Mr. CK is a 50-year-old married unemployed man who presented with suicidal ideation.

History of the present condition

He increased drinking in recent months since he became unemployed. His increased consumption of alcohol was up to two large cans and two small cans of beer per day, with half a bottle of local wine or white wine per night, which he claimed was for his insomnia. He reported that sometimes when he was drunk he felt even more hopeless and ruminated more about his loneliness and what he felt was past unfair treatment by his family. He tended to downplay his drinking problems. He denied craving or having any withdrawal symptoms.

His mood was further lowered by his housing problem. He could not provide his wife's signature for the income statement form, which was required to be handed in to the housing authority. He needed proof of the pending divorce if the requirement for her signature was to be waived. He was informed how to do so, but he found it "too bothersome and complicated." He was passive in resolving this problem. Mr. CK reported that if he failed to provide the proof of divorce by late June 2019, the lease would expire. He reported he just planned to live in his public housing unit until he was evicted, but he did not have a further concrete plan.

Mr. CK came across his mother in the street 2 or 3 months ago. He informed her about his divorce and housing problem, and his mother invited him to a family lunch. During the lunch, he drank local wine and felt irritated because he perceived that his family were "nagging" him about his drinking. His mother offered that he could live with her. He felt touched but also ashamed that he had to rely on his mother for a place to stay. He felt surprised that his mother was so kind to him but at the same time was worried that she may be hostile toward him as she had been in the past. He talked about the ways in which his brothers had bullied him on the family message group because he wanted his brothers to feel embarrassed. His brother told him to forget the past and to focus on the future. He felt angry at his response. He expressed his loneliness and death wish to his fifth sister because he felt she would understand him.

On the day of admission, he had a tea gathering with his family. He drank beer and wine and vented about his stressors toward his family. His family was worried about his previously mentioned suicidal ideation and brought him to the accident and emergency department; subsequently a voluntary admission was arranged.

Family history

There is no family history of mental illness.

Personal history

Mr. CK was born in the city. He lived with his parents, siblings, and maternal grandmother during his childhood. He was the fourth out of seven children. He has three older brothers, two younger sisters, and one younger brother. He reported that his relationship with his family was poor in childhood. His grandmother and father had died a number of years ago.

He felt that his parents hated him and treated him unfairly; they beat him more than they did his siblings and blamed him for his siblings' misdeeds. He reported that his mother often scolded him and perceived that she hated him because he had a stubborn personality that clashed with his father. He reported that his brothers bullied him. He never told his parents and sisters about this. He felt hurt and angry about his family's unfair treatment of him for many years. Despite this, he always paid his mother a monthly allowance and even gave her a large proportion of his salary. His relationship with his mother worsened as she had conflicts with his wife over household matters. His mother moved out 8 to 9 years ago, and since then, his mother ignored his telephone calls and they had no contact.

He married his wife from the country in 2004. His wife moved to live with him and his mother in the city. The relationship between his mother and his wife was poor, and his mother moved out in 2009 because of the conflicts with his wife. He had no contact with his mother since that time. He still cared about his mother and would check on her condition through other family members.

His relationship with his wife became distant in recent years. She had gone back to the country 2 years ago and had not returned. He lost contact with her then. He tried to contact her through her family, but he failed. Two years ago, he started living alone in a public housing unit. He filed for one-sided divorce and expected the legal procedures to be completed the following year. She often went back to the country for long periods of time.

He was educated up to Form 2. He initially worked as a manual worker. He then worked in pipe work for about 30 years. In recent years, he was given several workers to mentor (his mentees). He had a good relationship with them. He stopped working 1 year ago due to elbow pain. He did not resume his work even after the pain was managed because "he got used to resting." He supported himself by using his savings.

Mr. CK started to drink in adolescence. Initially he was a social drinker and mainly drank beer. In recent months he started to increase his alcohol consumption. He drinks every day and consumes beer, the local wine, and white wine. He sometimes felt more depressed after drinking and ruminated more about his loneliness and his past unhappy experiences. He mostly spent his spare time drinking and became more socially withdrawn recently. He denied craving or having any withdrawal symptoms.

Since living alone, he started reporting periods of low mood, low motivation, insomnia, and poor appetite. He withdrew from social gatherings and mostly idled at home. He ruminated that he had been lonely all his life and that he would continue to be lonely. He felt hopeless about his future and had a fleeting death wish. He gave up his job as a pipe worker 1 year ago because of elbow pain. He did not resume his job even when the pain had been managed.

Past medical and psychiatric history

Mr. CK enjoyed good past health. He is new to psychiatric service. He has arthritis elbow.

Management and progress

Mr. CK was diagnosed with dysthymia and alcohol dependence. Mr. CK's mood improved quickly after admission. He reported that on the day of admission his family already helped him to obtain the proof of divorce so that he could renew the lease to his public housing unit and to apply for transfer to live closer to his mother. His family (mother and younger sisters) visited him daily, and he felt the love and care from the family. He reported he was no longer angry toward his mother. He wished to start a new relationship with his mother and siblings. He planned to live with his mother temporarily, after discharge, so that they could provide mutual support. He was motivated to work as a pipe worker again.

He was started on citalopram 20 mg, which he tolerated well. He was referred to a clinical psychologist, who shared the case formulation with him and helped him to reconcile his anger with his family. His sleep and appetite improved. He was in "contemplation" of change to stop drinking. He was discharged late in July 2019.

Consultation   JM thanked the doctor for the thorough presentation and then asked the doctor in what way had Mr. CK's thinking changed since his admission. Following a discussion, it appeared that although Mr. CK was aware that his drinking was excessive and damaging, he became clearer about this after his admission. In particular, he had become more aware of how damaging his excessive drinking was to his relationships with his family.

JM then asked about the absence of withdrawal symptoms despite his high and regular consumption of alcohol. He was consuming about 5 L of beer a day plus a bottle of wine 3 to 5 times a week. The absence of withdrawal symptoms put doubt on the accuracy of the history provided by Mr. CK.

JM then referred to the two separate issues of *tolerance* and *dependency*. JM pointed out that alcohol is an enzyme inducer. Because of this function, chronic alcoholics can metabolize a large amount of alcohol much faster than a nonalcoholic organism. In fact, many alcoholics manage to function reasonably well despite consuming such amounts. This is different from a process through which withdrawal symptoms develop following a sudden withdrawal of the alcohol to which the organism has grown to be dependent to. The conclusion of this consideration is that Mr. CK does not seem to be a reliable historian. In contrast to the usual habit of alcoholics who usually underreport the amount of alcohol they consume, Mr. CK probably overestimated how much he drank. This may be linked to his wish to present himself in a way that is likely to elicit a helpful response from his treatment team. It is also possible that he "treated" early signs of withdrawal by consuming alcohol much earlier in the day than he admitted.

JM asked if Mr. CK's statements were backed up by actions. For example, was his statement about the wish to return to work backed by any actions of his that would lead him to return to work? The doctor responded that Mr. CK had contacted his mentee who told him that there was a new project starting and that there would be a role for him in that. JM questioned his relationship with the mentee, and the doctor clarified that his experience had been recognized at work and he had been appointed as a mentor to several people over the years. JM pointed out that he must have done well at work to rise to the position of being responsible for the training of younger workers. This progress over the years indicated quite firmly that Mr. CK did have the potential to make a better life for himself in the future.

JM then asked the doctor if Mr. CK had accepted that the future for him involved "total abstinence." The doctor responded that Mr. CK had managed, in the past, total abstinence for about 1 year. He had the experience of doing well at work during that year. The doctor confirmed that Mr. CK had accepted this truth about him.

JM then pointed out that Mr. CK did not seem to be identifying any difficulties in his life that were arising from within himself; he tended to attribute his problems to agents or events that happened to him and not events that he caused to happen. One example was the relationship with his family. Unless Mr. CK understood that he played a part in making the family relationships problematic, he would not be likely to work toward making them better. JM pointed out that Mr. CK would be more likely to accept criticism if this is matched with praise for the good actions that he had been taking toward his family. One example is that he was supporting his mother financially over many years. This is a real and genuine caring act. This can be used to point out to him that he is capable of positive action and that he is not only causing problems. The doctor can highlight for him that he has the potential of being a good worker, a good son, and a good family member and that it is not inevitable that he will only cause problems.

The essence of therapy would be, on the one hand, to support him as a person able to do good things but also, on the other hand, to point out to him that he was also who had been making things worse for himself. One example of his actions is his decision not to return to work even after his elbow healed. That was purely his action, his decision and he suffered as a consequence.

JM then suggested that Mr. CK requires close monitoring after the discharge from the hospital because he seemed vulnerable to relapse into drinking. JM reminded the doctor that there are objective tests to measure alcohol consumption and that these are used routinely by alcohol treatment services. This is because the temptation for alcoholics to give erroneous histories is always present.

JM then suggested that Mr. CK had regressed from a competent adult who had a good work record and who was having the responsible job of mentoring junior colleagues into somebody who was seriously dysfunctional. In terms of attitude, he changed from seeing himself as a responsible adult to thinking of himself as dependent on others and particularly his mother. Not seeing himself as the agent of his destiny (Bandura, 2006) was closely associated with the despair that he felt which led him to contemplate suicide. The tasks ahead for Mr. CK are to restore his work record, to restore his family relationships, and to restore his housing situation, which is linked with the divorce.

Thinking about Mr. CK's responsibilities, JM asked whether Mr. CK had children. He had been married for many years and the absence of children was an important factor deserving thorough understanding. The doctor reported that his wife often spent long periods of time in the country, but it was not clear if the marriage had been consummated nor was it clear if the couple had taken active steps to avoid pregnancy.

JM then asked about the sources of "warmth" for him. JM pointed out that every person needs to be loved, and it was not clear how Mr. CK was having this natural need met. He was obviously getting some of it from his mentees, but that is no substitute for love from his partner or wife and could not be confused with love from his mother and other members of his family. This lack of warmth may be close to the pathology that led him to alcoholism. The doctor pointed out that the only source of affection for him seems to have been his mentees. JM responded that this is a problem because not only is the source restricted, but there is also a tendency or a risk of Mr. CK seeking affection from his mentees that he should be seeking from his wife or partner, his mother, or his family.

JM pointed out that there are appropriate channels for each separate kind of affection. The maternal love is one channel, the erotic/romantic love is another, and the friendly or colleague affection is yet another. JM pointed out that seeking one kind of affection from the wrong source is not only going to be unsatisfactory but may also lead to serious complications. JM pointed out the example of doctors who inappropriately get drawn into having their romantic needs fulfilled through a relationship with a patient. This is so often a cause of serious adverse consequences for both parties. This matter raises also ethical issues, which are addressed by both the American Medical Association and the (British) General Medical Council. They illustrate that such relationships carry the risk not only of becoming exploitative but also lose the focus of the original relationship, which was treating the patient.

JM then asked if the reason why Mr. CK did not have friends had been explored. JM stated that work with Mr. CK needs to be focused on how he can work at developing appropriate sources of warmth for him and to do so separately from his mother, his siblings, his friends, a possible lover, and finally separately from his work colleagues. He has something to offer to each of these so that the relationships with these separate people are fair and not one-sided and not one in which he expects to be a recipient of affection without offering something equivalent.

Reference

Bandura, A. (2006). Toward a psychology of human agency. *Perspectives on Psychological Science*, 1(2), 164–180.

David

Presenting complaint

David is a 23-year-old vocational institute Year 1 student who presented with repeated suicidal threats and a suicide gesture of jumping from height 2 weeks ago.

History of the present condition

David started to encounter interpersonal problems in his extracurricular activities this year. He was thought to be too dominating and too critical of others. He felt more emotionally unstable and required more frequent venting to his friends about his feeling. Because of these complaints, he had been offered follow-up by a social worker.

David had a more marked emotional disturbance in the past two months after he witnessed a protestor committing suicide in recent political unrest in the city. Since then, he had low mood, which he associated to the political situation, but he denied that the low mood was pervasive. He enjoyed "hanging out" with friends. Motivation and energy levels were reasonable. He maintained similar performance in his studies and his extracurricular activities at school. His sleep and appetite were good. He was pessimistic about the future of the city, but he denied negative thoughts about himself. He reported that he intentionally mentioned suicidal ideation to seek friends' attention but denied genuine suicidal intent, plan, or attempt. He had not written a "final note."

David showed affection to a girl but was rejected by her a month ago. Afterward, he gave his credit card and password to a friend. He denied that this was a final act, but he had asked that friend to buy the girl a gift using his money on behalf of him because he felt that that friend was more familiar with the girl's interests.

Two weeks ago, after drinking a can of beer, David walked near the edge of a garden, which was a few floors above ground. He recorded and posted the video clip on social media. He reported that he tried to gain others' attention and to gain support from his friends on his political stance. Also, he repeatedly mentioned, on social media, wrist slashing and hanging. For this episode, he posted on social media again, mentioning being unhappy and having thoughts of suicide. A friend noted his post and notified the patient's social worker; his mother was also informed. On the day of admission, a friend and a social worker met David in a shopping mall where he appeared emotionally unstable. He tried to escape from them and claimed that he would attempt suicide no matter what or even after discharge from the medical unit. He was then sent to accident and emergency department, and psychiatric admission was arranged. David did not present any psychotic or manic features.

Family history

David's mother suffered from depression and had been followed-up in the public sector. It was also suspected that she abused hypnotic medication. She had a history of a suicide attempt by hanging 3 months previously. A maternal aunt (mother's younger sister) suffered from depression and alcohol abuse. A paternal uncle (father's elder brother) suffered from psychosis and had been admitted to a mental hospital previously. He committed suicide by self-immolation 6 years ago. A cousin (daughter of maternal aunt) suffers from dyslexia.

Personal history

David was born and bred in the city. He is the only child of his parents. He had normal developmental milestones. His father is a 43-year-old construction site worker, and his mother is a 43-year-old house-wife. His father's parenting style was strict and authoritarian, and he was indifferent to David's emotional needs. They had little interaction. David recalled an episode in which his father hit him with a chair when he was in kindergarten. Otherwise, there was no other history of abuse or childhood trauma. His parents divorced when he was 6 years old. David was once "triangulated" between his parents for the alimony settlement. He lived with his mother after the divorce. His mother was almost an absent figure in his childhood, and David had to seek help from neighbors when he needed it. His mother sometimes took him to bars and internet cafes. He regarded himself as a counselor to his mother. Currently, his mother contacted him whenever she could not sleep and felt upset. He reported that he would counsel her for a few hours each time. After his parents divorced, David seldom had any interaction with his father; contact was limited to religious festivals. His father remarried and has two children. David was emotionally attached to his paternal uncle who committed suicide 6 years ago by self-immolation.

David reported a happy school life and made several friends in primary and secondary schools. He reported fair academic results except in English where he achieved poor results. However, his academic results in junior secondary school deteriorated as he was actively involved in extracurricular activities (including student association, martial art, volunteering, chess, drama, etc.). He obtained just fair results in the public examinations but failed in English. He reported that he repeatedly left his seat without permission during primary school, so his conduct achieved a grade C in primary school but grades A-B in secondary school. He had no other major behavioral or conduct problems except an episode of fighting in Form 2, which resulted in a probation order for 1 year.

He had been living with his maternal grandparents since Form 6 because his mother did not want her mental illness to affect him. After the public examinations, David worked as an activity assistant in a community center for 9 months and as a real estate agent for 6 months; he used his income to fund his studies, which his family could not support. He then studied toward a foundation diploma for 1 year and a higher diploma in a vocational institute to the present. When he was studying in Year 1, his major was related to community service planning and navigation. He aspired to become a social worker to help others. He was still active in extracurricular activities in the institute. Financially, he was dependent on his family and to a government grant for his studies. His mother was receiving social assistance, and the family was in debt of US$1,000 to a financial company.

David has had five relationships. The longest courtship lasted 6 months while the shortest 2 weeks. He broke up most of the relationships. He broke up with his girlfriend 2 months previously after 4 months of dating.

David had experimented with smoking before but was not currently smoking. He was a social drinker. He had no history of substance abuse. He had no forensic records except the probation order for fighting in secondary school. He had no history of cruelty to animals or of fire setting.

Regarding his premorbid personality, he tended to seek attention from others by mentioning negative emotions on social media and longed for care from others, but he denied a chronic sense of emptiness or of repeated self-harm. He thought he was an assertive, extroverted, and sociable person. He was active in undertaking different leadership roles in school and enjoyed teachers' and peers' attention on him. He had no problem in establishing trust with others. He tended to bottle up his feelings toward his family, but readily "vented" to friends. He had a few friends. He liked jogging, singing, cycling, and board games. He is a Catholic.

Past medical and psychiatric history

David was known to child psychiatry since 2005 when he was 9 years old. He was diagnosed with attention deficit hyperactivity disorder. He could not recall his hyperactivity or attention deficit symptoms except sometimes he lost his belongings and left his seat without permission in class. He was once put on stimulant medication, but he did not take medication since he had been in secondary school and defaulted follow-up afterward. He reported to be mentally functioning well until this year, except during a week of low mood after his uncle's death when he was studying in Form 4.

He denied previous suicide attempts but recalled an episode of deliberate self-harm by scratching his forearm when he felt that his social worker ignored him due to her heavy workload when he was in secondary school. Otherwise, he had no other self-harm behaviors. Physically, his past health was good.

Present treatment and management   Organic workup, including urine toxicology, was unremarkable. David was diagnosed with adjustment disorder with prolonged depressive reaction and attention deficit hyperactivity disorder. He refused pharmacological treatment but agreed to receive psychological therapy. He was kept for drug-free observation. After admission, he remained stable in mood and settled in the ward. Sleep and appetite were good. He was observed to have good social interaction with other patients and staff. He had no more suicidal ideas. He trivialized his act of walking on the edge of a "podium" but showed remorse for seeking attention by this risky act. He was referred to a clinical psychologist for personality assessment. His personality was assessed by the Minnesota Multiphasic Personality Inventory-2. It showed elevated clinical scales of psychopathic deviate and hypomania. These elevated scales are thought to be typical among individuals who are seeking excitement and are risk-taking; individuals who tend to question authority and who have difficulties with trust and emotional closeness. These people can be charismatic, narcissistic, manipulative, and power-oriented, to focus on their goals, and may rationalize their behavior and externalize the blame. Assessment results were shared with David. He accepted some of them; he agreed that he enjoyed others' attention and recognition, but he did not accept that he was manipulative. Strategies for coping with stress were discussed. He proposed that he should take a break from the engagement in protests and political issues. He was eager to return to school and resume his internship work. He planned to found a new society at school to avoid further interpersonal problems. He was more motivated to adapt to the social and political situation.

Consultation   JM thanked the doctor for the thorough assessment. JM then asked for the doctor's understanding of why David, who had obviously suffered some trauma, became so dysfunctional at this time. The doctor responded that David's difficulties had been longstanding even from his school days. The doctor thought that his recent promotion at the institute and the greater freedom that he had were contributory factors. Furthermore, the disagreements that developed between him and his peers played a significant part. The doctor pointed out that there were conflicts, particularly in his extracurricular activities. It was difficult for the doctor to give specific examples of conflictual situations. JM commented that David was evasive about what happens in his interactions with his peers.

David was providing his impressions, opinions, and feelings about what happened without giving the actual description of the encounters; thus, he made it difficult for any independent observer to form a separate opinion. David says what he thinks but keeps to himself what happens. On further questioning, the doctor was able to explain that the conflict arose when David was in a position of leadership. His peers found him too domineering and authoritarian. JM suggested that it would be more helpful if the episodes of disagreements were gone into some detail so that the psychiatrist could form an independent opinion about what actually happened and in what way this was dysfunctional.

JM then moved to the previous traumatic events such as his uncle's suicide. This was obviously a traumatic event but had taken place several years previously. One needs to understand the connection between the event of 6 years ago and his present psychological state. There was no doubt that the event of an uncle's self-immolation was enormously traumatic. What was not certain was why an event that took place 6 years previously was not only traumatic but was also damaging a number of years later. The doctor reminded us that David had a close attachment to that uncle. This was particularly so because his parents were divorced and absent in his life. The parenting gap was filled in by that uncle. Even though that uncle was an immensely important figure in his life, David presented that he was upset only for 1 week after the uncle self-immolated. It seemed that after the loss of the uncle, David did not have a parental figure to turn to for support. It would be more useful to David, if, during the consultation, the psychiatrist invited him to connect the traumatic event with the feelings that make him dysfunctional at present.

David seems to have a difficulty in connecting previous events with his function at present, and his therapist can help him deal with this difficulty. He seems to connect events with changes in his mood but not to differences in his function, and his doctor can help him make this connection. David needs to be helped to realize that people with variations of mood are nevertheless able to function. Depressed people are not always unable to deal with the tasks of life. Low mood is not always incapacitating. David has not only become depressed, but he has also become incapacitated. Although the uncle's self-immolation took place 6years previously David's dysfunction began between six months and 1 year ago.

JM then asked if there were other intervening events that contributed to David's dysfunction. The doctor added that the recent demonstrations in the city had a major impact on him. The doctor explained that David became pessimistic about the future of the city. JM pointed out that it seemed that although many people in the city were pessimistic about the future of the state, few had become dysfunctional and certainly few indeed became as dysfunctional as David.

The doctor explained that David had been working as a counselor trying to help people with emotional needs. His studies were connected with social sciences. David seemed to be overwhelmed by the material brought to him by his clients who were involved in protests. JM suggested that it would be impossible for David to help others overcome their painful feelings if he himself had not overcome the same feelings himself. In this situation, he was facing an impossible task. The most David could do was to agree with his clients that the prospect is grim and confirm their and his own despair.

JM suggested that David should be helped to give up counseling others at present until he sorts out his own feelings and his own thoughts. He should give priority to sorting out his own emotions first and consider taking up counseling after he has overcome his own difficulties and after being more functional. JM pointed out that there are several people who take on the role of therapist to sort out their own difficulties but who in the process, simply accentuate their own difficulties. There is a difference between appropriate concern, which most people in the city feel about the future, from the dysfunctional state in which David had sank into. Although being concerned about the future of one's country is realistic and healthy, being dysfunctional is a matter for therapy. Because David attributes his difficulties to the external situation, he makes it impossible for his therapist to help him adjust and improve his own emotional issues. JM suggested that at some level David may aspire to imitate his uncle although, thankfully, he has not gone to the extreme of killing himself in a public and demonstrative way.

This case demonstrates two particular issues.

The first is the case of people with serious personal problems who choose the profession of counseling (or related professions of social work or therapist or even psychiatry) to address their own difficulties. Such persons find themselves in great difficulty and in need of greater help for themselves. They need to address their own problems before they can begin to take on those of others. Some professional groups have many members in this category. See review by Nielsen (2010).

The second important issue is that of the role of therapists in times of social uncertainty or upheaval. The role of the therapist is to disentangle the appropriate concern from the pathological and dysfunctional response of some to the same and inevitably unsettling social situation. The therapist has the task of helping those who become dysfunctional in the social setting to become functional and even play a constructive role in their community. Readers of this consultation may find of interest the article by Lyons (1971), which refers to the psychiatric sequelae of the Belfast Riots in 1969.

References

Lyons, H. A. (1971). Psychiatric sequelae of the Belfast riots. *The British Journal of Psychiatry*, 118(544), 265–273.

Nielsen, Y. (2010). Therapist motivations. *Psychotherapy in Australia*, 16(4), 14–20.

Jenny

Presenting complaint

Jenny is a 27-year-old married new immigrant who presented with low mood and suicidal ideation.

History of present condition

Jenny reported that she experienced periods of low mood with crying spells since August 2018; she complained that she found it difficult to adapt to life in the city. She came to the city to live with her husband and her in-laws after her husband convinced her to reunite with him. She did not enjoy the life in the city because she did not enjoy spending excessive time with her in-laws despite having a normal relationship with them. Furthermore, she could not get used to living in a small flat, as she felt "congested."

In addition to the change in living environment, she was also troubled by her father's extramarital affair and her mother's mood problem. Her mother had been in a low mood since finding out about his affair 2 years ago. Her mother lives alone in the country and Jenny calls her regularly to check on her. She found it irritating that her mother cannot let go of the preoccupation with the marital problem. She said that her mother had threatened suicide before; even though she had not acted on it, she had once disappeared and finding her required calling the police. Jenny's mood deteriorated further, and she became constantly anxious about her mother's well-being.

Jenny lost volition and interest in daily activities. She had poor concentration and low energy level. She had not been able to find a stable job since August 2019. She had worked as a waitress in the city for 2 months as her first job; she coped well at first but gave up her job after one of her colleagues resigned, and she was worried that she could not handle the increased work demand. She then went to another restaurant to work as a waitress, but the job didn't last long because she felt she was incapable to carry out the job duties due to her poor concentration. She was frustrated that she could not sustain her job as a waitress, and as a result, she had to spend more time at home with her in-laws.

As a result of these stressors, her mood further deteriorated. She had difficulty in initiating sleep at night. Her appetite was fair but felt that she had lost weight. She felt worthless and considered herself a burden to her husband due to her mental illness. She harbored fleeting suicidal ideas of jumping into the sea. No attempts or plans were made. She denied any substance misuse. She suffered no perceptual disturbances and held no irrational beliefs.

Family history

There is no family history of mental illness.

Personal history

Jenny was born in the country in 1992. She is the eldest of four children and has two younger sisters and one younger brother. She reported to have close family relationships with her siblings. She described the history of her childhood as unremarkable. She has a strong bond with all her siblings and maintained close contact with them despite being away from home. She commented that her parents had a good relationship when she was young, and she described her father as a reliable person. Jenny studied up to elementary school and she worked as a waitress and a salesperson before coming to the city. Jenny met her husband when she was 19 years old through her friends, and they got married in 2014 after dating for 3 years. She considered her husband to be the perfect husband as she reported that her husband had been treating her well and had gone through her mental illness with her when she was first diagnosed. They maintained a good marital relationship the whole time. She also described her relationship with her parents-in-law to be good and that there was no major conflict when they were living together. Since she arrived in the city, she had been in charge of taking care of household duties in which she found the work to be simple and easy to handle since the apartment is small in size. She is a nondrinker, a nonsmoker, and has no history of substance abuse. There is no forensic history. She described her premorbid personality as an emotional person who cries easily. She is introverted and compliant to others. She has a few close friends in the country but does not have many hobbies.

Past medical and psychiatric history

Jenny was physically well and enjoyed good past health. She had been mentally stable until 2011. Jenny switched work from waitress to salesperson at a shoe shop, which was owned by a relative. She suffered from high stress working there because her relative had set a sales quota for her to meet, which was a high requirement for her and she was the only staff in the shop. Moreover, she felt even more stressed to maintain a good performance in the shoe shop as her family was financially "tight" at that time, and she was one of the breadwinners in the family because all her younger siblings were still in school. Subsequently she attempted suicide by slashing her wrist; she attributed this to work and financial stress. Jenny was accompanied by her husband, who was her boyfriend at that time, to a private psychiatrist in the country. She was diagnosed with depression and was prescribed an antidepressant. She then developed euphoric mood, felt more energetic with decreased need for sleep, increased appetite, and increased spending after taking antidepressants for 2 to 3 weeks. Jenny consulted another psychiatrist, and her diagnosis was revised to Bipolar Affective Disorder. Lithium 250 mg nightly and olanzapine 5 mg nightly were prescribed. She refilled the medications without psychiatric follow-up over the past year.

Present treatment and management   Jenny is currently an inpatient. Since admission she complained about the ward environment and insomnia for a few nights. She blames herself for this admission, for underreporting her symptoms shortly before this admission at the accident and emergency department, and for allowing her symptoms to deteriorate further. She worried about how she may recover from depression and whether she will become more of a burden to her husband. Organic workup was performed and was unremarkable. Treatment was resumed with lithium CR titrated up to 800 mg nightly. She was also started on mirtazapine (Remeron) up to 45 mg at bedtime with as needed use of hypnotics. She has been attending appointments with a clinical psychologist while an inpatient and has joined a mindfulness class; she continues to attend activities in the ward.

Consultation   JM thanked the doctor for the thorough presentation and proceeded to clarify some details of Jenny's history. For example, it was confirmed that the owner of the shoe shop in which Jenny worked was satisfied with her performance, but it was Jenny who was not. The same pattern was repeated at the restaurant where she worked as a waitress. The owner was satisfied with her performance, but it was she who was concerned about it. The same pattern was repeated at a different restaurant in which the employer wanted to convert her temporary job to a permanent one, but she felt she would not be able to fulfill the demands of it. JM pointed out that the doctor had identified that the reason for her distress was that her expectations were beyond reasonable as expressed by employers or seniors in the same context.

JM then asked the doctor if she had any thoughts on why Jenny should have these excessively high expectations of herself. The doctor said that Jenny felt that because she was suffering from a mental illness she was less capable than she should have been. Jenny saw herself as an inferior person because of her mental illness. JM then summarized that Jenny did not feel that the work stress was making her ill but that her mental illness was causing her to underperform and, therefore, be stressed at work.

JM repeated that Jenny's notion that there is something wrong with her is not the employers' notion but her own. JM then asked if the doctor understood the origin of this major discrepancy between her view of her performance and that of reality as represented by her employers. As this was a gap in understanding Jenny, JM suggested that this be explored further with her. Her employers consider her to be good enough, but she herself underrates her ability and her performance.

JM then considered the role of the diagnosis of mental illness on her self-esteem. JM suggested that the evidence on which the first diagnosis of mental illness was made was not safe. The picture of Bipolar Affective Disorder was also complicated by the fact that it appeared after medication was taken. JM suggested that the possibility of iatrogenic contribution in this matter: first the rather, perhaps, hurried diagnosis of a depressive illness and the subsequent diagnosis of bipolar disorder on a clinical picture that may have been precipitated by medication. JM suggested that the initial and subsequent diagnoses were reconsidered in a much more rigorous manner at a ward round with the present psychiatric team. One needs to disentangle the clinical picture that was presented after the first diagnosis from that which presented after the first prescription of medication from the clinical picture that occurred before the first encounter with a psychiatrist. These three different phases may require a different diagnosis. JM suggested that the main factor that was driving the first episode of distress was her underrating of herself and the feeling that she would not meet the expectations of others against all evidence.

JM returned to the issue of the reason for her excessive expectation of herself. The doctor suggested that this may be related to the fact that she was the eldest child in the family and one of the expectations on her was to look after all the other siblings. JM added that although this may be a factor; it could not explain the whole picture because expecting to look after others does not lead inevitably to feeling inadequate. The different arguments are exposed in the literature (for example, see Easey et al. (2019), Stannard et al. (2019), and Granville Grossman (Granville-Grossman, 2018)). The matter of birth order and mental health is complex and unresolved. Jenny's case confirms that although birth order may have played a part, it cannot by itself account for her difficulties.

JM then repeated the position that the diagnosis of manic depressive illness was not secure or a sufficient explanation of her suffering and, then added that even if that was the case, that could not account for the reason why she is so dysfunctional because there are millions of people with mental illness who function much better than she does.

JM then expressed the view that the therapeutic target for Jenny should be to help her establish a realistic and positive self-esteem and a positive sense of self-worth. In trying to assess her value of herself in different functions JM asked about her esteem as a wife. The same pattern appeared in the sense that she considered herself to be a burden, while her husband did not think that. The same pattern was revealed in her estimation of herself as a family member. She underestimated her importance in relation to her family so far. Furthermore, Jenny did have a circle of friends in the country, so there was a group of people who valued her, again more than she valued herself. The therapist could help Jenny restore her sense of self-worth based on her value as a wife, as a worker, as a family member, as a friend, and as a daughter-in-law. Based on these things, Jenny could begin to value herself in a realistic way and begin to build a sense of pride in who she is and what she can offer.

References

Easey, K. E., Mars, B., Pearson, R., Heron, J., & Gunnell, D. (2019). Association of birth order with adolescent mental health and suicide attempts: A population-based longitudinal study. *European Child & Adolescent Psychiatry*, 28(8), 1079–1086.

Granville-Grossman, K. L. (2018). Birth order and schizophrenia. *British Journal of Psychiatry*, 112(492), 1119–1126.

Stannard, S., Berrington, A., & Alwan, N. (2019). Associations between birth order with mental wellbeing and psychological distress in midlife: Findings from the 1970 British cohort study (BCS70). *PLoS One*, 14(9), e0222184.

Amy

Presenting complaint

Amy is a 25-year-old woman who was admitted to hospital following a suicidal attempt using a broken wine bottle and scissors to cut herself.

History of presenting condition

Amy is a single woman living alone in a public housing unit. She was working as a part-time bartender. Amy's mood had been low for the past 1 month before admission. She attributed this to stress in relation to her debts.

Amy was cheated by her business partner with whom she planned to set up a "bubble tea" business in March 2019.She had borrowed around US$10,000 from a "loan shark." In order to repay it, she tried to work on three part-time jobs in a bar; this provided her with an income of around US$5,000 per month, which she intended to use for repaying the debt. Unfortunately, another friend again cheated her a month ago. Her debt had accumulated to around US$20,000; she was in financial stress to repay the debt in recent months.

Amy suffers from interrupted sleep and reported bad ruminations and reactive low mood. She has fleeting suicidal thoughts. She is worried that her family would find out of her debt problem. Unfortunately, the loan shark started to disturb her family with threatening words and by sending messages to them and photographs. Amy was shocked about these threatening actions. She felt ashamed and worried that she would be a burden to her family. Amy reported that she was muddled in thought and had fleeting suicidal ideas. She drank whiskey to fall asleep and then continued to drink cheap wine when she awoke in the morning. On the morning of admission, she wrote a suicide note addressed to her family and to the business partner who cheated her and cut herself on impulse by a broken wine bottle pieces and scissors. She said that she had not considered the lethality. Her parents found her locked inside the flat, and she refused to open the door. They were worried about her condition, and the police and firefighters were summoned. Amy was then sent to the emergency unit.

Family history

No family history of mental illness.

Personal history

Amy was born in the city in 1994. She is the second of three siblings. Due to father's work abroad, she was raised by and lived with her maternal grandparents since she was a baby; they are no longer alive. Her elder sister lived with her parents abroad; her younger sister lived with paternal grandparents in the country. For this reason, Amy has distant relationships with her siblings. She always believed that her father favored her older sister. Her parents moved back to live in the city when she was 6 years old. She described her father as having strict academic expectations and that he frequently used physical punishment, using belt or bare hands to hit her, ever since she was young. Her mother was also demanding in daily discipline. Under such strict parenting, Amy dared not express any emotions in front of her parents. She felt a strong need to fulfill irrational demands of her parents to gain their attention. Despite a lot of invalidating comments from her parents, Amy believed that she should love her parents but had ambivalent feelings toward them. When Amy was in Form Senior 1, she was bullied by classmates after she was pointed out what she considered to be their wrong behaviors. This bad experience made her sad for a few years.

Amy started becoming rebellious in secondary school because she could no longer suppress her emotions, and several times she fled home. She started to develop the habit of wrist-slashing whenever she was stressed or encountered emotional outbreaks. She felt wrist-slashing helped her to calm down and relieved her heightened emotions. She once impulsively attempted to strangle her mother and fetch a chopper against her elder sister in Form Senior 4. From that time on, she stayed in a children's home, a girls' home and, later, back at her grandparents' home.

Amy used to achieve good academic results in primary school but had a history of truancy for 6 months in Form Senior 4 and she gave up school afterward. She had worked in sales as a clerk and in causal work before. She usually gave up jobs that she did not like and felt she was forced to work on by her family.

Amy has had five relationships. The longest one, lasting for 4 years, was her first when she was 18 years old. The other relationships lasted about 6 months each; she felt that she did not really love them much. She always tried to have an independent role in a relationship for the fear of being abandoned. Currently she is not in a relationship. Amy's parents live in the country and had been visiting Amy about twice a week.

Past medical and psychiatric history

In 2005 (when she was 11 years old) Amy was once seen by a child psychiatric team in the pediatric ward after making suicidal threats, without an actual attempt. She was thought to have behavioral and emotional problems resulting from inconsistent parenting.

Amy has been formally known to adult mental health services since October 2015 (when she was 21 years old). She had been referred for impulsive behavior and repeated wrist-slashing. She was diagnosed with dysthymia with underlying personality difficulties. She had irregular follow-up and defaulted repeatedly on appointments with a clinical psychologist. She has been tried on several anti-depressants including fluoxetine, sertraline, and desvenlafaxine; these caused a number of side effects and she had poor drug compliance. She complained of emotional blunting with selective serotonin reuptake inhibitors (SSRIs), restlessness with fluoxetine, and mental dullness with desvenlafaxine.

Amy had been attending psychotherapy intermittently since 2016. It was thought that her emotions heightened easily and that she had polarized thinking about herself. She has also made many self-critical comments. She had difficulties in handling the ambivalent feelings toward her parents who she felt invalidated her when they were present but also admitted that she would feel lonely when they were out of town. Her condition had been improving in the recent year. She is more aware of her emotions and of how her personal history contributed to the present distress. She was treated with mindfulness therapy and dialectical behavioral therapy. She had much less frequent self-harm/ wrist-slashing behaviors in the past year. She has had fewer conflicts with her parents since they started to live separately.

Present management   After admission, Amy was able to calm down. She felt remorse for her suicidal acts and realized that there could be other solutions to the debt problems. She had strong guilty feeling for becoming a burden to her family and felt ashamed. She was started on mirtazapine for better sleep. She was referred for psychotherapy for emotional regulation. The plan is to continue the psychological intervention in the outpatient setting. Family meetings were held with parents and Amy, and time was allowed for Amy to vent her emotions so that her parents could understand her better. She was referred to the medical social worker for assistance with the debt problem. The discharge plan was considered jointly with Amy and her parents, and they agreed to live temporarily in the country until the debt issue settled down while Amy would continue psychotherapy and psychiatric follow-up in the city.

Consultation   JM thanked the doctor for this thorough assessment and congratulated her for knowing her patient so well. On discussing one of the precipitants of her depression, the unfortunate loan, it was clarified that although the sum was reasonable for the business she was planning to set up, the way she set it up made her vulnerable to exploitation. Amy borrowed the money then handed it over to her "partner" who disappeared and Amy could no longer trace him. As a result, Amy was not able to set up the business she was planning to open. Instead, she tried to earn the money by taking on three part-time jobs. Amy had not sought the advice of any debt agency and had not tried to come to some arrangement with the "loan shark." JM pointed out that the increasing debt will not be addressed as a problem by psychotherapy but needs to be addressed by a financial advisor. The doctor informed JM that Amy had been referred to a social worker who was advising her on this matter. The doctor felt that with her parents' involvement, Amy feels relieved that the problem is no longer escalating, and she is beginning to have some hope that this troublesome problem is nearing some resolution.

JM asked if Amy had a plan for her life: if she had some idea of how she would like to earn her living, where she would like to live, etc. The doctor added that her parents advised Amy to stay with them away from the city until this matter is sorted so that, at least, she is safe. JM asked the doctor if the opinion of the psychiatric team was that Amy was mature enough to manage her life on her own. There were many doubts about this. Amy seemed to be vulnerable to exploitation. The doctor added that Amy was easily led and easily influenced. It seemed that the parental wish for Amy to live with them is a hopeful approach because this will, at least, give her a period of realistic security.

Regarding Amy's intellectual ability, the doctor had formed the opinion that Amy is of average intelligence. The doctor explained that Amy gave up her education at Form Senior 4 because she had difficulties with her parents at the time, and she had become rebellious. One of the reasons for dropping out of school was the bullying to which she was subjected.

Arguments with her parents were often around their expectations that she should have better academic grades than she was achieving. The doctor felt that the parental expectations were reasonable because Amy's achievement at primary school was good. It was not clear why a girl who was doing so well in primary school should start failing in secondary. JM asked about Amy's experience with parenting figures. Amy was parented by her maternal grandparents until the age of 8. The doctor felt that the parenting her maternal grandparents offered was adequate (not neglectful or abusive). Amy continued to do well for the ages 8–11 when she was being parented by her own natural parents who had returned to the city. A detailed exploration of the transition from primary to secondary school indicated that parenting changed as she became more of an adolescent in the sense that the parental expectations for contribution to chores at home was increased, and the supervision about time-keeping and time at home also became stricter. Amy's parents would also restrict access to the phone and keep a much closer eye on her behavior. The doctor felt that the parents were too restrictive by city standards. JM suggested that during the family meetings the doctor explores the family relationships in a way that enables her to form an independent view regarding the sharing of the household workload. JM pointed out that in a household under stress, everyone is expected to "chip in" according to their ability. Sometimes, the parents end up being exploited by the children, and at others, the parents exploit the children. It would be helpful if the psychiatrist was able to form an independent opinion about this. Both parents had jobs outside the house. As both parents were working outside the house, it would be reasonable for them to expect that their 11- or 12-year-old daughter contribute in some form or other. JM suggested that it would be worthwhile exploring if Amy's view of what her contribution to family life should be was realistic. The picture that emerges is that the transition from childhood to adolescence was not handled in a constructive way by both parents and Amy.

JM then inquired about Amy's understanding of her deterioration of general adjustment with her transition to secondary school. The reason why this problem is addressed in the consultation is because that when Amy's life took a rather dysfunctional trajectory. As an overview, it seemed that with the transition to secondary school and the onset of adolescence, her parents became more controlling, her adjustment at school became more problematic, she started being bullied, her performance deteriorated, her ability to sustain school was reduced, she dropped out, and because the conflict at home was escalating to the point of even attempting to strangle her mother once, living at home was no longer tenable. She lived in a children's home and undertook a series of part-time jobs. Furthermore, her only long-term relationship had broken down, and she had a series of short-term affairs. The relationships with her parents had deteriorated to such a degree that she felt she hated them, and her grandparents were no longer alive (at least not all of them).

JM then pointed out that part of Amy's immaturity is the way she attributes her misfortunes only to other people. If Amy is to develop a better adjustment in life, she needs to start thinking of her own contribution to her misfortunes and how she could address the life tasks in a more constructive and functional way. JM pointed out that there is some strength in Amy as she does go out and does get jobs and, even at time, managing three part-time jobs concurrently. Although she does have that strength, she undermines the good result by developing dysfunctional and immature relationships. JM pointed out that it is fortunate that the psychiatric team has set up a series of family therapy sessions because the parents seem to have a useful role to play (in providing safety for Amy), but they also need to become more tolerant so that Amy's residual strength can be developed.

JM pointed out that the therapeutic "package" would need to include what they have already set up, which is an element of support and direction. Amy still needs some supervision so that she does not fall again victim of exploitation. The second therapeutic measure that has been undertaken is that of family therapy, which could advance the relationships within the family toward a more functional way. The third measure could be individual psychotherapy with aim to get Amy to consider how her approach and her reaction to other people could be more functional than previously. She needs to appreciate, for example, that her parents will have their own needs and their own expectations of her and that she would have some responsibility and something to offer them. The family therapist could facilitate the communication so that parents and daughter can come to an understanding of what is expected of each other. In this way the combination of supervision, family therapy, and individual therapy can have a positive outcome.

For an exploration of the issues around multiple therapies, see Maratos (2000, 2015, 2016).

References

Maratos, J. (2000). Combined therapies—A group analytic perspective. In S. A. Brooks & P. Hodson (Eds.), *The invisible matrix* (pp. 128–148). Rebus Press.

Maratos, J. (Ed.) (2015). *Foundations of group analysis for the twenty-first century*. Karnac.

Maratos, J. (Ed.) (2016). *Applications of group analysis for the twenty-first century*. Karnac.

Mr. Man

Presenting complaint

Mr. Man is a 47-year-old divorced bus driver who was admitted because of suicidal ideation.

History of present condition

Six months ago, Mr. Man's mood started to deteriorate because of a worsening relationship with his family and debt problems. He had increased gambling on soccer matches in the recent 6 months because he claimed that he felt bored during work breaks. He was lent more than US$10,000 from a financial company and around US$3,000 from his friends and relatives. He also suffered from chronic work stress, which he attributed to long working hours and customers' complaints. His ex-wife and children became indifferent toward him and to his debts, which in turn made his mood more depressed. In response, he spent more time gambling. He had reduced volition. His sleep and appetite had worsened. He was drinking up to 10 cans of beer on the rest day, and he attributed this to his low mood. He could still maintain his job as a bus driver.

Two days before admission, his ex-wife expelled him from their home because of his gambling. Mr. Man then went to a hotel to try to find a solution. He then thought of suicide by jumping from a height. He tried to look around the hotel for any stairs that could lead him to the rooftop. But he worried that the debtors would disturb his family and that his pension would be lost, so he abandoned the idea; he went to the accident and emergency department by himself seeking psychiatric admission.

Family history

His father had been observed to have self-muttering and grandiose ideas, but there was no formal psychiatric diagnosis. Otherwise, there is no known family history of mental illness.

Personal history

Mr. Man was born in the city. He was brought up in the family with uneventful childhood. He was educated up to Form Senior 2 level, at which point he gave up his education because he had a romantic relationship with a female friend. Since then, he gambled on horse racing, soccer, and cards. He had symptoms of pathological gambling including primacy, salience, tolerance, compulsion, psychological withdrawal, and rapid reinstatement. He married in his 20s, and he has two children (a 19-year-old son and an 18-year-old daughter). Family relationships fluctuated due to his gambling problem. Eventually his wife decided to divorce him, and he had been bankrupted once due to his gambling. He had to give US$1,000 per month to his wife and children for daily expenses. He rented a place for himself after divorce and maintained his job as a bus driver. In the last year he moved back to live with his ex-wife and children because they believed Mr. Man had corrected himself. Yet he described the relationship was not as close as before because the family seldom talked to him, and he found himself like renting a room from the family. The relationship became more distant in the last 6 months as his gambling increased, and he was eventually expelled from home 2 days before admission. He is a chronic smoker. He smokes around 1.5 packs of cigarettes per day. He drinks around five to five cans of beer per week on his rest day. He has no history of substance abuse or forensic history.

Past medical and psychiatric history

Mr. Man has mild allergic rhinitis and eczema, which do not need regular medical attention.

Mr. Man has been known to the psychiatric services since 2015 when he presented to the clinic for depressive symptoms arising from marital problems. He was diagnosed with depression. He has one previous psychiatric admission in 2015 when he presented with persecutory delusions about his ex-wife and following a suicidal gesture to jump from height after drinking a bottle of red wine and having conflicts with her. He was diagnosed with alcohol induced psycho-is and pathological gambling. He was put on a low dose of an antidepressant and an antipsychotic. He had regular follow-up in the clinic but defaulted the latest appointment in October 2019, before admission. His diagnosis is depression and pathological gambling.

Management and progress   Mr. Man was placed on his usual dose of antidepressant after admission. His mood soon improved, and he gave up the suicidal ideation. He came up with a plan to reformulate his debts, and he continued to work settle the problem more promptly; he was keen to gain back the trust of his family. His son visited him once a few days after his admission, and this made him feel positive toward the whole situation. He expected his son and other family members would keep visiting him and give him support, but since that visit by his son, no one else visited him for a whole week. His mood became depressed again, and he did not want to carry out the plan. He tried to phone his ex-wife, his son, and his siblings, but no one answered his calls. He felt upset by the fluctuating attitude from the family. He believed that his ex-wife and his siblings had already given up on him, but he would like his children to care more for him. He gradually understood and started to accept that the family relationship was irretrievably broken and that it was impossible for him to regain their trust in a short period of time. He started to think of an alternative plan, and he now thinks of early retirement so that he could use the lump sum of his pension to pay off his debts and to minimize the disturbance from debtors to his family. He plans to move to a private hostel after discharge where he could get support; he would then find a new job as a van driver, which he thought would be less stressful. He also plans to make some new friends from the gambling service in the community and to develop new interests. He knows it would be difficult for him in terms of finance if he chooses this plan, but he thinks that if he could start a new page in terms of job, living environment, and personal interests, his mood would be better maintained.

His son later also turned up every 1 to 2 weeks when he did not need to attend school, and his son also promised to accompany with him on the day of discharge. He believes he could still maintain regular contact with his son after discharge. He requested to try a higher dose of the antidepressant to make his mood more stable. He is more motivated to give up gambling. He also requested nicotine patch to help him stop smoking during the admission. His mood and volition are gradually improving.

Consultation   JM thanked the doctor for the thorough presentation and then asked him to expand on the relationship Mr. Man has with his previous wife. It was not clear whether they are emotionally divorced or whether one still has an influence on the other. The doctor responded that the divorce had taken place 11 years before. After the divorce, Mr. Man lived on his own for 1 year but then returned to live with his ex-wife until 2016. Mr. Man's ex-wife would still feed him and look after him in a way, but they did not have much emotional interaction. JM asked if they were financially linked in any way. The doctor responded that Mr. Man had been bankrupted a few times and had been instructed by law to hand over to his ex-wife US$1,000; although their finances are separate, Mr. Man is still expected to pay that amount to his ex-wife for the expenses of the family. The doctor confirmed that Mr. Man had kept up with his payments.

JM asked the doctor to clarify his earliest statement about "symptoms of pathological gambling" including primacy, salience, tolerance, compulsion, psychological withdrawal and rapid reinstatement." The doctor replied that this was copied from prior admission summaries, and he was not in a position to expand on them. The doctor added that salience meant that gambling had become an important aspect in Mr. Man's life; this was in agreement with his own self-perception of being greedy for money. The doctor also explained the term "tolerance" by the fact that Mr. Man required an increasing amount of gambling to gain similar satisfaction. The doctor added that although

Mr. Man had managed to be abstinent of gambling for a year or two, he was quick to reengage with this activity.

JM asked the doctor to clarify his statement that Mr. Man's mood improved after admission and explain how soon after admission that happened. The doctor explained that this was 1 or 2 days after admission. JM responded that if his mood improved in 2 days after admission that could not be attributed to medication. This timing of improvement is a valid indicator that medication is not the agent that improved his mood. The doctor informed JM that the hospital had increased his antidepressant medication. JM summarized that as his improvement took place before the antidepressant medication had time to act, and as his mood became more depressed on a higher dose when his family failed to visit, these are two strong indicators that his depression (i) is not likely to improve on medication and (ii) is not protected from becoming more severe when he is on medication. In summary, JM expressed the view that the use of antidepressants seems to be of doubtful benefit to him.

JM then added that there seemed to be two sides to Mr. Man. The first is that he is a competent person who held his job for many years, and this was a responsible job. The doctor clarified that Mr. Man had held his job for 25 years. JM pointed out that being a driver of people is a responsible job and Mr. Man seemed to have acted with responsibility. This reflects that there is a side of Mr. Man that is mature and responsible.

JM then added that there was another side that was less mature. The first indication was that he dropped out of school "because of a girlfriend." He dropped out of school at age 15 and that was the age when he and his friends began gambling. The doctor explained that Mr. Man gave up school for two reasons; the first was that he was losing interest in his education and second was that his girlfriend had also given up schooling. The doctor explained that the year after giving up education, he was idle for most of the time. He started working with the bus company after that year. After leaving school and before starting work at the bus company, he wasted several years doing little to no work.

JM asked if Mr. Man had given an account of his behavior, and the doctor replied that he had explained that he had acted selfishly not thinking of the needs of his family but only of himself. JM pointed out that for a selfish man, he did not serve his self-interest well. He left himself without money, without his family, without a career, and without the security that a career gives one.

The doctor informed the meeting that Mr. Man married in 1998. It was not known how this marriage took place, whether this was an arranged marriage or whether it was a marriage of convenience or following a love affair. JM pointed out that we understand why the marriage broke down (this was related to his gambling), he was wasting the family income on gambling. The doctor clarified that although in his early days he got into gambling influenced by his friends, currently he is gambling on his own because it is such an easy thing to do through his telephone.

JM asked if Mr. Man had an explanation for his gambling. The doctor explained that he accounted for this based on his love of money. JM responded that rather than giving him money, his gambling has landed him into debt and bankruptcy. JM pointed out another aspect of his dysfunctional approach to his needs: Instead of having a functional way of earning a living, he adopted a way that moved him further from his objective. JM pointed out that one needs to look further into why his love of money led to him being without money.

JM pointed out that for someone who describes himself as selfish, he does not manage to look after his own self-interest. Somebody who wants more money does not make himself bankrupt. And this is not the result of any lack of intelligence as this is indicated by his ability to hold a skilled and responsible job for 25 years. Furthermore, he is planning to make himself redundant, which means that he may be able to repay some of the debt, but he will make himself unemployed at the age of 47. JM suggested that Mr. Man was considering only short-term benefits, and this consideration was often against his long-term advantage. JM gave the additional example of him thinking short term when he abandoned his education. Had he thought what would have been to his long-term benefit, he would have stayed at school and gained some qualifications. JM added that immediate pleasure does not have to be in conflict with long-term benefit, but in his case, his choice for immediate pleasure was often at the disadvantage of his own long-term gains.

JM pointed out that Mr. Man had a difficulty in tolerating the frustration of the present, which could give him a long-term gain. Mr. Man could have connected in his mind the immediate self-interest with the long term. For example, he would have had a greater immediate and long-term pleasure if he looked after his wife, and if instead of spending his earnings on gambling, he invested it into looking after his family. That would have given him greater happiness in the present and in the future.

JM then addressed the issue of therapy. If Mr. Man could have a professional relationship with a therapist with whom he could feel secure, with whom he would be helped to tolerate the uncertainty and the stress of thinking of what is best for him and rethinking with the purpose of developing. Development for him would be to have the ability to combine the short-term with the long-term benefits. In the context of therapy, he can learn "efficient selfishness". Within the context of therapy, Mr. Man can be supported by having his own track record pointed out to him. His own track record includes holding a responsible job for 25 years and earning a reasonable salary during that time. He could be encouraged if this realistic ability was pointed out to him. He can be helped to see himself not only as a failing gambler but also as a person who has a mature and strong side to himself.

In therapy, Mr. Man can be encouraged that it is worthwhile putting up with some immediate frustration because he does have the potential of building a better life for himself and for his family.

For dynamic aspects of pathological gambling, see Maniaci et al. (2017) and Mallorqui-Bague et al. (2018).

References

Mallorqui-Bague, N., Mena-Moreno, T., Granero, R., Vintro-Alcaraz, C., Sanchez-Gonzalez, J., Fernandez-Aranda, F., Pino-Gutierrez, A. D., Mestre-Bach, G., Aymami, N., Gomez-Pena, M., Menchon, J. M., & Jimenez-Murcia, S. (2018). Suicidal ideation and history of suicide attempts in treatment-seeking patients with gambling disorder: The role of emotion dysregulation and high trait impulsivity. *Journal of Behavioral Addictions*, 7(4), 1112–1121.

Maniaci, G., La Cascia, C., Picone, F., Lipari, A., Cannizzaro, C., & La Barbera, D. (2017). Predictors of early dropout in treatment for gambling disorder: The role of personality disorders and clinical syndromes. *Psychiatry Research*, 257, 540–545.

Mr. Lo

Presenting complaint

Mr. Lo is a 65-year-old man who presented with low mood and suicidal ideas.

History of the present condition

Mr. Lo had been mentally stable until around October 2016. He was incidentally found to have a low platelet count when he was assessed for cataract surgery and was later diagnosed with idiopathic thrombocytopenic purpura (ITP). He had repeated admissions to hospital for both emergency and due to his low platelet count. He was required to have many investigations and intravenous immunoglobulin transfusions. However, he felt that the investigations were inconclusive and that the treatment he was provided with had limited effect. Due to his repeated hospital admissions, he was unable to work any longer or to make commitments to his hobbies. He used to own a trade company with his two brothers, selling plastic household appliances, but the company had to close after he was unable to work. His mood began to worsen, and he became easily more irritable over trivial matters. He was ruminative and anxious when he thought about his physical condition. He felt that because his condition was considered "idiopathic" (which meant that the cause was unknown), it was the doctors who did not know what they were doing. He felt that he was a burden to his siblings because they often had to visit him in hospital. He felt his siblings were supportive and did not blame him for the company closing, but he felt guilty about his health affecting others. He had feelings of hopelessness and had lost interest in sports he used to enjoy or in cooking for himself. He felt guilty making dates with his friends to do sports because he was afraid to break the commitment since he often had to be admitted to the hospital unexpectedly. He had worsened sleep and appetite. He lost 40 pounds in weight over 2 years. Subjectively he felt gradual memory impairment the past few years, and he was more forgetful and misplaced things at times.

His mood further worsened the past few months as he was admitted to the hospital once almost every month. He bought a pack of over-the-counter hypnotics and planned to overdose a few months ago. He also attempted to get hit by traffic by walking out on a busy street to end his life. But the cars stopped in time. He ruminated about committing suicide, including jumping from a height and slashing his wrist. He attempted to go up a building several months ago and thought about jumping but stopping himself because he felt he had to finish something for his friend. He claimed that each time he did not go through with his suicide attempts was because he always felt there was something still left to do or to complete before he could die.

He attended his first psychiatric clinic assessment in December 2019 with his eldest brother and a social worker, and an inpatient admission was arranged.

Personal history

Mr. Lo was born in the city. He was the sixth of 12 siblings. He reported he had constantly good relationships with his siblings and his parents. His father also worked in trading and was a hardworking man. They were not rich, but he had a happy childhood. He studied until Form 5 and obtained average grades. He worked in different trading companies until he set up his own company with his two brothers 3 years ago. He claimed that his brothers contributed money, but it was he who was the one involved with the actual business transactions. He claimed that the business was profitable. Because he was repeatedly admitted to the hospital, the company had to be closed.

Mr. Lo claimed that he had a good relationship with his parents. He had a chance to work overseas, but he refused the offer because he wanted to take care of his parents (despite his parents being physically well at that time). Mr. Lo's mother died at around the age of 70; he claimed that she had been quite weak prior to her death and that she died at home peacefully. His father had some chronic disease but was still up and about prior to the final admission to the hospital. His father was in hospital for a month prior his death; he claimed that the doctor attributed his father's death due to organ failure. He claimed that especially his younger brothers could not accept the cause of his father's death and had a tough time dealing with the grief because they felt unsure about the exact cause of death.

Mr. Lo had never been married and had been living alone. He reported having several romantic relationships with the longest relationship being for 10 years. Mr. Lo said they had a good relationship, but he was fearful that he could not support her financially in the future, and he made an excuse to break up. He reported that he felt remorseful afterward because his brother told him he should have discussed with her the financial situation first before deciding the breakup by himself. He claimed his girlfriend was working and was better off than him at that time. After that long-term relationship, he no longer committed to anyone else. There was no history of family illness.

Mr. Lo reported liking helping others but disliked being helped or relying on others. He claimed he had high expectations of himself but did not have high expectations of others. He liked being organized and have things scheduled; hence, he felt it was difficult to accept that he often needed to be admitted to hospital without notice because of an emergency. He reported being outgoing and having many friends and hobbies (i.e., soccer, basketball, traditional dancing, cycling, hiking, etc.).

Past medical and psychiatric history

Mr. Lo was new to the mental health service. Mr. LO suffered from refractory ITP; he was anti-hepatitis C positive and was on medication; he had a history of an ischiorectal abscess and septicemia, and history of acute renal failure, abscess of spleen, lactic acidosis, and septic shock, which required resuscitation in intensive care in January 2019.

Present treatment and management Mr. Lo is now an inpatient and is on antidepressants. He was still on suicidal observation because he still had fleeting suicidal ideas. He was referred to a clinical psychologist for psychotherapy.

Consultation JM thanked the doctor for the thorough presentation and proceeded to ask him how Mr. Lo responded to being admitted to hospital. The doctor responded that Mr. Lo was cooperative in the hospital and walked unaided. Mr. Lo tended to be quiet and spend a lot of time on his own. There was no significant change in his mood. He still believed that there was "not much hope in living." JM then asked if the doctor knew what was giving him hope to live 3 to 6 months previously. The doctor responded that it was his belief that he needed to do certain things for others and that was usually in connection with his work. His purpose for living was his work and his ability to offer a service. By closing his business he lost one main purpose for living. It seemed that what kept him alive was the notion of service and being useful to others.

Since his work closed, he lost one significant motivation to be alive and since his illness was diagnosed, he lost his ability to maintain the relationships with his friends and his hobbies. Mr. Lo suffered three major losses in his life that he has not replaced with any other objectives. The doctor clarified that Mr. Lo needed frequent admissions because he needed replenishment with platelets and immunoglobulin but also because he was in a vulnerable physical state and likely to develop septicemia or other life-threatening conditions. The doctor added that it is interesting that Mr. Lo is incapacitated even though he does not have any physical symptoms; he is not in pain and he is able to move. In other words, his physical condition is compatible with a more functional way of living than he has at present.

JM suggested that it may be useful for the doctor to speak directly with the physicians who are involved in his treatment because it is possible that Mr. Lo himself has blown out of all proportion the threat that his condition posed to him and the danger that he believes that he is in. Such contact with physicians may help Mr. Lo adopt a more realistic and balanced view of the threat that his condition poses to him.

The other losses that Mr. Lo has suffered are the retirement from his business, the onset of the thrombocytopenia, and the hepatitis C. JM pointed out that although these losses and threats were real, they did not absolutely exclude the possibility of a better life. Even if service was a pillar in his existence, there is no reason why the residual health that he has could not enable him to be of some sort of service that would be different but still important to others. Mr. Lo could be helped to develop a different plan for his life considering his illnesses and his age. He could develop a life of a "retired" person with some activities that would be compatible for a man of 65 years of age with his conditions. More specifically, there is no reason why, despite his conditions, he could not meet his friends although, naturally, there is a good reason why he should not play football. After all, there are few 65-year-olds who play football as a hobby.

The doctor added that Mr. Lo was withdrawing from contacts because he felt he could not make a predictable commitment to his friends. It was not so much the risk of injury to himself. The fact that he is financially secure would make his position a lot easier to manage. For a person, like Mr. Lo, it is a great advantage not to have to depend on other people for his survival. Mr. Lo could also be reminded that he does have people, his friends, who value his presence, so he can continue to be a valuable member of a friendship despite his health problems. This notion may help him restore the friendships that he has now withdrawn from. Because of the intricate relationship between his physical and psychological state, it would be helpful if the doctor communicated with the physicians and alerted them or help them become more aware of the psychological implications of his conditions and the need to make with him a plan of treatment in which his absences are more planned and predictable (to the extent that his ITP permits). Such an arrangement will go some way toward helping Mr. Lo realize that he is still a valuable member of society and that he is not someone to be rejected because he is not earning and that he is not able to contribute equally in the physical activities with his friends.

Mr. Lo can begin to see himself as someone who has a mind of his own, who has a functioning brain, who is somebody who does not depend financially on anyone, and who is somebody valued by friends and family. In this way Mr. Lo can be helped to **look forward to a life of retirement** instead of feeling depressed because he can no longer continue with his previous level of activities.

As a second thought JM suggested the involvement of an occupational therapist who would guide him to engage in activities that would be compatible with his conditions.

The present case illustrates the impact of a series of losses and the failure to mourn them as a first step toward planning a new life for the future. It also illustrates the interaction between physical conditions and mental state, as well as, physical conditions and incapacity. It also illustrates that patients with this level of complexity of problems require a multidimensional approach and a coordination of interventions by the medical and psychiatric teams. See Balint (1957), Rahe et al. (1967), Susser (1990), and Shoenberg (2007).

References

Balint, M. (1957). *The doctor, his patient and the illness*. Pitman Medical.

Rahe, R. H., McKean, J. D., Jr., & Arthur, R. J. (1967). A longitudinal study of life-change and illness patterns. *Journal of Psychosomatic Research*, 10(4), 355–366.

Shoenberg, P. (2007). Psychotherapy with psychosomatic patients. In P. Shoenberg (Ed.), *Psychosomatics; the uses of psychotherapy* (pp. 27–54). Palgrave Macmillan.

Susser, M. (1990). Disease, illness, sickness; impairment, disability and handicap. *Psychological Medicine*, 20(3), 471–473.

Section II

Neurotic Presentations

5

Low Mood: Suicidal Attempt

Ms. Y

Presenting condition

Ms. Y is an unemployed woman, aged 42; she is an ex-piano tutor, who presented with chronic dysthymia and hypnotic dependence.

History of present complaint

Ms. Y lives with her estranged husband in a public housing unit. She suffers from chronic low mood, which she attributes to an intense and ambivalent relationship with her husband. Her maternal grandmother, who brought her up, died earlier this year. Her mood has deteriorated since. She also experienced a change in social worker recently. She found her new social worker to be more critical of her condition, and she made Ms. Y feel stressed. On attendance to the psychiatric clinic, Ms. Y was distraught and reported to have harbored ideas of reference that pedestrians knew she suffered from a mental illness. She also had an increase of death ruminations of jumping from heights, taking a drug overdose, or self-poisoning by carbon monoxide by burning charcoal. She was therefore voluntarily admitted to hospital.

Ms. Y also became socially withdrawn. She had no daytime regular activities. She suffered from interrupted sleep at night. She became reliant on hypnotics, and at times, she used vodka as well. She often came before the date her next appointments to receive and hoard hypnotics. She had three episodes of withdrawal fits in 2005, 2006, and 2007.

Ms. Y. reported that her grandmother could not remember her at the end of her life. She pined for her grandmother after her death. She claimed her new social worker was critical of her. She felt distraught. Ms. Y started hearing inner voices making brief hostile comments. Ms. Y started experiencing increased ruminations of committing suicide by drug overdose or by jumping from heights. Eventually she attended the psychiatric clinic and was admitted to hospital.

Dynamic Consultations with Psychiatrists: Understanding Severely Troubled Patients, First Edition. Jason Maratos.
© 2022 John Wiley & Sons Ltd. Published 2022 by John Wiley & Sons Ltd.

Personal history

Ms. Y. was born in the city. She gave a history that was inconsistent at times. She reported that she never met her biological parents. Her father left her before she was born. Her father also left her half-sister who grew up with her. Her mother left her at age of 2 or 3 years of age. Ms. Y revealed that she and her sister were later sent to an orphanage. Her maternal grandmother first brought her half-sister out of the orphanage. She was visited by maternal grandmother in the orphanage and was eventually brought out of the orphanage when she was a teenager. She had a harmonious relationship with the family until she met her current husband. She said her family did not accommodate their relationship because they felt the man was too old for her and would put her studies at risk. She then moved out of the family home and cohabited with the boyfriend. She maintained a good relationship with her boyfriend for 10 years until he had an affair with another woman.

Ms. Y said that her husband was her first love; they met when they were teenagers. They had a good relationship until she discovered his affair with another woman. They had episodes of physical aggression (intimate partner violence) at that time and that caused her to seek refuge in a shelter. She said she never really forgave the boyfriend even though he ended the contact with the other woman. She withdrew from sexual contact, and they began living in separate rooms. She then became emotionally unstable. She made suicidal attempts by taking a drug overdose with alcohol and bought charcoal for burning, but this was discovered by her husband. No genuine harm had been inflicted.

Two years later, her husband suddenly proposed marriage. She agreed, but she still did not forgive him. Her relationship with her relatives became more distant because they still did not support this relationship.

Other relevant items of history, which she did not reveal at the time of admission, were the history of a spontaneous miscarriage in 2005 and a history of theft in 2011. These were multiple episodes that were perpetrated when she was not suffering from psychosis. Ms. Y claimed that they were carried out of impulse. Ms. Y also reported that her husband was once sentenced to prison in 2012–2013 for breaking his family's furniture. She had been sexually assaulted once by a correctional officer at that time.

Past psychiatric history

Ms. Y had been attending the psychiatric clinic since 2008 due to her dependence on hypnotics. She has a history of hypnotic withdrawal fits in 2005, 2006, and 2007. The diagnosis at clinic was chronic dysthymia and dependence on hypnotics.

Ms. Y had been treated with agomelatine and quetiapine to limited effect.

Present treatment and management of case   Ms. Y's mental state improved on admission. She was referred to a clinical psychologist for psychological intervention. She claimed she had a complete attitude change during the admission. She felt she was able to forgive herself and her husband. She believed her past hurt was completely healed. She wanted to confront reality and try to become reconciled with her husband. If that was not possible, she would like to break up with him completely.

Currently, Ms. Y is still being followed up at clinic with a clinical psychology referral. She had complete change of attitude compared with when she was first seen. She put on makeup and looked cheerful and bright. She was optimistic toward her interpersonal relationships. She often made glorifying remarks to previous medical staff during her admission. She experienced no more auditory hallucinations and had no further suicidal thoughts.

The treatment plan is for her to continue her engagement with clinical psychology so that she could work on underlying personality issues and on her intense and ambivalent relationships. Ms. Y will continue attending the psychiatric outpatients at about six weekly intervals and may also maintain contact with a community psychiatric nurse.

Consultation   After thanking the doctor for the thorough presentation JM asked her to clarify what the patient's expectations were of her. The doctor responded that Ms. Y's expectations were limited. The doctor added that the patient had commented that she had received generous support from the previous staff and that she no longer needed that high level of support. The doctor felt that Ms. Y had idealized the ward staff and the level of treatment that she had received. It was clarified that Ms. Y desired to have contact with doctors who she thought of in idealized terms. The doctor pointed out that Ms. Y was expecting the relationship with her to be long term and the doctor agreed with this expectation. The doctor added that she will move due to her rotation and that Ms. Y will then be allocated to another psychiatrist. The doctor pointed out that Ms. Y is used to the change of doctors. JM pointed out that because Ms. Y had idealized the doctor, the change of doctor will have a different effect on her. The doctor pointed out that it was not only she who was being idealized but all the medical staff and the clinical psychologists and nurses. Ms. Y tended to idealize any professional with whom she contacted during admissions.

JM asked the doctor to clarify the last time when Ms. Y functioned "normally." The doctor responded that Ms. Y had worked full-time as a piano teacher and later changed her job to part-time teaching (after she discovered her husband's affair). Ms. Y lost her job in 2004. JM asked the doctor if she knew the reason why Ms. Y changed her job from full- to part-time. The doctor replied that Ms. Y attributed this to the emotional torment that she went through when she discovered her husband's indiscretion. Ms. Y's relationship with her husband deteriorated in 2006. The marital relationship has continued to be problematic, and the situation has never been properly resolved. The relationship is still asexual, and they live in separate rooms. JM commented that although they live in separate rooms, they do share the same house. The doctor pointed out that the husband does all the household jobs, cooking, and shopping. He has undertaken these activities to compensate for the harm he caused through his affair. JM asked the doctor to clarify that Ms. Y is completely dependent on her husband, the state, and the medical services. She does not seem to contribute anything herself. The doctor confirmed this and added that Ms. Y had also withdrawn from her church. JM asked the doctor to state what Ms. Y's thoughts were for her own future. The doctor responded that her view of the future was "very bleak." The doctor added that Ms. Y contemplated divorce to begin a new life, but this was never actioned. Ms. Y felt that any such attempt may lead to her becoming so unwell that she would not be able to build her life again.

JM persevered in trying to get a clear picture of what Ms. Y felt her life would be if the situation with her husband was resolved. The doctor pointed out that she wished she was a friend with her husband but not to sustain a full marital relationship. She felt that she should share in the household chores and wished she could make some commitment to the couple. She also felt that she should be contributing toward the family finances.

JM pointed out that Ms. Y is an able woman, a pianist, and was a piano teacher. JM asked for Ms. Y's explanation why she does not use her talent to improve her own life. The doctor replied that whenever this subject is raised, Ms. Y reverted to the difficulties in the marital relationship and the grief over the loss of her maternal grandmother. Ms. Y claimed that she wanted to normalize her emotions first and start applying herself after. JM asked if Ms. Y feels that she is still in mourning for the loss of her grandmother and the loss of the relationship with her husband. The doctor added that Ms. Y's relationship with her grandmother was mixed because her grandmother did not approve of her own relationship with her husband. This mixed quality caused Ms. Y to feel guilty about her grandmother. Her grandmother had died earlier in 2017. JM pointed out that the loss of her grandmother could not be the cause of Ms. Y's under functioning because it took place well after Ms. Y had begun withdrawing from active life. Ms. Y had been dysfunctional for 5 years while the grandmother had died only a few months previously. Ms. Y has ambivalent feelings about her grandmother who was effectively in the role of her mother. The doctor added that the relationship was further complicated by the fact that grandmother used to take her out of the orphanage only occasionally and effectively took care of her when she became a teenager and was brought to live with her out of the orphanage.

JM pointed out that Ms. Y, despite the institutional upbringing and the interrupted family relationships, had managed to complete her education and additionally to learn a musical instrument to the degree that she was able to teach it. The doctor pointed out that Ms. Y had prematurely interrupted her piano studies because of the relationship with her husband. Her family stopped funding her studies when she developed the relationship with her husband. The doctor clarified that Ms. Y initially taught piano by working at a shop selling instruments. She later acquired individual pupils. JM tried to clarify if Ms. Y, who had less than an ideal upbringing, had managed to complete her education, acquire the skill of playing the piano, and work full-time as a tutor. JM summarized that despite her difficulties, Ms. Y had been managing her life constructively with education and learning the piano and later working as a pianist and then the deterioration started with giving up part of her work and then stopping working completely. JM then invited that the focus of the thinking should be the change in this young woman from coping with adversity to giving up. Ms. Y started becoming less independent and less self-reliant. The doctor added that a fact that was contributing to this change was the ambivalent relationship that she developed with her grandmother on account with her relationship with her husband. Ms. Y feels guilty that she did not listen to her grandmother's advice.

JM then asked why Ms. Y had chosen to stay with her husband when she now feels that he is not the right person for her. The doctor reported that this was not an area that had gone into thoroughly and that Ms. Y appreciates that her husband carries out all the household duties and physically supports her. JM pointed out that her feelings toward her husband are still ambivalent and unresolved.

JM raised the issue of the feeling of dependency and the feeling of anger in Ms. Y's mind. The doctor added that when Ms. Y discovered her husband's affair, she expressed anger and that led to a physical confrontation with him. Ms. Y was angry with her husband because she felt she sacrificed everything for him and then he went to have an affair. She had sacrificed her relationships with her family of origin and the relationship with her husband had cost her the financial support of her family. Ms. Y attributes the estrangement from her family and her loss of family financial support to her husband. She blames her husband for her not continuing her education; although the husband repented and tried to compensate for his behavior, Ms. Y has not felt able to forgive him. JM asked if there were any thoughts on why Ms. Y had failed to resolve the mixed feelings about the marital situation. Many couples go through crises, and they resolve them either by divorcing and separating or by reconciling to the fact and moving forward. It is worth understanding why for so many years the situation has not been resolved. JM asked how the nonresolution of the situation contribute to her deterioration and increasing dysfunction. The doctor gave the practical reasons for why divorce was not practical for her, and then JM asked why, in that case, they had not reconciled. JM pointed out that her husband had "served his sentence" and that he had actively shown for several years that he repented by looking after her even more than any reasonable couple would expect a husband to contribute. JM asked why Ms. Y was unable to reconcile her own feelings of ambivalence toward her husband. The doctor replied that Ms. Y had chosen to portray herself as a victim and, as such, her husband owed her to look after her emotionally and financially. JM asked if the understanding is that Ms. Y is manipulating or taking advantage of her husband.

JM asked if there was a connection between the way Ms. Y handled the current rejection and the current trauma, with earlier life experiences of rejection. JM clarified that he was referring to Ms. Y's early rejection from the family who placed her in an orphanage. JM pointed out the three major hurts in Ms. Y's life: the loss of her family and placement in an orphanage, the loss of the marital relationship, and the loss of her grandmother. JM asked if it was possible that the way she handled the previous losses affected the way she dealt with subsequent ones.

JM brought up the matter of Ms. Y's understanding of why she was put in an orphanage in the first place. The doctor pointed out that Ms. Y did have a half-sister but that she did not know why it was she who was placed in an orphanage and not her half-sister. JM inquired further about the feelings that Ms. Y has had about being the one who was placed in an orphanage and was not kept at home as her sister was. This is an area that has yet to be explored. JM then asked about Ms. Y's experience of being in an orphanage. This is another area of her life that is significant and, therefore, needs to be explored further. One could make more sense of the present difficulties if they are seen in connection with her life experiences, which we know are less than ideal and possibly quite traumatic. JM summarized that Ms. Y had the trauma of rejection from the family, the trauma of being brought up in an orphanage, the alienation from the family because of the relationship with her husband, the trauma of her husband's infidelity, and finally the trauma of the grandmother's death. In parallel to that, there are the positive signs of some resilience on her part (the resilience that enabled her to complete her education and develop her piano talent) but also some support, financial and otherwise, by the family, including the grandmother. JM pointed out that at some stage she had been able to develop a relationship with her husband to the point that led to their marriage. JM pointed out that there were considerable positives both within her and within her life experience. JM pointed out that the dynamic task ahead was to help Ms. Y resolve the ambivalent feelings toward her life experiences and to reconcile the traumatic and negative influences with the positive ones, which were both real. The resolution of these feelings would lead to an acceptance and would enable her to address the needs of her present life more constructively than she did.

JM indicated that Ms. Y's traumatic experiences had an impact not only on the way she established relationships but also on the way she saw herself. There was some indication that she felt guilt. She may also feel shame and certainly have her own sense of self-worth being diminished. Resolution of the ambivalence would not only lead to her having better relationships but would also enable her to work effectively and, that in turn, will contribute to building her sense of self-worth.

Miss MA

Presenting condition

Miss MA was voluntarily admitted from an accident and emergency department following a suicidal attempt.

History of present complaint

Miss MA is a 25-year-old woman who was admitted suffering from chronic low mood; she had been experiencing a feeling of chronic emptiness and of a vulnerable unstable self-image. She had crying spells with fleeting suicidal ideas and used to slash her wrist for "venting." Miss MA has had no real long-term suicidal ideas.

Miss MA's mood fluctuated since she became acquainted with the current boyfriend 6 months ago. She felt that he is not a caring boyfriend. She described their relationship as "stormy" and complained that it leaves her with a fear of abandonment. She could not leave him, even though she felt that he is not caring enough.

Miss MA would ruminate with suicidal ideas and have low mood whenever they had a conflict. She has never had any auditory hallucinations, but she admitted that she had an inner dialogue in which she was blaming herself whenever she felt unhappy. She often had negative cognitions and ruminated on suicidal ideas but never made an actual plan because she is not "brave" enough to do so. Miss MA denied having any abnormal perceptions or beliefs. Her appetite was maintained, her sleep was fragmented, and her function was maintained.

Miss MA's mood suddenly deteriorated 2 days prior to admission after she quarreled with her boyfriend. She claimed loudly that she wanted to leave home late at night, but her boyfriend had no intention to soothe or stop her. Instead, her boyfriend asked her to return his home key to him and told her to leave. Her mood became even lower because she felt that her boyfriend did not care about her. She then went to her neighborhood alone and drank some red wine near the harbor side. She cut her wrist there, resulting in superficial wounds, with a cosmetic sharp implement for eyebrows. She then went to rent a room in an hourly-rate hotel and took an overdose of benzodiazepines (20 tabs of Dopareel according to consultation liaison notes). She claimed she did it because she wanted to have a better sleep and that she had no suicidal intent. She called her sister on the night of the event and mentioned her suicidal wish. She was sent to hospital as a result.

Family history

Miss MA's younger sister had been admitted to the psychiatric ward of a hospital for mood disorders many years ago, and she was not sure of the exact diagnosis. She defaulted follow-ups after discharge.

Personal history

Miss MA is a 25-year-old woman and a higher diploma student and part-time sales lady. Miss MA reported that she had an unhappy childhood and that she had been abandoned shortly after birth. Miss MA is the second of three children. Her parents divorced when she was 1, and she had been raised by different relatives until she was 11 when she moved back to live with her father who lives in the country. She then went to a boarding school until tertiary level. Miss MA returned to the city at age 18 and lived with her mother and elder sister. The family relationships were described as "poor all along," with her mother only talking to her to ask her for money or to scold her.

Miss MA has had three previous relationships. The current one had been for 6 months. Miss MA described herself as pessimistic with no friends. She was a nonsmoker and nondrinker. There was no history of substance abuse. Miss MA is currently living with her boyfriend and his family in a public housing unit. She is new to the mental health services.

Past psychiatric history

There is a history of cutting wrists "for stress release." There was no history of cutting of wrists when she was with the previous two boyfriends.

Treatment and progress   This was thought to be a depressive episode in a person with an underlying Borderline Personality Disorder trait. Symptoms were controlled with medication, psychoeducation, and cognitive therapy. She had not been thought to meet full criteria for a specific diagnostic category at this present. Her ways of coping with stress, her problematic self-image, and emotion regulation were considered. She was discharged to a relative and continued to live with her boyfriend and his family as before.

Consultation   JM thanked the doctor for the thorough assessment, knowing the patient well, and communicating that equally well. The doctor replied that having considered this case, they would like to find out ways in which to help her through psychological means.

JM inquired what the doctor's thoughts about psychological interventions are. The doctor responded that the patient is young and has psychological capacity to benefit from psychological help.

JM asked how the doctor felt that Miss MA could be made emotionally receptive to the cognitive input. Breaking up with a boyfriend is an almost universal phenomenon in early adulthood, but this does not lead to breakdowns in most people. It needs to be identified why it led to Miss MA's breakdown and what made it impossible for her to deal with her breakup in a more constructive way. Additionally, in view of the feelings of emptiness and fear of being abandoned, he asked what psychological intervention would be appropriate for this patient.

The doctor responded that this patient is 25 years old, was able to study, is intelligent, and has some capacity to use psychological interventions. She has the capacity to change her negative behaviors.

JM asked what the doctor thought would help Miss MA become emotionally ready to become receptive to these cognitive interventions. JM needed to expand on this question. He reminded the doctor of Miss MA's vulnerability to rejections (like the rejection from her boyfriend). JM pointed out that in young adulthood the experience of breaking up with a boyfriend is universal, although it is not universally followed by a breakdown. This was meant to direct the doctor's thinking to Miss MA's specific vulnerability. JM then asked specifically, "what has made it impossible for this particular woman to deal with the separation more constructively?"

The doctor replied that this woman needed her boyfriend to be there immediately for her to rely on him. She was not able to contain her feelings until a different boyfriend was found. JM asked the doctor to confirm if Miss MA could not cope with feelings of being alone. This was confirmed, and JM then asked what was specifically difficult for this woman to cope with the state of being alone for time.

JM then expanded a little on the two meanings of "why" (meanings of causality). One meaning of why is "how did this something come about;" in other words, it refers to the origin of a response of a condition, why did it start? The second meaning of "why" is how does this person deal with the onset and, therefore, why this condition develop in this way. The two aspects of causality are how a development started and why did it continue? I am referring here to the psychoanalytic concepts of genetic causation and dynamic causation (Kohut, 1980, p. 508).

The first "why" refers to the origin some time ago, and the second "why" refers to the present processing of the situation by her. Then JM pointed out that the two dynamics that are causing pain to her are (a) the being alone and (b) the being rejected. JM pointed out that the dynamics of being alone are rather different from the dynamics of being rejected and then pointed out that being without is generating separate feelings from being deprived of something that you had previously.

JM pointed out that being alone or being without something is usually associated with depression, while being deprived of something that one previously had is associated with feelings of anger (Bowlby, 1973). JM pointed out that the other dynamic is that of anxiety, and specifically in this young woman, anxiety related to feelings of uncertainty that she would be able to cope (or not in this case) without the presence and support of another person.

JM then expanded that the "genetic why" is related to the origin of a condition both historically (in the distant past/the early childhood) and more recently to the origin of this episode of poor mental health or of dysfunction.

JM then asked the doctors to address the present dynamic causation, and specifically, "how does Miss MA process an event currently in a way that makes it impossible for her to cope with it? What is the meaning of being alone for her emotionally?" The doctor replied that Miss MA felt that she could not cope with her studies.

JM asked what was stopping her from studying? The doctor replied that it was her low mood and lack of motivation disturbing her study. She skipped her lessons because of lack of motivation. JM then asked the doctor to explain what "lack of motivation" meant for her. If she did not want to attend lessons, why did she enlist in the course? The doctor explained her ambivalence because, on one hand, she wanted to complete the diploma, and on the other, she was skipping lessons.

The doctor clarified that this was not a case of straight negative motivation but one of mixed feelings of wanting and not wanting the same objective. JM then asked the doctor to explain what the reason Miss MA wanted to get a diploma. The doctor replied that Miss MA felt that by gaining a diploma, her chances of getting a promotion and better salary were increased. JM responded that this seemed a realistic motivation. JM then asked the doctors to expand on the negative aspect of this ambivalence and what was it that was making her avoid doing the work that would get her to her chosen objective. JM felt that the doctor's response did not explain why Miss MA was failing to join up the positive aspect of her motivation with the negative one. She had not realized that to reach her objectives, she needed to do things that were awkward or difficult for her. JM gave the metaphor of a ship floundering and explained that this lady was swayed by feelings of anxiety and sadness of the moment rather than being directed by her long-term objectives. Miss MA was forgetting her wishes for her long-term benefit, which were equally strong with the anxieties about her present performance.

JM explained that this is a difficulty often encountered in people who have not had the experience of their emotions being, constructively and nontraumatically, contained. JM then suggested that this young lady's psychopathology, which seems to have arisen out of lack of containment, would require exactly this containment to be provided by her therapist or the therapeutic setting. If she is given the experience of being constructively contained by the system, she will be able to cope with her feelings, the painful feelings, of anxiety and depression to address the tasks ahead of her.

JM returned to the issue that the therapeutic services needed to provide containment, which would provide her the experience of staff staying with her on the same issue until she has a deep insight into her difficulties and more realistic appreciation of her present and of her future. This young woman has a healthy part that is that she is young, intelligent, has some healthy positive motivation, and wants to improve her life, but she resorts to dysfunctional behaviors when painful feelings arise. JM then pointed out that once Miss MA feels that she is contained by her therapist she can then explore why, emotionally, the classroom situation is not only stressful but unbearably so for her.

JM then pointed out that by asking this young lady to think on her feelings, the stressful feelings, during the time in the classroom she could begin to explore her feelings of anxiety, failure, rejection by the others, or criticism by the other pupils for not doing well. Once sad feelings emerge in the session, then the therapist can begin to address them. For example, if she feels a fear of rejection then the therapist could ask her to explore why this fear of rejection is incapacitating and not something that all of us experience but deal with in a more constructive way. For most healthy people, the fear of rejection is motivating. Such fears motivate most students to work harder and to contain unpleasant or painful feelings. The emotional presence of a therapist would play a big part in enabling Miss MA to contain the painful feelings during the stressful situations of being in classroom and of exams. The stressful feelings that she, up to now, dealt with by avoidance. JM then suggested that one level of insight is achieved then she could be helped to develop even more realistic expectations for her future. She may not achieve a top mark, but it is likely (on her past track record) that she will achieve at least a pass. Having more realistic expectations would enable her to cope with sad feelings more constructively than if she had unrealistic and usually excessively high expectations. In doing so, the therapist would give her the feeling that it is acceptable to have realistic and not excessive expectations. There is somebody in her life who expects her to do reasonably well rather than to excel.

References

Bowlby, J. (1973). *Attachment and loss volume 2: Separation: Anxiety and anger*. Penguin Books.

Kohut, H. (1980). Selected problems in self psychological theory. In P. H. Ornstein (Ed.), *The search for the self. Selected writing of Heinz Kohut 1978–1981* (pp. 4). International Universities Press Inc.

Mary

Presenting condition

Mary is a 17-year-old girl who was voluntarily admitted from the pediatric service following a drug overdose.

History of present complaint

Mary reported that she experienced low mood, on and off, in the last year. She felt that life was meaningless and that there were many unsolvable problems in her life. She had a chronic sense of emptiness. Mary worried about maternal grandmother's poor physical condition; her maternal grandmother, who lived in the country, had repeated hospital admissions following falls. Mary reported some vague persecutory ideas involving her parents; she was worried that her parents would harm her but could not elaborate further on this. She admitted to hearing voices from devils asking her to "die in her heart," especially when she had low mood or stress. She had a reduced energy level and experienced loss of interest. Her sleep became fragmented, and she was troubled by nightmares in which she was seeing herself falling down. Her appetite was reduced. She suffered anxiety attacks, which were precipitated by even minor events, and these were associated with palpitations, sweating, nausea, and shortness of breath especially in crowded places. She had negative cognitions of hopelessness. She had reduced self-esteem and fear of abandonment. She had fleeting suicidal ideas in the last month, which were preceded by the admission of her grandmother to hospital following a fall. Mary went to the seaside and thought of drowning herself about 1 month ago but gave up the idea when she received a phone call from a medical social worker.

On the day of admission, Mary was worried about her maternal grandmother's condition and developed the idea that she may commit suicide by a drug overdose. She took 10 tabs of a benzodiazepine (Xanax) impulsively at school. She did not believe that that act was lethal. She had made no preparation and had not written a final note. She told her secondary school teacher about the drug overdose and was advised to seek medical attention.

Family history

There was no family history of mental illness or suicide. Her father is a construction site worker and her mother is a kitchen worker. Her parents are supportive, but both are busy in work and lenient in parenting. Mary felt that her parents were not emotionally sensitive toward her. She felt that her father frequently gave her negative commands. Mary tended to bottle up her feelings and felt that her parents did not understand or care enough about her. Her elder brother (6 years older) was described as easygoing; he had a good relationship with Mary.

Personal history

Mary was born in the city following a planned and wanted pregnancy and a normal delivery. Her developmental milestones were passed at about the right time. Mary was brought up by mother and her maternal grandmother in the country until the age of 3; she then came to the city and was looked after by her paternal grandmother. Mary had a good relationship with her maternal grandmother, who was of advanced age and in poor physical condition; Mary was worried that her maternal grandmother would die soon. Mary is currently living with her father, mother, paternal grandmother, and her elder brother.

Mary studied in mainstream primary and secondary school. Her academic performance at primary school was average. She was sociable and loved chatting with friends. Mary presented with no conduct problems. Mary moved to the city secondary school where she attended forms F1–F5. The teachers had commented that she was "hardworking, well-disciplined, presented no conduct problems but was of below average academic performance." Mary repeated F5 in a private school where she developed only superficial relationships with her classmates.

Mary enjoys playing with children, cooking, and exercising. She has had three relationships, each lasting a few months. Mary thought there was a "personality mismatch" between them. She is not in a relationship at present. She is a nonsmoker and nondrinker. She has no forensic record and does not use illicit drugs. Mary tends to be introverted, well-disciplined, and has high expectations of herself. She wishes to improve the family financial condition in the future but felt disappointed with her underachievement in academic results. Mary aspired to become a nursing student in the city university. She has enjoyed good past health.

Past psychiatric history

Mary became known to the department of psychiatry in February 2017. She was then thought to be suffering from a "moderate depressive episode." It was then noted that she experienced gradual deterioration of mood since she was in the second term of Form 4 (June 2016). This was triggered by academic stress, a drop in academic performance, and the death of her paternal grandfather. She had episodes of crying and frequent complaints of being bitten by insects. Mary developed anxiety and low mood; she experienced declining self-confidence and had negative cognitions. Mary had become more avoidant of friends, was less talkative at school, and was less able to concentrate in class. Her sleep and appetite were reduced. She also developed multiple somatic complaints including a feeling of gastric bloating, shortness of breath, and palpitations. Mary's motivation to go to school was reduced, and she often needed to go to the sick room due to some somatic discomfort; she started "skipping" many classes. Mary complained of being "pinpointed" (harassed) by some teachers and requested to go to the sick room during their classes. Mary was required to repeat the fifth form because her exam results were poor. She decided to change school because she disliked some of the teachers.

Mary's attendance was regular at the private school and she denied being bullied or "pinpointed" but reported that the relationships with her classmates were superficial. Her friends made friends with a classmate who gossiped about that classmate behind her back. Mary felt that she could not trust her friends. She felt that the lessons were boring and that she was being taught material already known to her from the previous school. Mary tried to cope with the stress by wrist-slashing, which she did for four to five times; she claimed that she felt relieved afterward.

Mary was seen by private psychiatrist in August 2016 and was told that she had been suffering from depression. She was prescribed antidepressants. After titrating a few kinds of antidepressants (Mary could not name the drugs), she was stabilized on the following regime: Pristiq 50 mg daily, pregabalin 75 mg nightly, quetiapine 50 mg nightly, Xanax 0.5 m twice daily as needed (which she used around two to three times per week), and clonazepam 2 mg nightly as needed (which she rarely used). Both mother and Mary reported improved mood and reduced somatic discomfort on commencement of drug treatment. Mary tried Zoloft with limited effect, later added Lexapro, and was taken off quetiapine (as it was thought it may have been causing oversedation). A trial of risperidone was initiated in July 2017 because she was presenting with ideas of reference and believed that her parents knew what she thought.

Mary was last seen in adolescent mental health service in December 2017 and was maintained on Xanax 0.25 mg twice daily as needed, clonazepam 0.5 mg nightly as needed, Lexapro 5 mg in the morning, pregabalin 75 mg nightly, Pristiq 50 mg by mouth, and risperidone 1 mg nightly.

There is no history of suicidal attempts or aggression. The wrist cutting in August 2017 had been attributed to problematic family relationships. Mary had been admitted to the pediatric unit.

Present treatment and management

During the examination, Mary appeared calm and with low mood; her affect was reactive. Her speech was coherent and relevant, but she tended to give vague and approximate answers; she frequently answered: "I don't know." Mary admitted to hearing vague voices from her heart asking her to die. She had persecutory ideas involving her parents. Mary had fleeting suicidal ideas. Her insight was limited. Relevant physical and laboratory findings were normal.

Mary was diagnosed as suffering from a recurrent depressive disorder, current episode severe with psychotic symptoms, and an evolving Borderline Personality Disorder. The differential diagnosis involved moderate depression with quasi-psychotic symptoms and psychosis.

After admission, Mary still complained of low mood and fleeting suicidal ideas. She got along well with coresidents and engaged in leisure activities, but she was reluctant to go to a Red Cross school. She had low frustration tolerance and poor temper control, especially in relation to her relationship with her father. She felt scared of her parents, believed that they could not be trusted, and was worried that they would harm her. She did not allow her father to visit her and refused to talk with him. Her father tried to visit her, and Mary threw a temper tantrum; she threw her mobile phone and left the visiting room. She hit the wall and bit herself. She claimed that her reaction was in response to her father saying, "I don't know how to talk with you or be your father." The doctor tried to get a clearer account from her father who claimed that he had told her, "You suffer from a mental illness but this doesn't mean that you can do anything you want." During that visit after work, her father had brought Mary food, but she did not appreciate his effort and did not talk with him.

Mary showed greater acceptance toward her elder brother and mother. When her mother asked Mary to accept father to visit her and be fair to her father, Mary developed low mood and fleeting suicidal ideas again. She disliked that her mother was asking her many questions, and she perceived mother as pressuring her. She preferred to stay in the hospital because she believed that hospital was safer than her home.

Family relationships were reported as "harmonious" until the last 1 to 2 years. Mary had reduced communications with her parents, but her parents could not identify any triggering events. She was only able to recall a few incidents in the past that made her feel upset about her parents. She felt that she was being "kicked out of her home" by her parents during primary school years 2–3. She could not recall the details. Her parents did not recall such an incident, but they thought that Mary was punished for doing something wrong. Mary felt that she was being "abandoned," and she recalled that incident on and off. She also remembered being hit by her father when she was young, but she claimed that she did not remember the details. Her parents reported that they treasured Mary a lot and never implemented serious corporal punishment with her. Mary also recalled her father mentioning, "I don't know why I gave birth to you" after Mary and her mother got lost about a year ago.

Mary was upset that her parents favored her elder brother. Parents asked her to give in when she had conflicts with her brother in childhood. But her brother treated her well and she had good relationship with him. She recalled that parents agreed to a "Do Not Resuscitate" before her paternal grandfather died. She believed that her parents were ruthless and that they would treat her the same way if she had an accident. She was taking risperidone 3 mg nightly and Pristiq 100 mg daily. She had shown some improvement on this regime.

Consultation

JM praised the doctor for the thoroughness of the assessment. JM then stated that he had several questions about Mary, the first one being her parent's decision to offer her private education, when she needed to repeat Form 5 because it seemed from their occupations that they were not affluent. The doctor confirmed that the parents did have some financial difficulties and then proceeded to state that her mother was asking the doctor if there was a way to avoid paying the school fees for the 2 months that the girl was in hospital. JM repeated the question of how these parents of modest means undertook this huge expense to educate their daughter at a private school. The family was making a big sacrifice on Mary's behalf. After some discussion, the parents' motives were still not clear. JM then asked if Mary had appreciated that her family were making this sacrifice for her. The doctor stated that Mary did not appreciate what the family was doing for her. JM rephrased that Mary did not think that her parents valued her a lot to make such a sacrifice for her. Because Mary had not interpreted her parents' action in a positive way, JM asked if the doctor knew what meaning Mary gave to this parental action. The doctor pointed out that Mary felt that her parents were negative about her and cited some negative comments that she claimed her father had made about her.

The doctor pointed out that when this matter was broached with Mary, she was reluctant to explore it further. JM pointed out that this represented an immature approach because Mary seemed reluctant to look at the whole picture; furthermore, her father may have a difficulty in expressing affection as affection directly and tended to express it indirectly by making sacrifices for her (in this case a financial sacrifice). An independent point of view is that both parents seem to care a lot about their daughter because they were prepared to make this enormous sacrifice for her.

JM then moved to consider Mary's academic performance. This was below average. JM asked the doctor if this below-average performance was in concordance with her ability or if it was below her potential. The doctor responded that the performance was below Mary's high expectations. She was underperforming in relation to her expectations. JM pointed out that usually one expects the performance to match the level of ability. On this point the doctor stated that she had no opinion on Mary's overall ability because this had not been formally tested. JM then suggested that in the absence of a formal psychological assessment one relies on the track record of a student's performance. For example, JM asked what Mary's track record of performance had been in primary school. The doctor thought that Mary's performance at primary school was "OK." JM asked for clarification that Mary's performance at primary school was at least average. This was confirmed. JM then pointed out that if there was a drop in performance and there was an absence of any organic reason for her brain to function less competently than previously, then the reason for Mary's underperformance must be sought in emotional or relational sphere and not in her innate ability. One would need to look at such issues to understand her drop in performance. The doctor clarified that Mary was performing at least at average level during the first 2 years of secondary school. It was clarified that Mary's underperformance started after the second year of secondary school. JM then suggested that one tries to understand the reason for this change in performance level after the second year of secondary school. The doctor responded that this underperformance may be related to her "mood problem." JM confirmed that this is exactly what needs to be explored and understood more thoroughly.

JM suggested that underperformance in a girl of 13–14 may have started a vicious circle. That the disappointment of performing *below expectations* would exacerbate the low mood, which in turn would further cause her to perform at an even lower level. JM suggested that there may be other events or developments that caused this girl to perform less well at 14 than she did previously.

JM further elaborated that underperformance has at least the consequence of it being a threat to one's self-esteem and also to changing the parents' behavior toward the child. They may be puzzled by this underperformance and may exercise greater pressure on her to perform at what she had shown previously to be her level. JM continued that her parents were not able to manage the change in performance constructively. This may be related to her absorption of the family's generating funds or their innate difficulty in dealing with family emotions, and there is the possibility that the parents may have allocated more of their restricted family funds onto her, out of some sense of guilt about her emotions and her performance. It was also possible that the parents shared Mary's unrealistically high expectations because they were perceived as critical of her.

JM then directed the conversation toward Mary's peer and other relationships—such as the relationship with the teachers—at school. More specifically, JM asked if Mary had the experience of being bullied at school as well as being "pinpointed" (harassed) by a teacher. The doctor pointed out that apart from feeling "pinpointed" by one particular teacher, she did not have other difficulties and that her peer relationships were "normal." The doctor clarified that Mary's underperformance was not only on the subject that that teacher taught but it was also a more global underperformance. JM pointed out that Mary attributed her failure to that teacher and that she thought that the solution to her problem would be to remove her from that teacher and place her in a different environment. The parents seemed to have colluded with Mary in accepting that it was the teacher's fault by removing her from that environment and placing her in a different school. They seemed to have been unable to stay with Mary and her problem to understand it better and help Mary pursue it in a constructive way. The problems continued in the new school indicates that Mary had not learned from the previous experience something positive about how one approaches the demands of work.

JM then pointed out that this family of limited means placed their daughter in an environment where the other children are members of families that were more affluent and this would create their own problems on a peer-to-peer level. JM pointed out that Mary would not have been able to invite her peers to her home because their living standard would have been different. Placement at a private school may give Mary other reasons to feel herself less valued than her peers. This may also generate feelings of dissatisfaction with her parents who did not provide for her the environment that other parents were providing for her peers. JM then addressed the issue of poor children placed in private schools. JM pointed out that in England there are many scholars, children who come from poor backgrounds who excel academically and are placed in public schools (in England, some schools that require fees are called public schools); some of these children cope well, especially leaning on their status as scholars, which is high in an environment where academic performance is of great value. This was not the case with Mary who was struggling on all fronts.

JM continued to state that such problems continued up to university level in the United Kingdom in the days where university education was paid for by parents. Two of the most expensive universities were Oxford and Cambridge, and some bright children who gained entry to those colleges often had difficulties at the social level. JM repeated that the parents' approach to Mary's difficulties seemed rather limited because they failed to contain Mary's sadness or anger and equally had a difficulty in helping her get a better understanding and develop with them a solution to the problem. Their main response was to allocate funds (which they did not have) to take her to what they thought would be a less stressful school environment. JM pointed out that the parental behavior showed that they did not act out of animosity against their daughter but out of concern and possibly guilt about her by allocating money to her that they could hardly afford. The difficulty was in connecting with Mary emotionally and helping her to cope with emotions and process some thinking that would lead to a better understanding and a more creative solution.

JM then addressed the role of the therapy services. JM pointed out that Mary had not developed a way of reflecting on a problem and of managing her feelings and thoughts to the point of arriving at a deep understanding and a constructive solution. Mary tends to present the problem and then claims to "not know" or "not remember." She has great difficulty in staying with the emotion and the thinking about the problem. JM pointed out that failure to get a more realistic and deep understanding of a problem often leads to development of paranoid or quasi-psychotic interpretations. This is the process through which unrealistic scenarios are developed. The therapist who undertakes to help Mary can offer the emotional containment that will enable her to address the painful and threatening situations more constructively. By "constructively," it is meant that she will develop an understanding that is realistic (and not paranoid or psychotic) and will also find a workable solution. Specifically in Mary's case, she will need to develop realistic expectations (meaning expectations matching her ability and not arbitrarily high ones) educationally and in this way move closer to resolving the vicious circle of disappointment leading to increasing underperformance and so on. JM pointed out that one needs to proceed gently with Mary because she shows a great fragility and a tendency to divert into quasi-psychotic thinking when her preconceptions are challenged.

JM gave an example of a gentle challenge in the form of "tell me Mary, why do you think your parents have made this financial sacrifice for you?" But this should not be in a threatening or challenging way but as a joint invitation to explore one aspect of her experience. This can only lead to constructive thinking if Mary feels secure and safely contained in the relationship with the therapist.

A second example of an area that needed to be approached constructively would be an invitation for Mary to explore the emotions that make it hard for her to apply herself to some lessons. The likelihood is that some lessons are threatening her sense of ability and that threat may even be a danger to her aspirations of becoming a nurse. The relationship with the therapist would make it more likely for her to accept an average career and an average performance as being good enough for a person of average ability. The therapist can offer this kind of containment (James, 1984; Zinkin, 1989), which would enable Mary to process her feelings and her thoughts and bring about a change in them that would enable her to reach more realistic goals.

JM then pointed out that this kind of work will require some consistent and predictable contact with a therapist over several months at least. The doctor confirmed that the treatment planning involved periodic contact with a psychiatrist and more regular contact with a clinical psychologist.

JM then pointed out that the doctor should not expect that a monthly psychiatric assessment would give this girl adequate containment to process her feelings and, therefore, that the doctor should not be disappointed if such infrequent contact did not bring about fundamental change. JM then added that this combination of psychiatric supervision and psychological input from a clinical psychologist had a good chance of bringing about the substantial change that Mary deserves.

References

James, D. C. (1984). Bion's "containing" and Winnicott's "holding" in the context of the group matrix. *International Journal of Group Psychotherapy*, 34, 201–213.
Zinkin, L. M. (1989). The group as container and contained. *Group Analysis*, 22, 227–234.

Ms. WB

Presenting condition

Ms. WB is a 31-year-old unemployed woman, living with her mother in a public housing unit. She was voluntarily admitted due to low mood and a drug overdose.

History of present complaint

Ms. WB felt that her mother was critical of her romantic relationship because she believed that her daughter was being mistreated by her boyfriend and his family. Ms. WB felt that she was not supported by her mother and, temporarily, moved out of mother's place. Yet, soon after, she encountered financial difficulties and had difficulty in purchasing her psychiatric medications and she asked for a reunion with her mother for support. She had low mood with feelings of emptiness. She had occasional tearfulness, poor sleep, and poor appetite. She had poor motivation. She maintained an interest in reading and in playing phone games.

Her relationship with her boyfriend was again severed in the last few days. There were more conflicts between the two. She stayed at her boyfriend's home the night prior admission. Her boyfriend reported that they had a conflict the next morning because he dissuaded patient from taking a taxi to work too frequently. Ms. WB felt distressed by the quarrel. She bought three to four small bottles of red wine from a convenience shop, and she drank the red wine with 10 tablets of over-the-counter Imovane. She sent messages to her boyfriend saying she took many tablets of hypnotics. She was brought to the accident and emergency department and admission was arranged.

Ms. WB was clean, tidy, calm, and settled. Her mood was on the low side. She showed reactive affect. Her speech was coherent and relevant. There was no formal thought disorder. Ms. WB was evasive about her interpersonal relationships. She tended to play down her hypnotics and alcohol use. She was not psychotic. She expressed little remorse for her suicidal act. There was no family history of mental illness.

Personal history

Ms. WB was born in the city; she is an only child. She described she had an unhappy childhood but without any major trauma. Ms. WB reported being isolated and bullied by peers in her childhood. Male classmates teased her about her appearance. She always had a few friends. She once stole a classmate's pen in primary school and annoyed a classmate by drawing on her textbooks in secondary school; she stated that she wanted to get others' attention.

She described herself as being continuously pessimistic, dysthymic, introverted, and dependent but felt that her mother tended, at times, to be overprotective.

Ms. WB's parents divorced more than 20 years prior to her admission. Ms. WB has lived with her mother since then. Her father supported her family financially and with regular visits to them. She longed for her parents' reunion. Her father died in 2011 from carcinoma of the lung. Ms. WB missed her father a lot and felt it was a pity her parents could not ever reunite.

Ms. WB often suffered from a sense of loneliness; she failed to develop a long-term friendship and a long-term romantic relationship. She tried to meet new people through the internet, aiming to meet someone she could marry before she was 30 years old. Ms. WB engaged in many unstable courtships. She was reluctant to breakup from her previous relationships, although she had frequent conflicts with her boyfriends. Her mother was protective toward the patient's relationship issues; she often forbade them from seeing or contacting her. Ms. WB felt that these interventions resulted in the breakups.

Ms. WB's current relationship had lasted for more than 1 year; this was the longest duration of a relationship for her. She described her current boyfriend as trustworthy but manipulative at times. However, she felt that it was difficult for her to meet her current boyfriend because he was busy with work most of the time. They usually contacted each other online. She mentioned she wished her boyfriend could be next to her whenever she needed help. She met her boyfriend through the internet; she often checked boyfriend's whereabouts and his phone messages.

Ms. WB had fewer than three close female friends. She had always been dependent on her mother. She needed to seek mother's opinion for all her problems from an early age. She had increasing conflicts with her mother in recent years, and she felt that her mother mistrusted her. One of her boyfriends asked her mother to guarantee that she would not reinstate alcohol use, which her mother refused. Ms. WB blamed her mother for her breakup. Ms. WB also felt that her mother was overinvolved in her relationship issues.

Ms. WB studied up to Form 5 with a fair academic performance. She has an unstable job record. She tried different jobs but gave up or was dismissed after a brief period. She worked as a travel agency clerk and a pet shop assistant. She often could not settle her credit card payments when unemployed and asked her mother for financial help.

There was no history of substance abuse. Ms. WB was a nonsmoker and had no forensic record.

Past psychiatric history

Ms. WB was admitted to the hospital in 2006 for "unstable emotions" following a quarrel with her mother. She was assessed by the consultation liaison service, was diagnosed to be suffering from a "situational reaction," relationship problems, and an immature personality. Subsequently, Ms. WB was referred to a clinical psychologist for interpersonal training, but she defaulted psychologist's follow-up sessions.

Ms. WB's mood waxed and waned after her father died of cancer in 2011. She was introduced to hypnotics and alcohol by her then boyfriend. She made regular use of hypnotics for years, overdosing on hypnotics at times of stress. She drank different kinds of alcohol.

Ms. WB was formally known to mental health services in 2014 after taking five tabs of Imovane following a quarrel with her then boyfriend; she was then brought to the accident and emergency department. She was later referred by to the psychiatry center for outpatient follow-ups by staff of the accident and emergency department. Diagnosis at the time was dysthymia. She tried bupropion, pregabalin, escitalopram, and Pristiq with suboptimal effect.

She had multiple attendances to the accident and emergency department due to suicidal impulses of drug overdosing/ingesting a mouthful of detergents, mainly after arguments and interpersonal tensions; Ms. WB displayed abnormal behaviors when under the influence of alcohol. She has had four previous admissions to psychiatric hospitals, due to overdosing with hypnotics or to making verbal suicidal threats at times of stress. Clinical psychologists diagnosed a "dependent personality disorder." This diagnosis was revised to "recurrent depressive disorder" with background of dysthymia."

She was last admitted from June to July 2017 for threatening to drink paint thinner as suicidal threat. She was discharged to private hostel on mirtazapine 45 mg nightly and thiamine 100 mg daily.

Ms. WB reported to have suffered with low mood from an early age. She used hypnotics, on and off, virtually all her life.

Following discharge from hospital, Ms. WB reported to have a "rocky relationship" with her boyfriend; she had quarrels with her boyfriend and her parents. On one occasion, she was pushed against wooden furniture, and this caused bruising over both eyes; following that episode, Ms. WB attended a private general practitioner for advice. Since discharge, Ms. WB did not live in a private hostel because she disliked the environment. She moved back to live with her mother. She reinstated the use of hypnotics and alcohol. She often displayed aggressive behavior that required police intervention when under substance influence (e.g., throwing things in public, pushing furniture, and pulling her mother's hair). She revealed to have a worsened relationship with her boyfriend and her mother because the two disapproved of her substance use. She once disturbed her boyfriend's family when intoxicated. Early in September, she was pushed, hitting her head on furniture, which caused bruising on both eyes.

Ms. WB was introduced to hypnotics and alcohol by a boyfriend. This was an attempt to cope with her distress after her father's death in 2011. Ms. WB made regular use of hypnotics for years, taking hypnotics sparingly from a clinic. This was at a level of two to three tabs per day, up to 7 tabs at times of stress previously. She took alcohol for many years. In the past, it was around two to three times a week, usually alternated with the use of 3 to 4 cups of either wine or beer. Ms. WB reported to experience no withdrawal symptoms. She felt that hypnotics and alcohol helped her with sleep at first. At a later stage, her sleep was not much improved with the use of hypnotics or alcohol, but she continued because she felt her mind could be relaxed so she could be free from her problems.

She enjoyed good physical health.

Present treatment

The clinical impression was that Ms. WB was suffering from a recurrent depressive disorder and a dependent personality disorder on a background of dysthymia. Psychiatric medications were resumed. She had mirtazapine 45 mg nightly and thiamine 100 mg daily. Her mental state improved in the ward. Ms. WB was offered motivation interview. She was motivated to give up hypnotics and alcohol use to salvage her relationship with her mother and her boyfriend and to enhance her chances of a future more stable employment. She joined occupational therapists' training and assessment. She planned to look for a job as a pet shop assistant after discharge. Psychoeducation was provided.

In summary, Ms. WB is a 31-year-old female with recurrent depressive disorder, dependent personality disorder, and dysthymia. She had multiple admissions due to low mood with ambivalent interpersonal problems. Her low mood was easily triggered by relationship problems with her boyfriend. She had poor stress coping skills. She had frequent suicidal threats or gestures during conflicts with others.

Consultation

JM thanked and complimented the doctor for the thoroughness of the presentation. The doctor clarified that Ms. WB had been admitted in November for a period of 3 weeks. The doctor had known Ms. WB since October 2017. JM then asked for some further information about Ms. WB's life from birth to the age of 10. The doctor said that Ms. WB reported that she had no major trauma or incident during that period of her life. The doctor stated that from birth to the age of 10 Ms. WB enjoyed a happy childhood, her parents were still married at the time, and she had no difficulties in making friends. The doctor mentioned that she felt that "her parents spoiled her a lot." JM asked that this matter be expanded. The doctor explained that she used to spend a lot of time with her father who aimed to satisfy her wishes whatever they were. JM then invited the doctor to expand on his understanding of the meaning of "being spoiled." The doctor explained that most of her wishes or demands would be satisfied by her parents. JM then asked what the effect of being spoiled was on the child. JM clarified that the question was "why was the parental attention being called with a negative name 'spoiled'?" Why was this parental attention considered destructive—which is what spoiling means? The doctor then added that Ms. WB felt that her mother was also overprotective. The doctor felt that the combination of spoiling and overprotectiveness affected her abilities to make relationships. JM asked that the doctor expands on the notion of "overprotectiveness." The doctor gave an example in which her mother would intervene in sorting out the difficulties that Ms. WB had with other children. For an exploration of cultural factors in this and similar families, see Kuotai and Jing-Hwa (1985).

JM then summarized the two unhelpful strands of her early life experience: being spoiled and being overprotected. JM then asked the doctor to reflect on the effect of indulgence and overprotectiveness on Ms. WB's development. The doctor responded that that would make Ms. WB more dependent on her parents and that dependency would be instead of her own development of abilities to cope with interpersonal relationships. JM then reiterated the issue that in the absence of major trauma there were two significant influences (the indulgence and overprotectiveness) that would limit Ms. WB's ability to negotiate relationships and tolerate frustrations.

JM then asked that the effect of the parental divorce be addressed. Following the divorce, the father left the family home but continued to support the family financially and to visit Ms. WB to play with her. The doctor stated that the parental divorce meant that Ms. WB lost a significant person from her life. JM then returned on the issue of Ms. WB's development and asked how her development was influenced to become different from what it would have been had the divorce not taken place. The doctor replied that she became more insecure and felt less able to trust future relationships. The doctor replied that Ms. WB started feeling that relationships with others may break up just as her parental relationship broke up. JM then replied that it is Ms. WB who breaks the relationships prematurely before sorting out the issues that emerge both at work and with boyfriend.

JM then returned to the theme of how the parental divorce could have influenced how Ms. WB herself handles relationships and summarized the three major pathological influences on Ms. WB's life (a) the spoiling, (b) the overprotection, and (c) the parental divorce that gave her the expectation that she is entitled to everyone fitting in with her demands, that everyone would protect and make her life safe, and that if these expectations were not met she had no experience of working through difficulties and became desperate. JM then reframed this as a difficulty for Ms. WB who has not had the experience of (a) addressing her own difficulties and (b) staying with a difficulty until she overcomes it and finds a constructive and age-appropriate solution.

The reason why she broke down and needed psychiatric help was because her expectations and her skills only led her to a painful life existence. Her expectations could not be met in the real life of a 31-year-old woman because a woman of that age needs to be able to negotiate relationships, to cope with frustrations, and to sort her own problems out rather than seek to escape when they are not resolved. A 31-year-old person needs to find solutions to difficulties rather than aim to achieve unrealistic aims by manipulating others.

JM then addressed the issue of Ms. WB's overdoses. He pointed out that these were communicated overdoses in the sense that after she had ingested the medications, she would let people know and do so in a complicated and convoluted way, which had an ultimate objective of ensuring others' compliance to her wishes. The overdoses were a way of controlling other people.

JM then moved to consider the diagnosis of recurrent depression about which he expressed some uncertainty. JM's reservation about the diagnosis of recurrent depression was that there was an implication of a biological process beyond the patient's control. JM asked if there was a family history of Bipolar Disorder and was told that there was no family history of any mental illness. JM stated that this was one more argument that weakened the diagnosis of a recurrent depressive disorder. Then JM asked if the clinical picture suggested a biological process and expanded asking if there was any of the biological markers of a depressive disorder such as diurnal variation of mood, sleep disturbance consistent with the disorder, loss of appetite with weight loss, and a pervasive mood disorder rather than a depression, which is reactive to events. The doctor replied that the mood disorder was mainly reactive to circumstances. JM then concluded that Ms. WB's depression is essentially reactive to events and to her limitations in coping with situations and suggested that the clinical picture is more akin to a personality disorder.

JM then asked about the plan of treatment. The doctor replied that during her hospitalization, he addressed the issue of mourning for her father's death. JM asked about the overall contract, and the doctor replied that he saw her regularly when Ms. WB was in hospital; after Ms. WB's discharge, the hospital doctor would see her once every 2 or 3 months. The doctor then explained that Ms. WB had additional consultations with the psychologist once every 1 to 2 months. JM replied that this was a disorder of personality, which has been consolidated for more than 30 years and, therefore, it is unlikely that it will be changed significantly with consultations of half-hour duration every 1–3 months.

JM then referred the impact of this therapeutic plan on the professionals and in particular that because the effect will be limited, the risk is that the professionals will be disappointed. The ingrained pattern of expecting to be spoiled, overprotected, or divorce would be unlikely to be shifted with this level of input. This condition would require something more intensive. This line of thinking was not followed up. JM had in mind the demoralization of staff who expect to succeed in the difficult task with limited resources (Maratos, 1996; Swensen & Shanafelt, 2017).

The doctor responded that he would try to get Ms. WB to think about ways of dealing with stress that are different from use of substances including alcohol and different from manipulating others. The doctor wanted to focus on the stress arising from the two important relationships with Ms. WB— that with her mother and her boyfriend. In trying to understand the mechanism through which the interaction with her mother and boyfriend become stressful, the simplified picture immerged of "unless you let me have my own way, I am going to kill myself." How would this person be helped when she had an attitude like this. The doctor responded that he would first encourage her to express her thoughts and feelings. The doctor then added that he would encourage Ms. WB to think of the consequences of her present approach in particular because the consequences were counterproductive so she would have good reason to rethink of her approach to relationships and frustrations.

JM then addressed the issue of the concept of "coping." JM pointed out that although Ms. WB may have thought of her behavior as attempts to cope, they were, in fact, maladaptive approaches that were doing anything but improving her situation. Therefore, they were not coping mechanisms and should not be addressed as such. Ms. WB should have no doubt that what she calls "coping" is a dysfunctional way that only makes things worse for her.

JM then pointed out that many people must have pointed out to her that this approach is not helpful. Nevertheless, even though this has been pointed out to her, she has been unable to alter it because the emotional pattern that has been ingrained in her mind since early childhood was that she should expect other people to meet her needs as they are, she should expect other people to make life safe for her, and that if that is not possible, divorce is the only solution; no adult cognitions can counteract this emotional conviction that has been part of her being from an early age.

JM then pointed out that one of the ways in which her approach is dysfunctional is that instead of achieving an aim of satisfying her needs, it leaves her separated, isolated, alone, and without any support. We then moved on to how this pattern could be changed. Ms. WB needs to feel safe with someone to be able to reexamine herself and develop new ways of really coping. Such an approach would help her consider herself a 31-year-old woman, which she is, instead of a person carrying a dysfunctional early childhood with her. The first element that Ms. WB needs is to feel that she is in a safe relationship with a therapist. By safe, she needs to feel that the therapist is on her side and is prepared to work with her to support her. The contact with the therapist every few months does not stand a good chance of counteracting the effect of more than 20 years' experience.

The different experience that would stand a chance of altering this pattern would need to be regular (weekly or more frequent) either in the form of individual therapy or in the form of group therapy. That setting would provide the safety and the continuity to offer her a different emotional as well as cognitive experience. In that environment, Ms. WB has a good chance of being understood and accepted for the sake of developing and not for the sake of being supported to maintain the present (dysfunctional) pattern. JM then expanded on the two different types of support. The unhelpful support is one which encourages somebody to maintain the dysfunctional pattern; offering sympathy and comfort sometimes has that unhelpful consequence.

The more helpful support is the one that stays with the individual but does so for the sake of development, and by development meaning more functional skills that would have positive consequences. JM then asked if Ms. WB had any hope herself about her ability to change. The doctor responded that he thought she did and that she had expressed some concern about the high number of admissions that she has had in the past. Ms. WB had expressed the wish to learn to solve her problems in a different way. The doctor responded that Ms. WB did have a hope that she could develop into somebody who could be more functional in the future. In trying to explore the foundation of her hope, it became apparent that Ms. WB's hopes were still placed on her being treated differently by her boyfriend and her mother and not by developing any personal skills. JM repeated the question if Ms. WB thought of herself as somebody who does have the potential to ever become functional or if she saw herself as being stuck in the present pattern. The doctor reported that Ms. WB feels herself as being stuck. JM replied that Ms. WB needs to develop a sense of direction in the sense that "I need to be able to cope with relationships and frustrations in a more functional way than the method I have been using up to now." And the second point is that Ms. WB needs to develop a sense of self belief that she does have the potential to achieve that. More specifically she needs to develop a sense that she is no longer a helpless 5-year-old and totally dependent on her parents, but a 31-year-old woman with her own abilities and personality.

JM then invited the doctor to reflect on what the real functional competent aspects of Ms. WB were. The doctor responded that she had good performance at school and work and JM confirmed that this is an excellent and real potential. JM reiterated that this is a solid quality on which she can begin to build a healthy sense of self-esteem.

The second real solid quality was intellectual capacity. She had completed secondary education and, therefore, had at least average intellectual ability. In summary, she does have a potential to handle difficult situations because she did at work and at least average intelligence. Finally, she has had boyfriends in the past, so she is attractive as a woman. In summary, we have somebody who is intelligent, who has an ability to handle situations at work, and who is attractive. These can form a solid basis for her to have hope that in the future she could build a better life for herself. JM concluded that the task ahead is substantial and is more likely to be fulfilled if she is given substantial support in the form of either individual or group therapy.

References

Kuotai, T., & Jing-Hwa, C. (1985). Chapter 11—The one-child-per-family policy: A psychological perspective. In W.-S. Ang & D. Y. H. Wu (Eds.), *Chinese culture and mental health* (pp. 153–165). Academic Press.

Maratos, J. (1996). Professional burnout. In J. Georgas, M. Manthouli, E. Besevegis, & A. Kokkevi (Eds.), *Contemporary psychology in Europe. Theory, research and applications* (pp. 301–311). Hogrefe & Huber Publishers.

Swensen, S. J., & Shanafelt, T. (2017). An organizational framework to reduce professional burnout and bring back joy in practice. *Joint Commission Journal on Quality and Patient Safety*, 43(6), 308–313.

Claire

Presenting complaint

Claire, age 14, was voluntarily admitted, accompanied by her mother, from the pediatric department following self-harming behavior (suspected drug overdose) and wrist-slashing.

History of present complaint

Her mother reported that Claire had deteriorated mood since May 2018 due to an ambivalent relationship with her then boyfriend. Claire said that her former boyfriend became less affectionate toward her and had an affair with another girl. They broke up in February this year and then her ex-boyfriend "badmouthed" her via Facebook and WhatsApp, accusing her of being a prostitute. The couple rekindled the relationship in May temporarily but separated shortly after. Claire reported that her former boyfriend continued to disturb her and once brought two other male friends of his to her home to seek revenge. She sought refuge at her friend's home 1 or 2 weeks before admission.

It was reported by her mother that Claire would vent her negative emotions by slashing her wrist. Her mother reported that Claire became more vigorous in the self-harming behavior in the recent few months. Mother said Claire felt that her mood uplifted when she saw profuse blood flowing out from her forearm. She would post the photos on Instagram to ask for "likes." She would seek for more public attention by hash-tagging the photos with popular terms, such as, "self-harm," suicide, and "bluewhale" (referring to the "Blue Whale Challenge").

Claire also expressed suicidal ideation in May after the breakup with her boyfriend. She prepared a suicide note addressed to her paternal uncles and a friend, accusing them of ignoring her emotional needs. She went to the rooftop with a friend and said she needed to save up for more courage to jump from height but afterward she denied any genuine plans.

Despite this, Claire was able to maintain her study at the new school. She was able to seek pleasure from her hobbies including internet surfing and seeing friends. She maintained good volition and motivation. She slept and ate well. She denied any abnormal beliefs or perceptual disturbances. Claire's mood had deteriorated in the past week as her friend did not reply to her WhatsApp messages. Claire suffered a surging sense of abandonment and, again, slashed her wrist and posted photos of her deep cut wound onto Instagram. She also posted photos of fluoxetine and Ampiclox and told her friend she had taken at least 94 capsules in total. Her friend informed her mother, and Claire was brought to general hospital by her mother as she suspected that Claire had taken a drug overdose.

Family history

There was no family history of mental illness. Claire's father was known to be an illicit drug user.

Personal history

Claire was born in the country by cesarean section at full term. She had normal developmental milestones. She came to the city after few months, she returned to the country for kindergarten, but she returned to the city for primary school. Her parents separated when Claire was young. Claire said she had no memory of parental conflict.

She enjoyed playing music games and "cosplay" very much. Claire was described as an introverted girl with low self-esteem and a sense of emptiness.

Claire is a 14-year-old girl who is now living with her mother. Her parents divorced when she was 5 or 6 years old. Custody was awarded to her father; however, her father showed carer stress and frequently asked his extended family to take care of Claire. Her father was imprisoned in February 2017 for possessing illicit drugs.

Claire had studied in mainstream school. However, she showed limited motivation to continue her study due to low mood, which was precipitated by interpersonal relationships.

Claire stayed with her father until primary school. She then lived with paternal extended family (including granduncles, grandparents) because her father was not capable of taking care of her. Claire said grandparents were harsh to her, and she was often physically punished by them. A joint conference was held and established the physical abuse by paternal grandfather, and a care/protection order was applied. Since November 2016, she had then lived with her father. She subsequently lived with boyfriend's family (grandmother, parents, and boyfriend) since February 2017 after her father was sentenced to prison for possession of illicit drugs.

Her mother moved back from the city in September 2017 to take care of Claire because she noted her emotional turmoil. The mother and Claire had previously only seen each other several times per year. They contacted each other mainly by phone.

Claire disclosed a history of nonconsensual and unprotected sexual intercourse by an ex-boyfriend at age 12. She said her ex-boyfriend took obscene photos of her at that time. The incident was not reported to the police.

Claire studied in mainstream school until Form 2. She said she was too introverted to meet friends in Form 2 and, for this reason, started to refuse school more frequently. She eventually dropped out school but resumed her study in January 2018 in another school. However, she left the school shortly afterward in February due to relationship discord with her last boyfriend. She resumed her studies in June.

Claire met her last boyfriend during a "cosplay" event. The relationship lasted 1 year. They separated as "incompatible personalities" and found that her boyfriend had become less affectionate.

Claire was noted to have a strong sense of emptiness and fear for abandonment since early childhood. Her mother reported that Claire would set up conflicts with her whenever her mother returned home late. She felt mother was going to abandon her. Her mother also said Claire would escalate her self-harming behavior each time after discharge from hospital. Her mother perceived this as Claire's revenge to those who sent her to hospital and to those who ignored her. Claire is a non-smoker, nondrinker, and makes no illicit substance use. She has no forensic record.

Past psychiatric history

Claire had many self-harm incidents since Form 1, by slashing her wrists or thighs; she also practiced head banging and hair pulling. She once prepared a suicide note to great-uncles and her close friend to accuse them of mistreating her. She expressed the idea of jumping from a height in May 2018. She was suspected of a drug overdose in June 2018.

She was first known to the psychiatric clinic in October 2017 after being admitted to the general hospital pediatric department, with low mood, after breaking up with her boyfriend. She was self-harming by wrist-slashing, head banging, pulling her hair, and self-strangulating after the relationship discord. She was started on fluoxetine 10 mg daily and arranged follow-up; she defaulted follow-up.

She had two further admissions in July 2016 and April 2018 to pediatrics due to repeated self-harming behavior, by wrist-slashing at times of low mood, which was precipitated by conflict with mother and relationship discord with her boyfriend. She attended follow-up in our child and adolescent psychiatric clinic on May 15, 2015. Claire was documented as stable and was prescribed fluoxetine. Next follow-up was arranged for July 2018 but she presented at hospital before that date with further self-harming behavior.

Present treatment

Mental state examination showed that Claire had many keloid laceration scars on bilateral elbows, wrists, and thighs. She had long hair and wore spectacles. Her self-care was maintained. Eye contact was good, and she had a good social smile. Her speech was coherent and relevant. She had no auditory hallucinations or delusions. She was thought not to be actively suicidal or violent. Claire expressed superficial remorse for her self-harming behavior. Claire was thought to be suffering from dysthymia with evolving Borderline Personality Disorder. She was resumed on fluoxetine 10 mg daily and offered psychological intervention in the hospital.

Consultation

JM thanked the doctor for the thoroughness of the presentation. There was little consistency and care in the life of this girl. JM pointed out that the family or social environment in which she lives did not offer her any security or any appropriate attention to her needs as a child. Perhaps the only setting in which her needs are being addressed is the hospital. And she responds to being in the hospital by being better overall; she has better mood and better communication. The doctor pointed out that while she was in hospital, she was visited by some friends who apologized to her for not responding to her messages promptly, and she was also visited by her mother.

JM then addressed the issue of Claire's sensitivity to the lack of an immediate response to her messages. JM suggested that this vulnerability was because these messages signified for her a repetition of previous rejections. JM pointed out that this girl had experienced rejections from her mother, her father, and her grandparents, and the present nonresponse was, for her, another indication that people found her too much to cope with.

JM summarized the case as being one of child neglect and abuse. Assuming that she has been living with the "boyfriend," this implies that she has been exposed to a setting in which she is subjected to inappropriate sexual experiences such as nonconsensual intercourse and exposure to almost pornographic photographing. JM repeated the notion of "nonconsensual" because a 14-year-old girl (and younger) cannot be considered to have capacity to consent to sexual intercourse. The doctor gave the history of this girl who had previously been associating with much older boys, and it was then that she was raped and had inappropriate photographs taken of her. The doctor also pointed out that this child did not wish to report the abuse to the police.

JM then asked the doctor what her thoughts were on effect these experiences had on Claire's self-image. The doctor responded that she would not feel herself as loveable. In response to JM's question, the doctor said that it is unlikely that this set of events would make Claire feel proud of herself. JM pointed out that one of the tasks of therapy is to restore this girl's self-image. Claire needs to find evidence about herself on which to base a sound self-image and feel proud. JM suggested that she needs to be clear that the abuse and neglect that she suffered are not her fault and, therefore, not experiences for which she needs to be ashamed of.

She could be helped to be proud of the degree of which she has survived these experiences. The people who failed are the people who should have been providing an appropriate environment for her—the people who failed her through acts of omission and people who failed her through acts of abuse (the grandfather who was physically abusive of her and the man who raped her). These are the people who are responsible in law and considered responsible by our society. The first task of therapy will be to undo the damage that has been done to her and to start rebuilding a healthy and more secure sense of who she is—a sense of self.

JM then asked the doctor what her understanding was about the reason why Claire has allowed herself to form sexual relationships with older men. The doctor suggested that she was seeking the approval and the care that her natural environment was failing to provide for her.

JM repeated that the danger is in thinking of this child as an adult when in fact she is a damaged and traumatized 14-year-old. JM then expressed the view that the therapeutic attempt cannot be only intrapsychic. One needs to address the environment that is supposed to provide protection and care for her. JM continued that Claire is still a developing child who needs to live in an environment that takes appropriate care of her and provides some continuity.

JM suggested that this is a case in which one should seriously consider involving social services to secure that an environment appropriate for Claire is provided. The doctor pointed out that Social Services were already involved, but that the placements that they had arranged for her found that they could not cope with her because of her self-harming behavior. JM then suggested that this recent experience suggested that what would make these placements workable was a parallel support of this girl and of the workers who cared for her by the psychiatric service. JM then proposed that a conference is essential in which the various agencies think together of forging a care plan that will provide for her needs for care and her needs for therapy. JM pointed out the vicious cycle in which the threat of abandonment or of rejection sends her to deliberate self-harm, which in turn precipitates the rejection and abandonment that she feared in the first place.

JM then pointed out the need of continuity of care for this girl. We are aware that this continuity is not always possible because of the rotation of junior doctors. In that case the continuity can be provided by the institution. She needs to be prepared that the doctors will change but that the service will have a continuous commitment to her. Although she will have to cope with the losses of caring doctors, she will not need to feel abandonment or rejected by the service as a whole.

The object of this preparation would be for Claire not to feel rejected when the time for a change in doctors comes. She should not then feel that she is being abandoned because she is not good enough. JM then pointed out that the analytical term for this relationship with the institution is called "transference to the institution." That this girl will continue feeling that the institution is in a role of a parent to her and not the individual professionals working within it. This limited continuity would offer her some security, which would play a part toward enabling her to cope with changes or other rejections in her life without resorting to self-harm.

The doctor responded that her mother had reduced her hours of work to be more available to look after Claire. Her mother would be working only for 4 hours per day. JM then questioned whether this mother is able to provide a caring and consistent environment for Claire. The doctor shared this view. JM then pointed out that if Claire is placed in a seriously suboptimal (neglectful) environment, therapy has a limited chance of bringing about a positive therapeutic development. JM repeated that if the psychiatric service has justifiable concerns about the capacity of her mother to offer parenting, then these concerns need to be shared with the other agencies and acted on so that Claire is not subjected to a continuation of the neglect that she suffered in the past 14 years.

JM praised the doctor for having enabled Claire to trust her and make it possible for her to disclose all the private details of trauma that she had not been able to disclose previously. A next help would be to support her in a way so that she is no longer exposed to neglect or to abuse, including no longer being exposed to sexual abuse.

Regarding the effect of premature engagement in sexual activities, see Stuart-Smith (1996). Those interested in institutional transference can refer to Martin (1989), Safirstein (1967), and Matarazzo (2012). The literature on the long-term effects of child sexual abuse is vast, but one useful publication is by Kendall-Tackett et al. (1993).

References

Kendall-Tackett, K. A., Williams, L. M., & Finkelhor, D. (1993). Impact of sexual abuse on children: A review and synthesis of recent empirical studies. *Psychological Bulletin, 113*(1), 164–180.

Martin, H. P. (1989). Types of institutional transference. *Bulletin of the Menninger Clinic, 53*(1), 58–62.

Matarazzo, B. B. (2012). Adaptive institutional transference in the treatment of individuals with borderline personality disorder. *Bulletin of the Menninger Clinic, 76*(4), 297–313.

Safirstein, S. L. (1967). Institutional transference. *The Psychiatric Quarterly, 41*(3), 557–566.

Stuart-Smith, S. (1996). Teenage sex. *BMJ, 312*(7028), 390–391.

Ms. Wendy

Presenting condition

Ms. Wendy is a 24-year-old woman who was voluntarily admitted from the general hospital accident and emergency department following a suicidal attempt by drug overdose and charcoal burning after breaking up with her boyfriend.

History of present complaint

Ms. Wendy presented with unstable emotions, which she attributed to relationship problems. Ms. Wendy had been longing for affection and love from her boyfriend. She reported experiencing unstable emotions and an urge to self-harm by slashing her wrists following relationship problems.

Ms. Wendy's mood worsened from December 2017. She expected her boyfriend to be more affectionate to her as it was her birthday month. She was disappointed because he needed to work. To secure the relationship, she kept seeking reassurance from her boyfriend for marriage. She was not pervasively depressed. Sleep and appetite were fair. She could cope with her work.

On the day of admission, Ms. Wendy had argued with her boyfriend who was reluctant in responding on "WhatsApp," on whether he would marry her. On impulse, Ms. Wendy took 18 tabs of prescribed Ativan and burnt charcoal when she was alone at home. She wrote a suicide note to her parents and to her boyfriend. She perceived the act as lethal. Her mother returned home 3 hours later and reported this to the police when she discovered her daughter unconscious. Ms. Wendy was sent to accident and emergency department and required intubation in the intensive care unit. She was seen by consultant in liaison psychiatry when physically fit and inpatient management was suggested.

Family history

There is no family history of mental illness or of suicide.

Personal history

Ms. Wendy was born in the city. She is an only child. Her developmental milestones were normal. Her father is a 54-year-old bus driver. Ms. Wendy claimed that he had been verbally abusive and critical of her; he never praised her academic performance or achievements. Her mother is a 48-year-old office assistant. Ms. Wendy claimed that her mother was irritable and ill-tempered and that she tended to displace her anger on her by physical punishment (this was denied by mother). There is no history of sexual abuse.

Ms. Wendy achieved above-average academic results in primary school, but the results at secondary school were only fair. Ms. Wendy studied for an associate degree and then studied up to Year 3 in university (bachelor linguistic course). Ms. Wendy dropped out in Year 4 in university. She attributed this to the break-up of a relationship with her ex-boyfriend.

Ms. Wendy has had many unstable and stormy relationships for more than 10 years, each lasting from weeks to months. The longest duration of courtship had been 3 years in 2013. Ms. Wendy started dating her current boyfriend (who was a 25-year-old insurance agent) in June 2017. She contacted him via a dating app. She reported that their relationship was harmonious in the first few months because her boyfriend was caring to her. Ms. Wendy has been in courtship with current boyfriend for 7 months.

Ms. Wendy has no forensic record. She is a single, insurance agent and freelance makeup artist. She is living with her parents in a private flat.

Ms. Wendy described herself as hot-tempered and impulsive. She has had longstanding mood fluctuations that are precipitated by interpersonal difficulties. She has had many unstable and stormy relationships since her teenage years. Her relationships lasted from weeks to a few months. Ms. Wendy tends to get easily attached to others. She has many friends and likes singing, playing piano, and hiking. She follows no religion. She did not smoke or drink. There is no history of illicit drug use.

Past psychiatric history

Ms. Wendy has a history of many episodes of self-harming behavior by wrist-slashing since her teenage years. There is also a history of drug overdose by taking 10 tabs of Ativan after a broken relationship in March 2017. She has been known to mental health services since July 2015. Previous diagnoses were of depression and Borderline Personality Disorder.

Ms. Wendy attempts to overcome the distress of a breakup by seeking another relationship. She has a strong sense of emptiness with increasing fear of abandonment. She has been self-harming by slashing her wrists and thighs since her teenage years. She has used cutting as a way of relieving stress.

Ms. Wendy had been followed up at the psychiatric clinic. There is a history of psychiatric admission to a hospital once (March 17, 2017–March 23, 2017) following a self-harm-harm gesture of drug overdose with 10 tabs of Ativan and slashing her upper limbs, thighs, and abdomen. Her last follow-up in the psychiatric clinic on December 21, 2017. There is no significant past medical history and no known drug allergies.

Present treatment

Ms. Wendy was treated with antidepressants; admission for monitoring suicidal risk, and referral to a clinical psychologist to be helped to develop better strategies for coping with stress.

Consultation

JM started by thanking the doctor for the comprehensive presentation. JM then proceeded to ask the doctor what was the understanding of why Ms. Wendy was resorting to self-cutting and making attempts against her life with either a drug overdose or carbon monoxide. More specifically, JM asked why she resorted to this form of response to stress rather than a more constructive and more functional way of responding. The doctor's view was that her present behavior may be related to the early family experience of her parents being critical of her and the pervasive feeling of emptiness that she has. JM then asked how the doctor made the connection between the experience of being brought up by critical parents 20 years previously and cutting herself when under stress. The doctor suggested that this response may be related to the anger that Ms. Wendy carries in relation to the abusive environment that she was brought up in. JM inquired if the doctor considered her behavior to be the result of anger and that these acts are angry acts, even the attempt to end her own life. JM then asked, "who is this anger directed at?" The doctor said that it was directed at herself because she was harming her own body. JM followed up with, "what is she angry with herself about?" The doctor responded that she was angry about being abandoned once again by her boyfriend. JM interrupted the doctor and asked him to return to the original question, which was: Why did he think that Ms. Wendy was angry with herself?

It was clarified that she was also angry with her boyfriend who was threatening to abandon her. The question was: How did that anger lead to her to attack her own body? JM returned to the question why would Ms. Wendy be angry at herself? The doctor responded that she may be blaming herself for her failure to have long lasting relationships. JM then repeated, "why should Ms. Wendy be angry with herself for not having satisfactory long lasting relationships?" This was a difficult question for the doctors to respond to and JM acknowledged this. At that point he summed up that the doctor had made a reasonable assumption that Ms. Wendy was attacking herself because she was angry with herself for failing to establish satisfactory relationships. JM added that she may additionally be blaming herself for her failure academically. In this way, Ms. Wendy was repeating the pattern of criticism that originated from her parents. JM then asked the doctor how a well-functioning person responded to stressful situations similar to those that Ms. Wendy was facing. The doctor responded that functioning persons would vent their feelings with others and make attempts to distract themselves. JM then added that functioning people would learn from failures so that similar encounters in the future did not lead to distress. Ms. Wendy resorts to attacking herself instead of learning from the experience for her own better adjustment with future similar events.

JM then expanded on the issue of "venting." One kind of communication is just to tell the other person what is on your mind and stop at that. The other kind of communication is one in which there is actual processing of thinking; there is a dialogue and new concepts emerge as a result—a new understanding of the encounter. It seemed that Ms. Wendy is unable to do the second type of venting. JM then asked the group of doctors if they had any views on what made it impossible for Ms. Wendy to process experiences in the second way of thinking. Did the doctors have any hypotheses on why Ms. Wendy was unable to learn from the adverse outcome of her experiences? The doctor responded that Ms. Wendy would immediately seek a different relationship instead of understanding why the current one went wrong. The doctor added that Ms. Wendy had claimed that she did not have time to process the experience but in fact she had decided not to use the time for that but to use the time and her energies to comfort herself by making the next relationship.

JM then asked "when you are a child and you are distressed, what is it that helps you to process the experience?" The doctor responded that in a child, a caring parent would offer that. JM confirmed that this is exactly what a caring parent would do. They would offer comfort, sympathy but would not stop there. After the comfort and the sympathy has had the effect of making the child less anxious and in less pain, then they would proceed to help the child reach a better understanding of what happened and finally to prepare to address similar situations in the future in a more constructive way.

The parents would help the child to see things in a more realistic perspective, help the child regain some hope for the future, and ensure that the unfortunate incident does not damage the child's self-0view. As a result, the child will not end up thinking anything less of themselves (for example, that they are not lovable and that they should only expect rejection from others). Obviously one single episode will not have that effect, but a series of such incidents with a series of lack of a constructive intervention by a caring adult would stand a high risk of seriously affecting the child's self-esteem and the child's capacity to deal with adversity. JM repeated that Ms. Wendy's parents had been described as those who were not able to offer support, sympathy, and advice. This has had an influence on making it hard for Ms. Wendy to process adverse events in a constructive way. Instead of having the containing and nurturing response, she has had criticism, which compounded the trauma of the adverse incident. As a result, Ms. Wendy's self-worth was reduced further and she missed the opportunity to learn how to cope with these situations in a more constructive way in the future.

JM then asked the doctor if this current formulation helped him in deciding what therapeutic intervention would be more appropriate for her. The doctor responded that the psychodynamic approach would be helpful. JM asked further if they could define which elements of that approach would be more helpful to Ms. Wendy. Because difficult question, JM expanded that the aims in the treatment for Ms. Wendy were to enable her to cope with the distress and pain of adverse situations and to be able to turn to appropriate others for help.

JM then gave a similar example of a stressful event happening to a junior doctor. He posed the hypothetical question of the doctor being the subject of a complaint by a patient. The first response would be personal distress and containment of this distress. The second step would be to share it with appropriate colleagues, and the third step would be to work out a way of appropriately responding to this complaint. Finally, the result of this process would be that the doctor would be better prepared so that, in the future, such complaints or similar complaints do not arise. This would be a functional response and a functional process. The difference of a functioning junior doctor from Ms. Wendy is that Ms. Wendy does not have the personal capacity to cope with the distress on her own, even for a finite time.

In conclusion, the therapeutic intervention needs to provide for her what she lacked in her real-life (growing-up) experience. This is different from "informing" her or "educating" her in a cognitive way; what is required is an actual lived experience of having these effects happen to you (Kohut 1984). Cognitions are important but not enough to effect a change. What has a bigger chance of effecting a change is an environment that would provide for her what she has not had growing up. Ms. Wendy needs acceptance, sympathy, and emotional support. Only when these are experienced can she find herself in a position of thinking through these experiences and developing a better way of responding to them. She will then be able to address stressful situations functionally and not dysfunctionally.

Reference

Kohut, H. (1984). *How does analysis cure?* University of Chicago Press.

Ms. M

Presenting complaint

Ms. M. is a 24-year-old woman, who has been suffering from panic attacks and multiple episodes of deliberate self-harm.

History of present condition

One week before admission, Ms. M had returned from the United Kingdom. She started to experience low mood and anhedonia. She had a sense of hopelessness and loneliness. There were some fleeting suicidal ideas of rushing out to traffic to kill herself, but these subsided spontaneously. One day before admission, she overdosed by taking 15 mg of diazepam and 1 g of parasol with 5 cups of vodka. She claimed that she used these to achieve better sleep and that she had no suicidal intent. The next day, when she went to work, she broke down at the Metro Station and called her friend for help. She was brought by her friend to the accident and emergency department and was voluntarily admitted in view of the recent drug overdose and suicidal ideation.

Ms. M is a medium-built woman with neat appearance and dyed hair; she was forthcoming and polite. Her mood was euthymic, and her affect was preserved. Her speech was coherent and relevant, and she was keen to share. No psychotic features were detected. There was no suicidal ideation. Ms. M did not perceive the drug overdose as lethal. Insight was good because she thought of herself as having a mental illness and was willing to receive treatment.

Family history

Her father is an alcoholic. Her mother had a history of drug overdose. No formal psychiatric diagnosis was provided.

Personal history

Ms. M was born in the United Kingdom. She had one older brother. Her birth and developmental history are unremarkable; she was brought up by her parents.

There is no history of childhood trauma or sexual abuse. She recalled her relationship with her brother as "OK." There were no frequent conflicts, but neither were they close. Ms. M recalled she felt scared when her father overdrank in her childhood. However, there were no episodes of verbal abuse or physical punishment. She described her mother as a gentle and caring person. Her relationship with her family was "OK." The bonding was not a close one, but they respected each other.

She studied at university and majored in French and Philosophy. Ms. M. came to the city after graduating in August 2015 to work as an English teacher. She coped well. Ms. M. works as a native-speaking teacher in a government secondary school and lives with friends in a rented flat.

Ms. M. described herself as an "introverted extrovert." She had many friends, but she easily developed a feeling of being abandoned. When a friend slightly disappointed her (e.g., canceling their date due to some sudden event), she felt abandoned and stayed away from that friend. As a result, she developed many brief and intense relationships.

Ms. M. felt chronically empty at heart even though friends accompanied her. She described herself as "needing time on my own but depended on friends to make me happy." She felt lonely on every Friday night as she ruminated she would become bored at the weekend. She would plan her weekend schedule so that she could have a packed day and meet her friends.

Ms. M. had always had an unstable self-image. There was a high school classmate whom she liked, and she cared for how he viewed her. She recalled one time she overheard a conversation by this boy with another friend of his. They were referring to another girl with whom she shared the same first name. When the friend verified if it was Ms. M about whom the boy was talking, the boy said "No, the thin one." Ms. M heard this, and she perceived this casual sentence as describing her as fat. She is weight conscious and has always wanted to maintain her weight, but there were no anorexic features. Her body mass index is in the normal range.

Since her teenage years, she "coped" with stress by self-harming. She would cut her wrist and her thighs for stress release. All resulted in superficial wounds. She felt much more in control when she did this. She admitted that she still had episodes of self-harm when she started working, but the frequency was lower. There were more than 20 episodes.

Ms. M. was having her first courtship at the time of admission. It was a long-distance relationship with a boy whom she had known for several years. They had "dated" for about 1 month at the time of admission. She described her boyfriend as a reliable figure. She would contact him by phone when any issues arose and depended heavily on him. Her expectation toward him was like what she had toward her friends. If any slight disappointment arose, she would become greatly distressed.

She is a nonsmoker and nondrinker with recreational trial of cannabis in United Kingdom. No history of substance abuse.

Past psychiatric history

Ms. M. reported to have had episodes of mood swings since 2012. She recalled that she would feel energetic and restless at the time of high mood, with overspending activities. These episodes would typically last 4 to 6 days. There was no hypersexuality, no racing thoughts, or psychotic symptoms related to these episodes. Daily function was not affected.

When she was in an episode of low mood, she would feel persistently upset with fleeting ideas of self-harm and insomnia. She would feel hopeless and empty. These episodes typically lasted for around 1 week. She recalled that every time she came back to the city after visiting her hometown in the United Kingdom, she would experience this. She would attempt to "cope" by cutting her wrists and thighs. Those episodes of self-harm resulted in superficial wounds. There was no suicidal intent.

Ms. M. was first known to the mental health service in United Kingdome in 2012. She then presented with fluctuating mood and multiple episodes of cutting her wrists. She was prescribed fluoxetine and sertraline. The drugs were discontinued in 2015 as she reported to have increasing urge to self-harm after taking them.

There is a history of panic attacks starting in 2013.

Ms. M. was maintained well after the selective serotonin reuptake inhibitor was discontinued. She became known to the psychiatric clinic in 2016 after she came to the city for panic disorder and was put on benzodiazepines.

Present treatment and management

A diagnosis of Bipolar Affective Disorder II was made in view of episodes of mood swings since 2012. Ms. M. was put on oral risperidone and responded well to a low dose. She remained mentally stable throughout admission and settled in the ward. Ms. M. was observed to participate in ward activities and enjoyed good relationships with other patients.

In view of traits of Borderline Personality Disorder, a clinical psychologist was asked to conduct a personality assessment. Stress coping and early signs of relapse were discussed. Ms. M was participating enthusiastically in the process, and she came up with a comprehensive mind-mapping of her probable factors of impulsivity and ways to stay well. She learned to adopt positive ways of stress coping. Insight was instilled.

She was keen to continue to see a clinical psychologist for psychotherapy as an outpatient.

Consultation

The doctor clarified that the objective of treatment was to prevent further attempts of self-harm and that the care of Miss M had been transferred to another team since her discharge from the ward. It was then clarified that her condition had a mixed biological and psychological basis. There was good evidence that manic-depressive illness is influenced by genetic and other biological factors as well as psychosocial stressors.

At this point, JM made reference to a new research study that showed that the risk of a manic-depressive illness is more than two times higher in people who had experienced childhood adversity (Palmier-Claus et al., 2016).

The doctor then pointed out that her mother's condition and the change in her body shape may have been additional contributing factors. The doctor pointed out that Ms. M's experience of being brought up by a mother with this pathology would have affected how Ms. M is coping with her life in the present. The doctor clarified that it was her father who had a drinking problem and that her mother had taken an overdose.

JM pointed out that although there is evidence that there were significant difficulties with her parents, Ms. M denies their presence. She claims that her childhood upbringing was OK.

The doctor agreed, saying she says that they were not close as a family but that she regarded her family as not unusual.

JM then asked the doctor to say how she thought her patient constructed her life experience as a young person. The doctor suggested that Ms. M was loyal to her parents and did not wish to say anything negative about them. JM repeated that there is a conflict between the fact of her father being alcoholic and her mother attempting suicide, and Ms. M denying all this and saying that her life was not unusual.

JM then went on to point out that Ms. M's defense mechanism was that of denial (Freud, 1936). JM also pointed out that this is a primitive form of defense. It seemed that the reason why Ms. M employs this primitive defense mechanism is to protect herself from the pain of the conflict that she experiences on one hand for not being brought up in an environment, which is conducive to good mental health, and, on the other, of feeling loyal toward her parents.

JM proceeded to point out that in handling denial therapeutically, one needs to proceed carefully. Challenging a primitive form of defense may expose the patient to unbearable feelings, may threaten the therapeutic relationship, or may precipitate different symptomatology. JM then explained how dysfunctional this defense is compared with more healthy ways of dealing with unpleasant or traumatic experiences. For example, a more functional response would have been to acknowledge the distress for trauma of the experience but perhaps give it the meaning of her parents having their own difficulties and having to cope with perhaps stresses and adverse experiences in their own background. A more functional person may have been able to see her parents more globally as people who tried their best but who also had significant difficulties.

It seemed that if Ms. M felt that the therapist is challenging her defenses too harshly, she may resort to producing other symptoms or making another attempt at her life. Her therapist needs to be mindful that if new symptoms surface during therapy they need to be more careful and proceed more cautiously.

JM then shifted the focus to the relationship between the patient and the doctor. The doctor responded that Ms. M was referring to her self-harm as a way of "stress relief." She told the doctor that when she harms herself she feels more in control. Ms. M is concerned to appear as a polite young woman and particularly that she is not someone who speaks ill of her parents.

JM asked the doctor to clarify what her therapeutic objectives have been up to now. The doctor explained that when Ms. M was an inpatient, she tried to get Ms. M to consider ways to which she tries to handle stressful situations and distressing feelings. The doctor pointed out that following their consultations, Ms. M was more prepared to search for alternative ways of dealing with stress.

JM asked the doctor to explain how she thought Ms. M was understanding her stress. What was it that Ms. M was considering as stressful? The doctor pointed out that Ms. M was stressed when important people to her did not respond to her approaches. An example was that when Ms. M would phone people and they did not pick up the phone, Ms. M tended to interpret this nonresponse as a rejection or as an indication that these people did not care for her when the reality was that they may have been unable to respond for different reasons not related to her.

JM underlined that the matter that the doctor elicited was the inability of Ms. M to tolerate feelings of rejection. Ms. M was interpreting nonavailability for whatever reason as a personal rejection of her.

JM then asked the doctor if she had been able to connect this pattern with any of Ms. M's experiences of her early life. For example, what were the experiences in her early life that set the pattern for her to interpret every nonavailability as an active rejection? The doctor was able to refer to experiences of rejection during Ms. M's school life. JM then pointed out that although the history is indicative of early life traumata with a father who is not available because of alcoholism and a mother who has her own difficulties as indicated by her attempt at self-harm, Ms. M does not refer to any early life experiences that would justify her present sensitivity to rejection.

JM then shifted the focus to the difficulty of the family environment to "contain her." JM then proceeded to elaborate on the concept of containment (James, 1984; Winnicott, 1965) and gave examples of natural containment in early life. JM gave the example of a child being distressed in a playground and then being "contained" by the parent. The parent would absorb the child's anxiety, comfort the child, and help the child to return to their playing. A parent, who is unable to contain the child's distress, will take the child, remove the child and themselves from the playground. This will be damaging to the child because it would not help the child learn to contain their own anxiety later.

Ms. M's parents also had good qualities. It is because of these good qualities that Ms. M feels loyal to them. The mixture of good and problematic qualities is what lies underneath Ms. M's internal conflict, and it is this internal conflict that needs to be addressed in therapy.

The consultation then moved to focus on the role of a therapist as a transitional object (Winnicott, 1953). The therapist needs to serve as transitional object for the initial stage of therapy, in the sense that they will need to be the ones who absorb this woman's distress and who will enable her to experience it as part of life without having a damaging effect on her psychological development. By sharing the experience with the therapist, Ms. M stands a better chance of understanding the process in a more realistic way and not give it the unrealistic and pathological extensions that she has been giving to her life experiences.

By misapplying the early experiences of her family and of the school to the present, Ms. M recreates the same early experiences in the present environment. In this sense, experiences that are not in themselves inherently traumatic become traumatic with the meaning that Ms. M gives to them. In a way, this is a transferential phenomenon.

References

Freud, A. (1936). *The ego and the mechanisms of defense.* Hogarth Press.

James, D. C. (1984). Bion's "containing" and Winnicott's "holding" in the context of the group matrix. *International Journal of Group Psychotherapy, 34,* 201–213.

Palmier-Claus, J. E., Berry, K., Bucci, S., Mansell, W., & Varese, F. (2016). Relationship between childhood adversity and bipolar affective disorder: Systematic review and meta-analysis. *The British Journal of Psychiatry, 209*(6), 454–459.

Winnicott, D. W. (1953). *Transitional objects and transitional phenomena. Collected Papers.* Tavistock Publications.

Winnicott, D. W. (1965). *The maturational processes and the facilitating environment.* Hogarth Press.

Mrs. W

Presenting condition

Mrs. W is a 77-year-old woman who presented with a panic disorder. She suffered from frequent and disabling panic attacks with somatic symptoms.

History of present complaint

Mrs. W suffered from panic attacks of increasing frequency and severity (felt palpitating, sweaty, dizzy, out of breath, chest discomfort, numb) since 2012 when her first son was going through a divorce. The attacks occurred usually when she was in crowded places; she had anticipatory fear and was only able to go out accompanied by her husband. There was hypervigilance with startled response to stimuli. She also had gastrointestinal symptoms (e.g., abdominal pain and diarrhea). She harbored excessive worries about her son remarrying, and she would have deteriorating health that would have rendered her unable to attend the wedding. There were also hypochondriac ideas that she may suffer from a heart condition; she had a checkup and was reassured. Her mood was not pervasively low, but she was irritable at times. Her appetite was maintained. She could sleep at night but was deeply disturbed by vivid nightmares. One recurring dream was that her sister's dead body was chasing her. She had deep-seated negative cognitions about herself thinking: "I am very weak and vulnerable."

Family history

There was no family history of mental illness. Her father was a landlord who tended to be authoritarian to her family. Her mother was her father's third wife. Mrs. W had one sister who was 14 years older and it was this sister who raised her and not her mother. This sister committed suicide late in her teenage years (10 or 20) when Mrs. W was aged 6. Her father committed suicide soon after. Her mother died more than 30 years ago.

Personal history

Mrs. W was born in the country and received no formal education. She came to the city at age 21 and worked at first in factories and then as a babysitter. She retired at the age of 60. She was married at age 30 and raised two sons. She enjoyed good marital and family relationships. Her baseline personality was rather anxious prone and introverted.

Past psychiatric history

When Mrs. W moved to the city from the country in her 20s, she started experiencing sudden onset of palpitations, a feeling of suffocation, generalized weakness, dizziness, restlessness, and abdominal spasm. At that time, she consulted many doctors who ordered many investigations that did not reveal any pathology. Through the years, the frequency of these panic-like attacks decreased, and she did not require any regular treatment or medical consultations. She became known to the mental health service in 2012 when she presented with these anxiety symptoms.

Mrs. W was treated with oral medications. On sertraline 50 mg daily, she reported to be more anxious and to experience more gastrointestinal symptoms. On flupentixol/melitracen she experienced extrapyramidal side effects. With mirtazapine, she suffered limb weakness.

Mrs. W received six sessions of individual psychotherapy (of the cognitive-behavioral approach) from January to October 2016. She had gone through memory reprocessing of the childhood trauma event. Mrs. W prepared a narrative script of her traumatic early life experiences; this was organized with a highlight on expressed emotions and reframed meanings. A summary of the script is as follows: The traumatic incident took place in 1950–1951 when Mrs. W thought she was aged 6. In fact, as she was now 77, she was born in 1942, and, therefore, she was 8 or 9 at the time her sister died.

As an exposure exercise, she was asked to read the script at home. Positive points of the incident and her strengths were discussed and emphasized. Interoceptive exposure was also conducted. Her conditioned anxiety response to physical sensations was reduced. She had fewer traumatic flashbacks of the trauma event (sister's suicide and discovery of body) and was able to adopt a more open attitude toward the incident.

Present treatment and management of case

Mrs. W was maintained on citalopram 10 mg daily and propranolol 10 mg daily as necessary.

Consultation

Mrs. W's history is closely linked with the recent history of unrest in her country. JM thanked the doctor for the thorough presentation. The doctor clarified that the new law introduced at that time required even family members to testify against members of their own family who were considered to be "landlords." Her older sister, then in her early 20s, initially resisted this with some strength. As a result, she was repeatedly interrogated. One day her sister disappeared and soon after that, her father took her to look for her. In searching for the sister, they reached a fishpond where Mrs. W remembered that many people had gathered looking at a body that had been found. This was the body of her sister, which she identified because her father did not feel he had the strength to face the body of his daughter. The body was removed from the pond and the father then recognized that this was his elder daughter. They then went to the police station for formalities. One month later, Mrs. W's father committed suicide in the same fishpond. During this brief time, Mrs. W had lost her sister, who she felt was like a mother to her, and her father.

JM then asked the doctor if she had explored with Mrs. W what connection did these events have, which had taken place about 60 years previously, with her present psychological distress. Since those traumatic events, Mrs. W had to make a major adjustment to her life, from living in rural life to living in one of the biggest cities in the world under a different regime. JM then asked if there was an understanding of the personal resources that this woman had that enabled her to survive this major adjustment. How did Mrs. W manage to live for more than half a century and develop these complaints only recently? The doctor connected the onset of Mrs. W's symptoms with her son's divorce (2012). JM's second question was: if the divorce was taking place 5 years previously, why should Mrs. W develop the symptoms at present? There was no clear understanding of why this should be, but the doctor added that Mrs. W was also concerned that she may not be well enough to attend her son's second wedding. There was little understanding of why the prospect of the son remarrying should lead Mrs. W not only to be concerned or even preoccupied but to develop incapacitating symptomatology.

In trying to understand this, JM asked for further information about Mrs. W's life situation. The doctor explained that she was living with her husband and that she was physically healthy and able to look after herself. The consultation highlighted a further area of Mrs. W's life that needed further exploration. The doctor made some references to the culture in the city and to some "negative cognitions." JM then suggested that it would be worthwhile if the negative cognitions and the cultural factors were identified and clarified. JM then speculated that the son's divorce and remarriage may have a negative reflection on how she saw herself as a mother. JM then further asked if Mrs. W felt in any way responsible for the failure of her son's marriage. JM then asked if Mrs. W was aware that her son had marital difficulties before his divorce. Did she consider herself responsible in the context of close family relationships within her culture?

JM then pointed out that in psychotherapy one aims to connect actual events with the meaning that a patient gives to them. Specifically, how did Mrs. W construct a personal narrative the major and traumatic events that had indeed happened in her life because it was this narrative that was causing her to suffer incapacitating symptoms. JM then pointed out that many parents in their 70s may experience their children's divorce but not all of them will develop symptomatology. What was the specific connection that Mrs. W was making that was causing her distress? JM pointed out that Mrs. W's distress was well beyond what one would normally expect to arise out of concern of an elderly mother for her adult child. It was not only that she was unhappy about the stress that her son may be going through but also extending this experience to mean something negative about herself. Identifying this connection would make it possible for the therapist to help Mrs. W first identify the connection and then develop a different understanding that would be realistic and not a cause for pathology. JM pointed out that his ideas were simple speculations, and the actual connection could be different and need to be discovered through open-ended questioning. It needed to be better understood in what way the events that were indeed traumatic negatively affected how she saw herself.

JM added the speculation that Mrs. W may feel a worse mother because she may be assuming that her son's divorce was the result of her neglect of his needs. Did she feel that if she was a better mother

her son would not be divorcing? If, for example, Mrs. W sees these events as a negative reflection on herself, it may be useful for her to be reminded that for her 50+ years in the city, she had been a dedicated mother and wife, and she worked and played an important part in the good functioning of her family. JM then further speculated that Mrs. W may have had the struggle to combine the needs for survival of the family through working and the needs of addressing her children's emotional needs. Mrs. W may have felt responsible for the children's well-being even after they were adults and were running their own life.

JM then distinguished the functional aspects of the cohesion of the extended family from that of a dysfunctional family. For example, the cohesion, on many occasions is quite functional with the allocation of different roles. The grandparents often play a useful role in maintaining the functioning of the extended family. On some occasions, the grandparents contribute to the life of the extended family by, for example, undertaking many roles of the family (such a cooking and looking after the grandchildren) so that their adult children can work and develop their own careers and their own life. The dysfunctional aspect of such cohesion may be an excessively intrusive and controlling grandparent who interferes negatively with the lives of their (adult) children. JM stressed the need to separate what is cultural and functional from what is cultural and dysfunctional. The definition of dysfunctional is if the culture causes a member of this extended family to become ill, as in the case of Mrs. W.

It is useful to remember that most members of any culture function well, and it is a minority who develop symptomatology. It is not appropriate to attribute to the culture, as a whole, the symptomatology that only a minority (within the same culture) develop. The cohesion in the family can be a source of direction and a source of support. The wisdom and experience of the older generation can be quite helpful to the subsequent generations.

Ms. D

Presenting condition

Ms. D was admitted to the psychiatric hospital in March 2018 for low mood and suicidal ideation.

History of presenting illness

Ms. D had been suffering from periods of varying low mood, with crying spells, since late in February 2018. These were thought to be a reaction to interpersonal problems with her supervisor and other colleagues. She harbored fleeting suicidal ideas and once wrote a suicide note. She then requested an early appointment at the psychiatric Center in March 2018 on account of her worsened mood. The dosage of desvenlafaxine was increased from 50 to 75 mg daily, but there was limited improvement in her mood. She was feeling sad, frustrated, and hopeless. However, she had maintained volition and interest in daily activities. She was able to concentrate at work. Sleep and appetite were maintained.

Later in the same month, Ms. D had a conflict with her brother over some trivial issues. Her sister-in-law joined in the conflict and sided with her husband. Ms. D. became emotional, grabbed a chopper, and voiced the idea of harming her sister-in-law. She put down the chopper after her mother and brother persuaded her. They asked her not to return home to avoid further conflicts. She felt abandoned and became even more upset. She thought of jumping from a height or of hanging herself with a rope. She stayed at her boyfriend's place for a few days. On the day of admission, she took sick leave from work "due to flu symptoms." Her sister-in-law advised her to attend the accident and emergency department for her mood problems. After discussing for some time, she agreed. Voluntary admission to hospital was arranged after assessment by the consultation liaison team.

Family history

Ms. D's mother suffered from Bipolar Affective Disorder and had been on medication for nearly 19 years. Her mother had gambling problems as well. Her father was a substance abuser with gambling problems.

Personal history

Ms. D was born in the country and came to the city at the age of 4. She had an older brother. Her parents divorced when she was 7 years old, and this was attributed to her father's substance abuse and gambling problems. She lived with her mother and brother since that time. They moved residences and changed schools frequently when she was younger to avoid her father's demands for money from her mother and his threats to the family. They had been on a state benefits until her brother and she started working. She is currently living with her mother, brother, and sister-in-law in a public housing unit. She stays at her boyfriend's apartment on the weekends.

Ms. D's brother was the person who she trusted most in the family. She described him as "the father at home." In 2012, she borrowed around US$30,000 from the bank and gave this sum to her brother for him to invest. She considered it a loan rather than a joint investment, but they did not discuss this issue clearly. Her brother lost a lot in the investment in 2013. Both were declared bankrupt. Ms. D blamed herself for making the wrong decision of borrowing the money for her brother. She did not know how to ask him to pay her back, so she just waited for him to make a proposal on how to settle the debt. Four years after the incident, her brother finally agreed to pay her US$200 every month until he paid back the money that she paid to the bank during the 4-year bankruptcy period (around US$16,000), but her brother paid for 1 month only. She was disappointed and became distant from him. She often had conflicts with him over trivial issues; this was her way of expressing her dissatisfaction with him.

Ms. D reported a longstanding disharmony with her sister-in-law, whom she described as impolite and disrespectful. Ms. D's brother got married in January 2018. Ms. D treated her sister-in-law as a guest after she moved in and expected her sister-in-law to show respect toward her and her mother. She said her sister-in-law was rather bossy when it came to allocation of household responsibilities. Her sister-in-law also advised her brother not to pay her back the money and considered it a joint investment. Moreover, her brother sided with his wife when Ms. D had conflicts with her, and this upset her even more.

Ms. D had been dating her current boyfriend for about 1 ½ years. They were planning to get married the following year. She had a fiancé 2 years previously, but they broke up 3 months before the wedding when she found out he cheated on her. She had a few close friends in whom she could confide.

Ms. D studied business at the university. She switched to biochemistry after a year because she found out she was not interested in business. She could not adapt to the new learning environment and subsequently dropped out. She started working at a law firm in 2008. After working for 3 years, she enrolled in the bachelor's program in occupational therapy because she wanted to further her studies. However, she could not cope with the study stress and dropped out again. She continued working as a clerk or an assistant in different law firms. Ms. D is currently working as a law clerk for the department of justice.

Owing to her bankruptcy, Ms. D could not be involved in certain lines of work in the department of justice. She felt worthless and guilty. Over the past 4 years Ms. D felt that, for most of the time, she had nothing to do at work. Although her senior gave her good reviews in the annual appraisal and she got a pay raise every year, she did not have a sense of achievement at work. She expected that her duties could be rearranged after the discharge of the bankruptcy order, but it remained the same. She felt frustrated and did not know how to communicate with her supervisor about her job aspirations. On the other hand, she did not want to quit the job because of the stable income it provided and the good working environment.

Past psychiatric history

Ms. D had been known to the mental health service in 2006. She then presented with low mood following a suicide attempt by hanging with a belt in front of her family; this was in reaction to study stress after she entered the university. She was admitted to the hospital. She was diagnosed with an adjustment disorder. She was admitted again in 2007 for fleeting suicidal ideas, which were triggered by examination stress. She was diagnosed with an adjustment disorder. Desvenlafaxine was prescribed. She has had regular psychiatric follow-up. Her mental condition remained stable over the past decade.

Management of the case

Ms. D was diagnosed with a moderate depressive episode. Desvenlafaxine was stepped up from 75 to 100 mg daily. She was referred to a clinical psychologist for psychological intervention. Triggers related to the current admission and relationship problems with her family were explored. Her mood became stable soon after admission. Sleep and appetite were maintained. No suicidal ideas were expressed. She was referred to the community psychiatric nurse for community support on discharge.

Ms. D's early life experience in a chaotic and insecure family influenced the way she undervalued herself, weakened her resolve to claim her rights, and established a lifetime of avoidance of conflict. Ms. D's condition was thought to be precipitated by frustration at work (and disappointment that her normal duties were not restored after she was discharged from bankruptcy) and by family conflicts (including brother's nonrepayment of her loan to him).

Consultation

JM congratulated the doctor for the thoroughness of the presentation. JM then asked for a clarification of the therapeutic contract with Ms. D. The doctor confirmed that Ms. D would be followed up but not by her. JM asked the doctor if she had a question in her mind about Ms. D. The doctor responded that she wanted to understand more thoroughly the combined effect of family tensions and work difficulties. Following on the issue of family tensions, JM asked the doctor if she knew how the house workload is shared in the family home. The home is shared between Ms. D, her mother, her brother, and his wife. The doctor responded that although every person living in that home is earning, the proportion of financial contribution of each member was not clear. Ms. D felt that the proportion of financial contribution was "fair." Regarding the work contribution, their mother was doing most of the work and that the sister-in-law was carrying out the least work. This unfairness is unresolved although frequently addressed. This leads to confrontations between the sister-in-law and Ms. D with Ms. D's brother siding with his wife.

The situation remains unfair for Ms. D and remains a constant source of sadness, irritation, and frustration for Ms. D. She feels exploited by her brother and her sister-in-law. This is in addition to the exploitation that Ms. D feels because of the loan of the US$30,000 which is not being returned. JM asked the doctor if the details of how this significant loan was negotiated were known. Ms. D gave this loan to her brother without going any deeper into the implications of it for her and without taking any advice from her how interest could be secured. After some discussion it emerged that Ms. D did not take due care in handing over this significant sum of money to her brother. She did not ask if he would contribute an equal sum to this potential investment nor did she ask of how and when she would begin to gain the returns from this. The doctor mentioned that Ms. D was not aware why the brother needed *her* to get the loan instead of getting the loan himself. She was aware that her brother was not eligible for a loan from the bank. Ms. D did not secure this loan with any paperwork. Considering the reasons why she did not ask for some security from her brother, this was explained by the doctor in terms of family dynamics. The brother, following father's departure, had assumed the role of head of the family, and it was he who had been taking most of the important family decisions. In this context, Ms. D felt it would have been inappropriate for her to ask for securities from her brother. Such a request would have led to a conflict.

JM pointed out the complexity of business transactions between family members, the complexity of family dynamics, and financial transactions. A functional family would consider the contractual safeguards of the financial transaction as normal and necessary; a dysfunctional family would confuse family relationships with financial issues, and in this confusion, when matters turn out in a disadvantageous way, the family dynamics become more painful for all (Rodriguez et al., 1999).

JM pointed out that in terms of Ms. D's psychopathology, Ms. D tends to make decisions impulsively and without considering all the implications first. She seems to have difficulty staying with the uncertainty of certain important moves in her life and to prematurely rush into decisions. This has been her pattern with her higher education, with her employment, and finally with the business transaction with her brother.

JM then focused on the difficulties that Ms. D had at work. The doctor explained that, on the one hand, she was restricted in taking work because of her status as a bankrupt person but that the matter of not taking on so much work as her peers was seen and commented on by her colleagues. They were accusing her of not sharing the workload fairly. The doctor informed JM that Ms. D had been discharged from bankruptcy in 2017. JM then asked for clarification if Ms. D was entitled to be allocated work like that of her peers from that year. Although Ms. D was entitled to undertake this work, she had not been allocated such work. JM asked if she had approached her seniors with this issue, asking them to allocate to her the similar range of work now that she was discharged from bankruptcy. The doctor responded that Ms. D had not undertaken such steps. JM asked for the reasons why she had failed to bring this matter to her seniors when this source of frustration was an important contributory factor to her becoming mentally unwell. JM suggested that Ms. D assumed that if she stated the claim for something that is legitimately hers, this would lead to a confrontation, which would be damaging to her. With this appreciation, she avoids taking steps that would improve her predicament. Ms. D did not think that highlighting her concerns could lead to a resolution and to an improvement of her life at work.

JM then asked the doctor about her understanding of the source of this pattern. The doctor responded that the early family experience was one in which if she made a request, this would be followed by conflict and destructive arguments. Resolution of arguments in a constructive way was not something that Ms. D was able to experience in her family when she was developing. JM pointed out that the doctor had identified the source of this dysfunctional pattern of relating. JM then pointed out that Ms. D was no longer a child dependent on her family but an adult with an independent job and an independent source of income.

There was also the possibility that Ms. D "felt" that she was given less work than she should and was able to carry out but that it was possible that Ms. D was not eager to undertake a heavier workload.

JM also pointed out that Ms. D had several adult capacities such as a good intelligence because she had been able to enter university. She could use her good adult mind to address her current issues in a more constructive way than she does at present. JM also pointed out that the feelings that Ms. D currently has about her family, and particularly about her brother, are based on factual inter-actions. Her feelings are not only historical but also contemporary because her brother has used her to get a loan that he is refusing to repay. This is an issue that she can address constructively as an adult who is equal to her brother. In Ms. D's case, the feelings of being hurt and possibly sad and angry are a natural consequence to the treatment she received by her brother in relation to the finan-cial transaction and not some neurotic symptom that arises from internal psychopathology. What would be therapeutic for Ms. D is to be supported emotionally so that she can relate to the members of her family in an "updated" way, like an adult to other adults and not an outdated way of being a child with older parents and parental figures. JM pointed out that there is no doubt that the brother behaved inappropriately by withholding the loan and by failing to repay it as it was agreed (US$200 a month). Although this failure to repay was not her doing, it was up to her to take constructive steps if this financial conflict was to be constructively resolved.

JM then asked the doctor how the department was intending to help Ms. D adopt the attitude of an independent 30-year-old woman so that she could tackle the issues that confront and will confront her in a constructive way. The doctor suggested that a first step would be to help Ms. D realize that avoiding issues was not something that was helping her. She needs to be clear that by attempting to avoid difficult issues she is only creating more difficult emotional and practical situations.

The second step in her therapy would be for the therapist to help her think through the consequences of actions and of inaction. JM responded that the issue between emotions and cognitions is relevant in this case because how Ms. D feels, influences how she thinks. In more specific terms, her emotions stop her from thinking through how she will address important issues in her life. JM pointed out that the presence of a therapist would enable her to use her intellectual ability when she feels emotionally sup-ported by their presence. Being emotionally supported would enable her to think more thoroughly and more constructively. JM repeated that a psychiatrist is well placed to offer a combination of emotional support and a prompt so that Ms. D can think her issues through to a constructive conclusion.

JM then highlighted the difference between *communication* and *negotiation*. Ms. D first needs to be helped to communicate, which is an exchange of information, but this will not be enough to bring about change. That exchange needs to be followed by negotiation, which has to do with transactions and factual measures taken. Work allocation at home and at work, financial transactions, and method of repayment of debt are examples that need to be negotiated and not just communicated about. JM pointed out the need for emotional support from the therapist so that she is enabled to carry out both the communication and the negotiation necessary for her improvement.

JM then pointed out that a therapist could encourage her by pointing out the realistic change in her situation: She is not a child dependent and relatively less able than the rest of the family; she is an adult who has a good (adult) mind and has the means to support herself independently. This would be empowering and encouraging for Ms. D.

Reference

Rodriguez, S. N., Hildreth, G. J., & Mancuso, J. (1999). The dynamics of families in business: How therapists can help in ways consultants don't. *Contemporary Family Therapy, 21*(4), 453–468.

6
Anxiety

Ms. G

Presenting condition

Ms. G was recently hospitalized on account of anxiety, low mood, and the suicidal idea of jumping from a height. Ms. G is a 20-year-old single woman who lives with her parents and a younger brother and who is studying for a high diploma since 1 year ago.

History of present complaint

Ms. G experienced low mood in the last 2 weeks because she felt that her classmates had started to boycott her and to gossip about her. She felt uncomfortable about their facial expressions. She felt scared and rejected when classmates told her that they did not want her to stay in their group for the year's final project. She tried to join in with other classmates but got rejected by them as well. Ms. G felt upset because she felt that she had done a lot to help her friends in the past, but she still lost their friendship. She felt distressed because she perceived that they had been expecting her to do and know about everything and to help them out.

  Ms. G felt abused by her family. She felt low in self-esteem and ruminated whether she had done something wrong. She pondered why her classmates would criticize her, but they would immediately reject her when she criticized them. She felt tired and frustrated. She enjoyed watching YouTube music videos. Sleep and appetite were maintained. There was no perceptual disturbance. One day, prior to admission, she still felt low in mood, blank, helpless, and thought of jumping from a height while she was staying at the seventh floor of her school, after a further rejection by her classmates. She called her parents and shared her feelings with them. She eventually gave up the idea of suicide after talking to them. The school social worker suggested that she should attend the accident and emergency department and postpone school.

Dynamic Consultations with Psychiatrists: Understanding Severely Troubled Patients, First Edition. Jason Maratos.
© 2022 John Wiley & Sons Ltd. Published 2022 by John Wiley & Sons Ltd.

Family history

Ms. G's younger brother suffers from depression and is on medication.

Personal history

Ms. G was born in the country and was brought up by her parents. There is a history of smoke inhalation and of a minor head injury when she was 8 years old during a fire accident. She came to the city with her family when she was of kindergarten age. Ms. G has one brother who is 5 years younger than she. Ms. G felt that her parents always favored her younger brother and that they had spoiled him; they kept praising him while they were criticized her for trivial matters. She was forbidden to dance and had other limitations put on her. Ms. G recalled that her mother became moodier and had stepped on her while she was on the floor after she had given birth to her younger brother. She felt that her younger brother was spoiled and had become easily irritable toward family, scolding her and using foul language, kicking the door when others were using the washroom, throwing things at home, etc.

Physically, Ms. G has history of complex partial seizures for which she had been on treatment for several years; treatment was discontinued in 2013 and she remained seizure free.

Ms. G studied up to Form 3 (age 15). She often got bullied and teased for having pimples and poor communication skills. She did not attend school for 1 year; this was following an agreed-on decision among her, her parents, and the school. The following year, in 2017, she took a part-time job and then studied for a diploma. Ms. G still had some disputes with her colleagues at her place of work (she worked as a sales assistant), after she told them to work harder and got scolded back.

Ms. G is single and not in a relationship. She is a nonsmoker, nondrinker, does not use illicit drugs, and has no forensic record.

Past psychiatric history

Ms. G presented with on-and-off low mood related to interpersonal problems. She felt boycotted and bullied by classmates at school. This condition was worst in 2011 and was attributed to poor relationships with her classmates; her mood was pervasively low for a year, with decreased sleep and appetite, anhedonia, social withdrawal, hopelessness, and fleeting suicidal ideas. She did not attend school for 1 year. Ms. G has been known to psychiatry since 2012. A previous psychiatric admission was for 1 month in October–November 2016, for low mood and suicidal ideas (to jump from height); this was attributed to disputes with classmates. The diagnosis then was of an adjustment disorder in a person with limited intelligence (FSIQ 70–76) and epilepsy. There is no history of other deliberate self-harm. Ms. G was seen by a psychologist for counseling. She is not on psychiatric medication, has been working part-time, and is trying to save money for a concert. Her mood was grossly stable.

Present treatment and management of case Ms. G was thought to suffer from an adjustment disorder with the differential diagnosis being between recurrent depression and anxious personality disorder.

The scenarios that led to her feeling rejected by others were explored as was the way she came to such conclusions and whether there were alternative explanations about others' behaviors or of her facial expression, their likelihood, her feelings, and coping strategies. Therapy with formal cognitive behavioral therapy (CBT) or psychodynamic psychotherapy was considered.

Consultation

JM thanked the doctor for the thorough presentation and then proceeded to query Ms. G's intellectual assessment. JM asked that if her IQ was indeed in the region of 70 to 76, how did this girl manage to attend school until the age of 15? A person with an IQ so well below the average would be expected to have serious difficulties in learning and to stick out as different from her peers. JM also asked how she, with such limited IQ, attend for a diploma. The doctor doubted the validity of this measurement and thought that Ms. G may have underperformed because of her emotional state. JM counterproposed that a psychologist would have detected that and would have stated some reservation about the validity of their findings. The uncertainty about Ms. G's IQ implied that if valid, then she had been put in a setting in which she will fail and, therefore, will have other difficulties as a result. If her real potential is above 70–76 and that the difficulties and the underperformance are a result of emotional or relationship difficulties, the whole approach will have to be different. In either case, this question needs to be thoroughly resolved. JM then asked if there was any information about Ms. G's school performance over the years. The doctor responded that Ms. G was performing within the average range. JM commended that if a girl of below-average ability performs at an average level, then this implies that she was performing at a level way above her potential. In any case, one needs to have a valid opinion of her actual intellectual potential.

It was not clear whether the diploma that she studied for was an appropriate form of education for somebody with an IQ of 70–76. The same issue was reiterated that if it was above her potential, then by enlisting this girl for that degree one may be setting her up to fail and would be responsible for bringing about all the adverse emotional responses that she has experienced.

It seemed essential to provide Ms. G with some guidance in the form of either educational or career so that her education and her expectations for a career are appropriate for her intellectual capacity. JM then pointed out that only if she is given a realistic education and career guidance can she be given a chance of succeeding and, as a result of this success, can she begin to build a positive view of herself.

JM then pointed out the relevance of a major difference between her IQ and that of the people around her. JM suggested that friendships are usually formed among people of similar educational or intellectual potential. If she is placed with other young people who are much more able than she is, she will inevitably compare herself with them and find herself to be not only less able but also less desirable. She will not be able to keep up with the more able peers and many social difficulties will complicate and aggravate her mental health.

Such a mismatch between her ability and that of her peers could account for a large part of the bullying and isolation (or scapegoating) that she has been subjected to.

JM then asked if she was treated less favorably by her parents not only because she was not a boy, like her brother, but also because the parents sensed that she was not as able as he is.

JM then, in discussion with the doctor, clarified that Ms. G's first experience was of being not wanted largely because she was female. That was her first experience of being found to be not good enough and to be rejected or, at least, not to be loved as much as her male sibling. The doctor clarified that Ms. G remembered her life changing when her brother was born. That was the time when her parents became more rejecting and critical of her. That was also the time when she was subjected to the physical abuse of being "stepped on the floor." JM then suggested that the attitude toward her that she was not good enough antedated the birth of her brother and was only aggravated by the birth. The attitude about having a girl existed before the boy's birth. Ms. G remembered the discriminatory way in which she and her brother were treated. He was indulged, and she was overcriticized and abused. If her brother was of average intelligence, which means higher than hers, this would complicate matters even further for her.

JM suggested that the first therapeutic task would be to help this young woman formulate and establish a healthy, realistic, and positive view of herself despite the limitations that she may have.

The doctor responded that the line of approaching therapy would be to try to identify these with her the strengths that she has. Such strengths are that she is hardworking, empathetic, is willing to help others, and is generous toward others. Furthermore, Ms. G has a good degree of resilience, persistence, and tends not to give up easily. She is kind and thoughtful of other people. JM responded that these were realistic, genuine, and positive characteristics that would help her form a view of herself of which she can be proud. Ms. G can feel good about herself for having these characteristics.

JM then asked how Ms. G is going to be helped to have a positive view of herself when her ability is below that of most people. The doctor responded that if she is guided toward a job in which she can succeed, she can feel proud of the success that she has made. JM pointed out the difference between the satisfaction that one derives from work and the sense of pride that one gains from doing a job well. The former has to do with implications on the mood and the latter with implications on the self. Although these two are connected and one influences the other, it is useful for them to be considered separately. JM then offered a simplistic example that could be considered in her case and that was that she may be a failure as a university lecturer but be a success as a hairdresser. This would enable her to have a positive approach to her limited ability. JM then suggested that the sense of pride is related to Ms. G's expectations. If her expectations are realistic, she is likely to succeed and, therefore, is likely to derive a positive view of herself. If the expectations are above (or even way below) her potential, then the result would be dissonant, frustrating, and the basis of a constellation of dysfunctional emotions.

JM then pointed out that the original expectations are influenced by parental expectations. Even if parents have average expectations this would be inappropriate to a child who has below-average potential.

JM then addressed Ms. G's need for security. He pointed out that if she has the expectation of doing a job that is appropriate for her ability, then that will mean that she will be able to earn a living, support herself, and form relationships as an equal partner. This will reduce her sense of insecurity and increase her ability to tolerate frustration and some of the inevitable rejections that she will encounter in her life. As a result, she is less likely to feel desperate and less likely to be preoccupied with suicide or self-harm-harm.

This case raises several issues related to disadvantageous discrimination: The first is against those of the female sex and the second against the less able. The literature is wide-ranging, and it is not possible to recommend one publication that does justice to all aspects. The selective termination of pregnancies with female fetus, the discrimination against women at work, and the pay gap between men and women for the same jobs are well established facts supporting this view. Discrimination against the less able is less well researched. The publication by Scott (1994) addresses some issues relevant to this young woman and others in her predicament.

Reference

Scott, S. S. (1994). Determining reasonable academic adjustments for college students with learning disabilities. *Journal of Learning Disabilities*, 27(7), 403–412.

Sally

Presenting complaint

Sally is a 42-year-old primary school teacher and single mother presenting with anxiety and shortness of breath.

History of the present condition

One day in mid-July 2019 when she was waiting for her daughter, who was having a swimming class, Sally experienced a sudden onset of vertigo on the street. She also experienced chest discomfort, generalized tremor, and shortness of breath. Her mother was with her at that time. No apparent psychosocial stressors were identified. Since that time, she has been experiencing shortness of breath and chest tightness whenever she felt the urge to take deep breaths. Such feelings occurred around the clock, and she was quite distressed. She was admitted to a private hospital with investigations including a computed tomography (CT) angiogram, which was normal. She consulted another general practitioner who gave her alprazolam and flupentixol/melitracen (Danxipress). In August, she went to the accident and emergency department presenting with the same symptoms. A chest x-ray was normal and she was given a salbutamol puff; this brought about no improvement.

In these 1 to 2 months, Sally had been anxious with a low mood and with marked concerns about her health. She wanted to find out the cause of her shortness of breath, which could not be identified. Sally lost her appetite and lost 10 pounds. She slept poorly at night. Her motivation and energy level were very low. She could no longer enjoy reading and listening to music. She had social avoidance and stayed at home lying in bed most of the time. It was the summer holiday and she did not need to work. Her mother would bring her downstairs for a daily stroll, which she was able to maintain. Housework and childcare were carried out by a domestic helper. She had no abnormal beliefs or perceptions. She had neither negative cognitions nor any suicidal ideas.

After the start of school term, Sally could not resume work. On September 6, she attended the clinic for a follow-up with her mother and agreed to hospital admission.

Family history

There was no family history of mental illness.

Personal history

Sally was born in the country in 1977 and came to the city when she was 1 year of age. She was the second child of her parents and has one older brother who works in the country and is distant to her. She reported having a happy childhood. She had a good relationship with her parents. Her mother was dominating. Sally attained a master's degree in education and worked as a primary school teacher teaching the local language since graduation. She had been in her current school for more than 10 years, and she coped well all the time. She reported herself as having a carefree personality. She enjoyed reading and listening to music.

Sally has had one courtship. She met her then-boyfriend during a trip in the country at age 21. They had a 10-year long-distance relationship. She had an unplanned pregnancy at age 32 and gave birth to a daughter who is now 9 years old. Her mother strongly opposed this relationship and finally Sally broke up with him. She brought up her daughter with the help of a domestic helper. She had been secretively meeting her former boyfriend occasionally in the country after the breakup without her mother's knowledge.

Sally lives with her daughter and a domestic helper in a public housing unit, and her parents live upstairs. Sally is a nonsmoker and nondrinker. She has no history of substance use.

Past medical and psychiatric history

Sally has had a good physical health.

Sally was known to the private mental health service after childbirth when she was diagnosed with depression. She started being followed up in the public mental health service in 2014. She had a regular clinic attendance and was mentally stable. She had been maintained on risperidone 1 mg nightly, mirtazapine15 mg nightly, lorazepam 2 mg nightly, and zopiclone 7.5 mg nightly as needed. The regime was continued from the private service. She had good compliance.

Present treatment and management   Sally was admitted to the psychiatric ward on a voluntary basis after the clinic consultation. The purpose of hospital admission was explained to her, namely, to observe her physical symptoms, to adjust medication, and to receive inpatient clinical psychologist consultation. In the ward, Sally did not experience any shortness of breath. She was able to talk and breathe normally. She was asked to chart her breathing difficulty on a scale of 0–10. It decreased from 2 on admission to 0 the next day and maintained 0 marks throughout her stay. She was calm and settled. Her mood was not overtly low in the ward. Her medication was revised to ease her anxiety and improve her sleep. Risperidone was switched to Quetiapine 25 mg nightly. Lorazepam was tapered down to 0.5 mg nightly and clonazepam was added and then tailed down to 0.25 mg nightly. Mirtazapine was kept.

A clinical psychologist saw her twice. Health anxiety was elicited: She was worried she may have the symptoms again, her parents would be worried about her, and her health would affect her family financially. There was no catastrophic thinking noted. She was thought to be suffering from a panic attack in July followed by anxiety and hypervigilance to breathing. The case conceptualization was shared with her, a stress-coping strategy was explored, and diaphragmatic breathing relaxation was taught. However, internal inconsistencies were noted during the consultations, namely that she denied work stress at first, but on concluding, she stated that she had much stress about taking sick leave. Her answers had been brief and nonelaborative. Finally, the case was closed with her agreement.

Sally demonstrated quite a drastic improvement in mood, somatic symptoms, and sleep shortly after admission, and she soon requested discharge home to resume work. Yet, when discharge plan was laid out, she exhibited ambivalence and requested to postpone it. She agreed to take a rest on discharge and was granted a few more days of sick leave. She was discharged from hospital on September 19.

Sally attended the clinic with her mother for follow-up on October 4. She reported deteriorated mood with more anxiety, tiredness, and poorer sleep shortly after discharge. There was no recurrence of shortness of breath or other somatic symptoms. She could not resume work. She went to see another private psychiatrist and was prescribed some more benzodiazepines, but she could still not sleep after taking them. She had been extending the sick leave with the help of the private doctor. On observation, she was anxious but able to maintain good eye contact and attention throughout. Her mother was worried and asked the case doctor to adjust medications for her. She wanted to extend her sick leave.

Conceptualization was once again shared that she suffered from anxiety and that she had an avoidance pattern that further perpetuated her anxiety. She was advised against use of excessive benzodiazepines, which did not seem to be effective, and could give her paradoxical agitation, long-term dependence, and memory impairment. She was encouraged toward behavioral activation (i.e., to start with simple tasks first, for example, in preparation of teaching materials). She was offered follow-up in 2 weeks' time.

Consultation   JM thanked the doctor for the thorough presentation. The doctor mentioned that Sally would come to the appointments with her mother and her mother did the talking and not Sally. The relationship with the dominating mother had not been explored adequately. JM then focused on the dysfunctional nature of the relationship of mother and daughter. JM pointed out that it was unusual for a woman of her age to have to hide her relationship with her boyfriend from her mother. JM pointed out that the enmeshment (Barber & Buehler, 1996) between mother and daughter is not only historical but is current. JM suggested that Sally's feelings toward her mother must be mixed and ambivalent. On the one hand, she appreciates mother's support and presence, but on the other, she may have some negative feelings about mother's intrusiveness, domination, and control. The doctor added that she was impressed by how compliant and obedient Sally had been toward her mother.

JM then commented that Sally did not seem to have moved from a childhood dependence on her mother to an adult dependence. JM pointed out that for a woman in her late 60s, her mother is approaching the age when the balance of care will be shifting and instead of mother caring most for daughter, there would be an increasing need for the daughter to care for her mother. The balance of dependency will shift. For Sally, to care for her mother, will be difficult because her mother tends to be domineering. JM pointed out that Sally was still functioning as primarily a daughter of her family rather than an independent young professional that she is. It seemed quite clear that Sally needed to renegotiate her relationship with her mother.

JM then asked the doctor to expand a little on Sally's teaching experience. The doctor responded that teaching did not seem to be difficult for Sally and that she seemed confident about her work. In view of this, JM asked further if there was an understanding of why Sally would be avoiding return to school. The doctor responded that Sally was afraid that if she had one of these episodes of panic, she would not have been able to cope in the classroom. JM summed up that Sally was suffering from chronic anxiety with exacerbations in panic.

JM then asked about the detailed history of the original panic attack in July 2019. The doctor responded that Sally was walking in the street with her mother going to pick up her daughter from a swimming lesson. The doctor said that there were no obvious precipitants. Despite the doctor's efforts, it was not possible to reach an understanding of what precipitated the first panic attack. JM then asked if there was anything in the interaction of mother and daughter that could have contributed to that attack, but this was not possible to establish. The only precipitating factor was the concern that Sally had that she was suffering from a physical condition. This concern persisted even after she was thoroughly investigated and was found to be physically well. JM then suggested the possibility of this fixed idea, which was against all evidence, of being a delusion and that Sally may be suffering from a hypochondriacal delusion.

JM asked if Sally had an explanation of why she was well in hospital and why she did not have any of the anxiety symptoms or the discomfort that she had experienced outside. The doctor replied that this had not been explored with her but felt that the absence of attacks was because Sally felt more secure and better looked after in the ward. JM pointed out that hospitalization is a complex experience. One component of this experience is that by being in the ward Sally was away from her mother. Sally's anxiety is not made better by her mother's presence. The doctor added that her mother seemed anxious as well. JM returned to the issue of enmeshment and how mother's and daughter's anxieties can be exacerbating each other's feelings. It would be useful to get Sally to reflect on how she manages at school not to have any anxiety attacks and why the anxiety attacks take place mainly when she is with her mother. JM then returned to the issue of mother-daughter enmeshment (Barber & Buehler, 1996; Lonardo et al., 2009; Werner et al., 2001). Sally felt "stuck" in that relationship because, on the one hand, she loved and was dependent on her mother but, on the other, she was controlled or dominated by her. She could not distance herself from her mother because of her love. JM also suggested that Sally was probably thinking in absolute terms in the sense that you either comply and obey your mother or you cut yourself off from her completely. Sally seemed not to have in her mind the notion that relationships change with age and that they do so through a series of small, negotiated steps. Sally will need to be helped to renegotiate her relationship with her mother so that it is maintained but also changed to be appropriate for Sally's age and development. JM pointed out that it seemed that renegotiation would be difficult without an external mediator. Sally has a difficulty of doing that with her mother, and her mother seems particularly set in her own ways. From this thesis, JM suggested that it would be useful for Sally to receive some individual help by the psychiatrist in relation to how she could renegotiate her relationship with her mother and then the same psychiatrist could see mother and daughter jointly to mediate so that the relationship can develop in a more functional way.

The impact of parent–child relationship in cases such as Sally's has been explored in a study by Parker and Lipsombe (1980). Those who are interested in a deeper understanding of attachment and dependency can read Mary Ainsworth's chapter (1969) on the subject.

JM then discussed the notion of adult dependency and adult independence. A child is dependent on their parents and has no control and no choice of who they will depend on. This is not only necessary for survival but also because the power differential between adults and a, say, 2-year-old is enormous. Adults also need to depend to other people but need to do so in a different way. Adults can *choose* who they depend on, for what, and for how long. They are free to engage and depend in a relationship under these parameters, and they are also free to bring the relationship to an end. Any adult relationship that has the characteristics of a child–parent relationship is bound to be dysfunctional.

References

Ainsworth, M. (1969). Object relations, dependency, and attachment: A theoretical review of the infant-mother relationship. *Child Development*, 40(4), 969–1025.

Barber, B. K., & Buehler, C. (1996). Family cohesion and enmeshment: Different constructs, different effects. *Journal of Marriage and Family*, 58(2), 433–441.

Lonardo, R. A., Giordano, P. C., Longmore, M. A., & Manning, W. D. (2009). Parents, friends, and romantic partners: Enmeshment in deviant networks and adolescent delinquency involvement. *Journal of Youth and Adolescence*, 38(3), 367–383.

Parker, G., & Lipscombe, P. (1980). The relevance of early parental experiences to adult dependency, hypochondriasis and utilization of primary physicians. *British Journal of Medical Psychology*, 53(4), 355–363.

Werner, P. D., Green, R. J., Greenberg, J., Browne, T. L., & McKenna, T. E. (2001). Beyond enmeshment: Evidence for the independence of intrusiveness and closeness-caregiving in married couples. *Journal of Marital and Family Therapy*, 27(4), 459–472.

7

Agoraphobia

Ms. E

Presenting complaint

Ms. E is a 38-year-old woman presenting with agoraphobia.

History of the present condition

The present condition is one of agoraphobia, which existed since early in 2017. The agoraphobia related to Ms. E's feeling of being unable to escape. At that time, the diagnosis of depression was considered. The agoraphobia was also related to some overvalued ideas of reference. The present episode seems to be associated with a loss of a friend who went to live with her own husband. Ms. E believed that other people called her "ugly, fat, and arrogant" and she hears all these comments when she is on her own outside of her house.

Personal history

Ms. E is a 38-year-old woman who lives with her father, aged 77; with her stepmother, aged 47; and with her sister. Her mother died in 2002.

Ms. E reported that when she was at primary school she was subjected to sexual abuse by a stranger; it was a one-time even. She did not disclose the abuse at the time because she was afraid of the consequences, which appeared to have no significant results.

Ms. E developed a second personal relationship which lasted 8 years. She felt guilty that she was not able to go out with her boyfriend on dates because she had to stay at home to look after her father. Ms. E is a Christian and has church friends who visit her at home.

Ms. E took a part-time job at a school but agreed to leave it and to take it up again after she improved with therapy.

Past psychiatric history

Ms. E became unwell following a fallout with her boyfriend in 2001. She was then prescribed Seroxat. She promptly improved and later became elated. Ms. E reentered the mental health system in 2003 with an admission to the hospital following work stress. The presenting picture was that of agoraphobia.

Her mood had been low since 2013 following another breakup with her boyfriend at the time.

During her childhood, she had developed absence epilepsy, and this was documented by electroencephalograms. These were considered to explain episodes of possible mutism. During such episodes, Ms. E believes that she was laughed at by her classmates and by her family. These symptoms improved over 3 years.

There is a past medical history of asthma.

Family history

There is a family history of depression; her brother suffers from it.

Present treatment and management   At the beginning of her therapy, Ms. E felt that the ideas of reference were real and objective, but since starting therapy, she has gained some insight that these experiences may be creations of her own imagination. Ms. E had devoted her life to looking after her father even though her father was married to a young woman. His wife (her stepmother) was going to work, and she (Ms. E) looked after her father.

The therapeutic contract involved short-term cognitive behavioral therapy of 14 sessions with the objective of correcting the cognitive distortions and working with the fixed objectives.

Consultation   The issue of whether it is acceptable in the prevailing local culture for a daughter to look after her ailing father, even when he has a competent and young wife, was considered. It was later clarified that Ms. E's life had been dominated by her father's illnesses and by her own agoraphobia. When her father was in the hospital (in an orthopedic unit), there was an opportunity for Ms. E to show some psychological improvement, but this opportunity had been lost. Since the time of his discharge, it was Ms. E who had to take her father to outpatient appointments.

Ms. E was giving in to her difficulties and accommodating them instead of addressing and overcoming them. She had decided to sacrifice her life for her father, and she had given in to agoraphobia and to other cognitions. This pattern led to a vicious cycle in which the sacrifice for her father and the agoraphobia led to the deterioration of her mental state, which then made her less able to pursue realistic and constructive goals for her life.

Therefore, the aim of therapy should have been not so much to offer support but to give her the opportunity to use the therapy to gain hope for the future that would encourage her to address her difficulties instead of accommodating them.

Points of Interest
Diagnosis   There was a need to reexamine the diagnosis of bipolar disorder on the basis that:

a.   the onset of the present condition followed a dramatic life event,
b.   the response to treatment was prompt on onset of treatment and before the antidepressant effect was due to take place,

c. the clinical picture was not a comprehensive picture of a depressive illness and the absence of biological criteria stated in the diagnostic and statistical manual, and

d. Ms. E tended to improve with support and deteriorate with further losses (or adverse events).

The possibility of a Borderline Personality Disorder was considered, and in addition to the depressive symptoms, there were transient phenomena that are normally associated with psychosis (such as auditory hallucinations).

Cultural dimension   Ms. E presented as a dutiful daughter who gave up important aspects of her life (work, peer relationships, intimate relationships, etc.) to look after an infirm and deteriorating father who was married to a young and able wife.

Although some care of a needy father is expected in the city culture, the same culture would not expect a child to sacrifice their life when their parent had a competent partner. This is valid even within the country culture of two generations ago and the city culture of the present time.

Interaction between cultural and personal pathology   Cultural expectations of a child looking after a needy parent is inappropriately distorted in Ms. E's case, so that it fits with Ms. E's individual psychopathology, which is influenced by her conviction that she will fail in whatever action she undertakes. With this present hopelessness, she tends to avoid tasks instead of addressing them and resolving and overcoming difficulties and problematic situations. The difficult situations were those that emerged in the school setting and in the "agora."

Interaction between physical and psychological parameters   Absence epilepsy (of which she had outgrown), a condition over which the subject is indeed helpless, has contributed to the feeling of helplessness when Ms. E was at a vulnerable young age. The misunderstanding of its nature by teachers and fellow pupils at school further traumatized Ms. E's value of herself. One consequence was that she felt that she would burden her last relationship, which she broke off out of concern for her partner. This consultation highlighted the interplay among social, cultural, personal biological, and psychiatric factors in promoting a vicious circle (or a vicious spiral) that led to (and can lead again) to complete dysfunction if not addressed properly.

How does the analysis inform the therapeutic intervention?   This young lady will need a combination of support and interpretative psychotherapy. Ms. E needs the support of an available person (like a counselor because she has limited support in her own life). Ms. E responds well to support and collapses when support is removed.

Psychotherapy needs to be offered in addition and not instead of support, and it needs to contain cognitive and emotional elements. Ms. E could be helped to see herself in a more realistic way (that she is a young, healthy, able, caring person etc.—a list of her real positive attributes) and, therefore, one who has the potential to build a good life for herself. Ms. E needs to regain a realistic hope for her future. Based on this hope, she needs to be encouraged to address her difficulties instead of avoiding them. Avoidance not only leaves her problems unresolved but also makes her life worse (as is the case with her agoraphobia and the teaching). Ms. E needs to learn that she can still be a good dutiful daughter without sacrificing her life. She also needs to regain the sense that she can be a good lover and wife if she invests some energy in the hopeful prospect of sorting out her social anxieties.

8
Obsessive-Compulsive Disorders

Mr. A

Mr. A is a 19-year-old single student with an associate degree, living with his parents and younger sister in a public housing unit.

Presenting condition

Mr. A presented at the outpatient clinic of the psychiatric center with the complaint of repeated handwashing.

History of present complaint

When Mr. A was a Form 2 student, he started to have compulsive handwashing of about 20–30 times per day, whenever he touched something he believed that it was contaminated with bacteria or dirt. He worried that he would contract an illness, such as gastroenteritis or flu. He also believed that he could be responsible for family members' illnesses.

Each time Mr. A would rub his hands with soap twice, according to the handwashing technique as suggested by the World Health Organization (WHO). It usually took him 2 minutes, and his emotional distress would readily be relieved by this compulsive act. He could temporarily suppress this ritual with mounting anxiety and restlessness. The recurrent unwanted obsessive cleanliness was not imposed by external force, and he considered the repeated handwashing to be excessive and time-consuming. With time, he developed pain and dermatitis of his hands. Mr. A also followed specific rituals in taking showers. He divided the body into 10 parts, rubbed the body parts with soap, and rinsed them separately. His parents criticized him for using excessive amounts of water and soap. Mr. A denied a pervasive depressed mood or suicidal ideas. No psychotic experiences were reported.

In school, Mr. A had briefly learned about Obsessive–Compulsive Disorder (OCD). He was referred to the school social worker for anxiety due to study stress. The social worker suggested that Mr. A might suffer from OCD after he revealed a history of repeated handwashing. He briefly searched for

Dynamic Consultations with Psychiatrists: Understanding Severely Troubled Patients, First Edition. Jason Maratos.
© 2022 John Wiley & Sons Ltd. Published 2022 by John Wiley & Sons Ltd.

relevant information on the internet. He did not seek active treatment until he was promoted to an associate degree. He worried that the debilitating illness would reduce his ability to work as a social worker.

Family history

Mr. A had no family history of mental illness. His father, in his 50s, worked as an internal decorator, and his mother, in her 40s, was a salesperson working in a supermarket. His sister, 2 years younger than he, was a Form 6 student. All family members enjoyed good past health.

Personal history

Mr. A was born in the city. He had an unremarkable postnatal history, and his developmental milestones were normal. He described his childhood as normal. However, when compared with his younger sister, Mr. A had more frequent illnesses, such as gastroenteritis or upper respiratory tract infections, during childhood. His father commented that he was "ill-prone." When he was a Primary 6 student, Mr. A was bitten by a red ant, resulting in pain and swelling of his prepuce. He considered himself to be too careless and thought that he should bear the sole responsibility for the injury.

Mr. A reported good relationships with his parents and sister; he felt loved by them and there was no sibling rivalry with his sister. Mr. A did not feel that he could express his emotions to his parents. The doctor felt that this was not unusual in traditional country families.

Mr. A studied in a local secondary school up to Form 6. He enjoyed the school life. He got fair results in the city diploma of secondary education examination. He was promoted to associate degree at the university if the city, with social work as his major. He would like to work as registered social worker after graduation. During psychotherapy, Mr. A had enrolled into placement training in a nongovernmental organization.

Past psychiatric history

Mr. A was first assessed in the psychiatric center in December 2016 and was diagnosed with OCD. He was prescribed fluoxetine. However, he soon stopped taking this antidepressant because he was troubled by side effects such as oversedation and impaired concentration. There was no history of a psychiatric hospital admission. Mr. A had not reported history of substance or alcohol misuse.

Past medical history

Mr. A suffered from community-acquired left-sided pneumonia in 2015, which required hospitalization for 1 week. He was also weak in color differentiation. He was health conscious and often presented himself to various family doctors and traditional medicine practitioners for various physical discomforts. Mr. A is a nonsmoker and nondrinker. He has no history of substance misuse. He has no known drug allergy.

Present treatment and management of case   Mr. A is a small-built young man. He has satisfactory self-care and hygiene He was cooperative and polite. His mood was normal. His speech was coherent and relevant. He harbored obsessive doubts about cleanliness with compulsive checking rituals and handwashing. He had no psychotic features. He was not suicidal or aggressive. His insight was good, and he was motivated for treatment. He had mild hand dermatitis. He was diagnosed with OCD.

Mr. A was treated with a full course of cognitive behavior therapy (CBT) to which he responded well and was discharged having achieved 90% improvement.

Consultation   The present series of consultations are meant to focus on the dynamic understanding of the presented patients and for this reason, the discussion that followed focused on the dynamics of Mr. A's suffering without undervaluing the achievements of his previous therapy.

JM thanked the doctor for the thorough presentation and moved on to examine Mr. A's family relationships, particularly the way in which emotions were communicated with his parents. The doctor felt that this was an area that needed further exploration. JM then asked about Mr. A's peer relationships from an early age, such as those at primary school. The doctor replied that Mr. A did have friends and that he even had a girlfriend a few years previously. He used to play with his friends, and he also had some relationships with fellow church members. In fact, he was able to talk about his OCD problems with another OCD sufferer. JM asked further about the nature of his relationship with his girlfriend and the doctor felt that this was an area that required further exploration, even though Mr. A felt that it was "normal." JM concluded that Mr. A had a difficulty in expressing his thoughts about his relationships both within his family and outside, such as with teachers, fellow church members, peers, and his girlfriend. This was one basis on which his OCD developed, a difficulty in becoming aware of the substance of his relationships at many levels. Mr. A had difficulty in communicating about genuine feelings such as those of fear, anger, or love. He operates in a mechanical way and because of this he "gets lost." He loses out on the human dimension of his relationships. The treatment offered to him may have been on the same cognitive level, giving less attention and significance to his feelings and the human or emotional side of him.

JM then returned to complete some data about Mr. A's illness. It started 6 years previously (2011) when he was in Form 3 at school and was 13–14 years of age. JM tried to obtain more information about the degree to which his OCD had interfered with his life. The doctor mentioned that Mr. A had been able to continue with his studies at college (he had not dropped out) and maintain his relationships with peers and fellow church members. It became clear that Mr. A had managed to live a fairly "normal" life despite his OCD.

JM diverted the focus to other aspects of Mr. A's life, but the responses were frequently in terms of his OCD. This reflected Mr. A's preoccupation with OCD rather than the other aspects of his life. This tendency deprived him of the opportunity to address his life issues more creatively or constructively. The doctor added that Mr. A had been an "average" student, and he was not at risk of failing at college. Despite his OCD, Mr. A was living a full and satisfying life. He is building up his career. He aspires to become a social worker. OCD had become a major part in defining his identity. Mr. A was reluctant to explore the more human side of his life because his sense of who was he directly linked with his OCD. His obsessions had become his identity. This was confirmed by the doctor who added that Mr. A felt that he had been "born" to be an ill person; he was born with inadequate immunity and a tendency to develop more illnesses than his siblings or peers. It was made clear that Mr. A views himself as a sick person. Mr. A held on to this belief despite a health track record that is no different from that of his peers or siblings.

Mr. A is heterosexual, but the doctor was not aware if Mr. A was active in searching for a girlfriend or if he felt the lack of one. JM asked about Mr. A's sexual life because this was an area that needed further understanding to know more about his sexual emotional world, his fantasies, his relationship with women in his course or the church, and his sexual activity.

It seemed that Mr. A tended to revert to talking about OCD whatever the subject was, and this led to him remaining static or returning to the same known themes and stopped him from moving forward to examine other aspects of his identity (his sense of self—of who he is), other aspects of his sexuality, and of his relationships with people. If he is to be liberated from this repetitive and stagnating pattern, he needs to be helped to explore his life as a human, as a whole, and not only as a sufferer of OCD. JM expressed the view that Mr. A may have some important difficulties in the area of relationships and in the field of his identity of his self-value that could be worked with to his advantage. It is possible that in a context where emotions were not acknowledged or explored, the early illnesses that he suffered gave him the feeling that he is vulnerable to illnesses that fed his compulsion to handwash. This traumatic view of himself dominated his existence and defined his identity.

Those interested in the psychoanalysis of OCD may start by reading Freud's account of treatment of two cases with the condition, who later became known as the case of the Wolf Man (Freud, 1955a), and the Rat Man (Freud, 1955b) even though many reservations have been expressed about the value of these cases in current treatment. These papers are more interesting as historical documents than as aids to present treatment.

A more contemporary point of view can be found in Kempke and Luyten (2007) because integrates elements from classical psychoanalysis with cognitive theory and behavioral approaches.

References

Freud, S. (1955a). The case of the wolfman. In *The standard edition of the complete psychological works of Sigmund Freud. Vol 17: An infantile neurosis and other works*. Hogarth Press.

Freud, S. (1955b). *The standard edition of the complete psychological works of Sigmund Freud. Vol. 10, Two case histories: (Little Hans and the Rat man)*. Hogarth Press.

Kempke, S., & Luyten, P. (2007). Psychodynamic and cognitive-behavioral approaches of obsessive-compulsive disorder: Is it time to work through our ambivalence? *Bulletin of the Menninger Clinic*, 71(4), 291–311.

Miss F

Presenting condition

Miss F is a 42-year-old single unemployed woman; she is currently living with her elder brother in a village house. She was admitted from the orthopedics and traumatology department for obsessive behavior, which caused significant impairment of her daily functions.

History of present complaint

Miss F. presented in the current episode with symptoms that had persisted for many years. She had been repeatedly washing her hands, having prolonged baths, and spending an excessive amount of time in cleaning her room. These behaviors were out of a belief that she would contaminate others if she was not clean enough.

Miss F was able to cope with these symptoms because she used to be taken care of by her mother. For example, her food was prepared, and housework was done by her mother or a maid. This was no longer the case after her mother died late in 2016 and no one else took up the responsibility of taking care of her. The functional impairment related to these symptoms, therefore, had become more prominent since that time.

On a typical day, Miss F would spend 1 to 2 hours on washing her hands, washing the toilet, and tidying herself in the morning. She would then eat prepackaged food with the need to wash her hands again after eating. Afterward, she would spend several hours tidying her room. If she had any free time left, she would watch videos from the internet. She was only eating biscuits or bread after her mother died because no one was there to prepare food for her. Miss F is slightly underweight. She avoided taking a bath because it would take her from half a day up to 2 days every time to take a shower; she would only bath when she felt she was dirty and then only have a bath about once a month. She also only went out once a month to buy daily necessaries and prepackaged food to sustain her basic needs.

Miss F carried on living in this lifestyle for several months. Eventually her poor personal hygiene and possibility of malnutrition lead to bilateral lower limb cellulitis. She was admitted to department at the orthopedic and traumatology department in May 2017 and she stayed there for 1 week. She was discharged with antibiotics, and it was suggested that she should have regular wound dressing in general outpatient clinic. However, she was only able to attend the clinic twice. She defaulted because she spent too much of her time performing washing and cleaning at home and was not able to get out of her flat. Her cellulitis recurred, and she needed to be admitted to orthopedic and traumatology department again. After learning about her mental condition, an admission to the psychiatric hospital was arranged.

Family history

Miss F has an elder brother who is suffering from schizophrenia and is currently living in a private hostel and under regular psychiatric follow-up. Otherwise, there is no other family history of Obsessive-Compulsive Disorder or of mental illness.

Personal history

Miss F was born in the city and is the 6th of eight siblings. Her parents both died. Her father passed away more than 10 years previously and her mother died in 2016. She described her mother as critical of her, and she recalled being tied up and hit with wooden sticks with her siblings during childhood. Miss F felt that her parents tended to compare her with other children. She felt they had high expectations of her; for example, they expected her to have a profession in the future. Her parents often blamed her for being lazy and incompetent and rarely praised her. She was previously educated up to Form 5 level and had poor academic results; she failed all subjects in open exams. She recalled that when she was young, her eldest sister often hit her when she sought her sister's help for her homework. Miss F recalled episodes of her sister hitting her head, slapping her face, and raising her temper at her. She had worked on and off as a clerk, and her longest employment lasted for more than 1 year, but eventually she gave up because she disliked working in an office. Miss F became unemployed at the age of 23–24. She is currently living with her elder brother in a village house owned by her family and is relying on the savings that she inherited from her late grandmother. She is neither a smoker nor a drinker. She had no history of illicit substance use or any forensic record. She described her premorbid personality as oversensitive and prone to anxiety.

Past psychiatric history

Miss F was known to mental health services in 2005 when she was diagnosed with Obsessive-Compulsive Disorder. She was reported to have had the onset of mental illness in 2003 during the epidemic of severe acute respiratory syndrome (SARS). She recalled numerous news and advertisements advising the public to clean their hands to prevent transmitting diseases to others. She started to have a fear that if she did not clean her hands well enough, her hands would contaminate others. She worried that others would get infected, become sick, and might even die from it. She then started to have repeated handwashing behavior, and she soon needed much more time in washing hands and bathing. She also started to clean everything she had touched with the fear of having physical contact with others. The whole situation eventually progressed to the need for locking herself inside the toilet because she spent too much of her time cleaning herself and the toilet; this also prevented contact with any other person. She received food only if it was given to her by her mother through a slip at the door. Eventually she was brought to the hospital in 2005 by police when the community psychiatric team visited her. She was given selective serotonin reuptake inhibitors and was subsequently discharged after a short stay. Her condition had improved with fewer obsessions toward performing her cleaning task, and she was able to attend follow-up regularly for 3 years. However, she eventually defaulted because she felt the medication was not useful for her condition, and there was a recurrence of her difficulties in going out of her home.

Present treatment/progress   Various antidepressants had been given to Miss F, augmented with anxiolytics or antipsychotics, but she showed a limited response only. One difficulty in selecting medication for her is that she was sensitive to medication side effects, and it was difficult to achieve a therapeutic dose that she could tolerate. In addition to the pharmacological management, she is currently seeing the clinical psychologist from the hospital and attends the rehabilitation service by occupational therapist and nurses. Her condition remained suboptimal, and she still reported a frequent compulsion in handwash. She also reported episodes of compulsive counting at times, which caused her great discomfort and distress. The plan will be continuing medication and psychological treatment and to look for a suitable supervised environment for her in the long run.

Consultation   JM thanked the doctor for the thoroughness of the presentation. He then pointed out that this woman who was so preoccupied with cleanliness would go for a month without a bath. The doctor explained that if she started a bath, then she felts compelled to continue with it for, sometimes, up to 2 days. This makes her reluctant to start the process of having a bath, and this is why sometimes a whole month lapses before she has one. JM then asked about the general state of the house, and the doctor's response was that it was "reasonable." JM then asked how the cellulitis was related to poor hygiene. It was clarified that the cellulitis was related to poor bodily hygiene and not necessarily to the state of the house in general. JM then restated the paradox that somebody who is so preoccupied or somebody for whom cleanliness is so important would neglect their own bodily hygiene. Miss F was claiming that she would only have a bath when she found the dirt on her body intolerable.

JM then asked if Miss F thought it "reasonable" to wash her hands for such a long period of time. The doctor responded that it was not clear whether Miss F considered handwashing essential part of hygiene or whether she thought it was an unnecessary act. JM pointed out that on this point rests the differentiation between a delusion and an obsessive thought. An essential element of an obsessive thought or of an obsessional compulsion is the conviction that the acts are unnecessary. If a person believes that they are still dirty and that they need to wash for 2 hours to be clean, then this thought is more akin to a delusion. The differentiation will influence the diagnosis and, therefore, the appropriate psychiatric and pharmacological treatment (O'Dwyer & Marks, 2000).

JM then suggested that the psychopathology of Miss F is more akin to one of delusion than to a simple obsessive thought and compulsive act: Miss F is convinced that she would infect other people if she did not continue washing for this length of time. Her thought does not seem to be amenable to change through argument. It is as fixed an idea as a delusion. JM pointed out if this is the case, the diagnosis needs to move on from that of a borderline disorder to a psychotic disorder.

JM then suggested that it is not only the psychological approach that needs to be different—in the sense that you do not expect conversations or discussions to affect fixed ideas. The general approach, including medication, also needs to be considered differently, because of treating a psychosis rather than a neurotic condition. JM pointed out that the presence of schizophrenia in Miss F's brother would make the psychiatrist more mindful that she may have elements of that disorder herself.

JM then moved to considering the nature of Miss F's psychosis. The differential diagnosis would be between that of a depressive psychosis and a schizophrenic psychosis. What would help in deciding the diagnosis would be deeper understanding of the content of her delusions as well as her other thoughts about herself and her environment. It would be useful to understand the contradiction that she lives with, which is that she neglects her body hygiene but is overexercised by her hand cleanliness. JM suggested that this is some of the work that needs to be carried out with Miss F in the next stages of her treatment.

JM then moved to the fact that her current treatment is being more or less dictated by Miss F's psychopathology. It is established that she cannot function normally in her own environment and that she poses a risk, at least, to her physical health. Miss F can only function safely if she lives in a context in which there are other people (professional or not) who can keep an eye on her and help her limit the compulsive behaviors. The recent experience has been one of discharging her to her home and then having to readmit her, and it is highly likely that the same pattern will continue, possibly with each admission requiring more drastic interventions. Miss F will require the services of a rehabilitation setting (possibly rehabilitation ward) and antipsychotic medication as well as occupational therapy. JM pointed out that although a dynamic understanding may be helpful, one should hold back from approaching this lady with deep interpretations that would only unsettle her in this fragile state of mind.

In a rehabilitation setting, Miss F will be given the opportunity to interact with other people—something that she lacks in her natural environment. She would not only be in a safer environment but in an environment that promotes her rehabilitation, her return to a better level of functioning, and that would safeguard her health (reduce the risk of reinfection).

JM then addressed the issue of causation of Miss F's condition. He felt there were no significant elements in her early history to justify a psychological onset of her condition at this age. Furthermore, there is a definite family history of schizophrenia, which indicates that there may well be a hereditary element in her condition. JM then expanded on the benefits of a therapeutic environment such as the opportunity to learn to live with and to enjoy the interaction with other people, the ability to develop a sense of perspective for her future, and to limiting of unnecessary compulsive behaviors. Although it is unlikely that she would be able to form an intimate personal relationship, she may well be able to coexist with other people either in some social, sheltered, or working environment.

Reference

O'Dwyer, A. M., & Marks, I. (2000). Obsessive-compulsive disorder and delusions revisited. *The British Journal of Psychiatry, 176*, 281–284.

9

Emotional Dysregulation

June

June is a 54-year-old divorced woman (born 1963). She works as a real estate agent and lives alone in a public housing unit.

Presenting condition

In March 2017, June accidentally came across a friend of "the man." She kept asking the friend where she could find him. She developed unstable emotions, sudden onset of headaches, dizziness, and a hand tremor. She feared she was going to die. She also recognized the need to seek help, so she attended the accident and emergency department. Voluntary admission to the psychiatric hospital was arranged on the same day.

Personal history

June was born in the country. She came to the city when she was 19. She is the eldest of four siblings. She has a good relationship with her family. Her sisters used to listen to her advice because she was the eldest daughter. Two of her younger sisters live abroad. One of them lives in the city. June has regular contact with her mother and sisters. Her father died in 2016 from a physical illness.

Educational and vocational history   June received her education in the country. She came to the city after graduating from secondary school. She became a housewife after getting married at the age of 22 (in 1985). She started working as a real estate agent in 1998 when she was 35. She changed to different real estate agencies over the years due to conflicts with her superiors or clients. However, she had a successful career with a stable financial status.

Medical History   June has good past health. She never smokes or drinks alcohol.

Dynamic Consultations with Psychiatrists: Understanding Severely Troubled Patients, First Edition. Jason Maratos.
© 2022 John Wiley & Sons Ltd. Published 2022 by John Wiley & Sons Ltd.

Relationship history   June married in 1985 when she was 22. Her ex-husband was an engineer. They have a 31-year-old son who works as a director and a 28-year-old daughter who works as a nurse. She had a good marital relationship. She described her ex-husband as loving, loyal, and supportive. Their marital relationship turned sour when she started having gambling problems. She was in debt for a few hundreds of thousands of US dollars. Her husband settled the debt for her. She had a lot of guilt toward her husband and children. Eventually the couple divorced when she was 35. She gave up the custody of her children because she could not support them financially. The couple still had feelings for each other after the divorce. They continued to live together. Her ex-husband planned to send their children abroad to study so he asked her to sign a document giving consent so their children could leave the city. She also signed another document giving up her right to the alimony so her husband could have more money to spare for their children's education. In 2003, she discovered that her ex-husband had a 17-year-old girlfriend in the country. She confronted him, and he said he needed to find someone to fulfill his sexual desires. She felt betrayed and devastated. On the other hand, she felt guilty that she tore the family apart. She attempted suicide by drug overdose in reaction to her ex-husband's "love affair." Eventually, she convinced herself that she should let go because the breakup was her fault. She remained single for years because she did not have the courage to start another relationship. Until recently, she had been keeping a wallet her ex-husband had given her.

Past psychiatric history

June has been known to the mental health service since 2003. She was admitted to the psychiatric hospital after a suicide attempt by drug overdose in reaction to her ex-husband's love affair. The impression was that she suffered from an adjustment disorder. She failed to attend psychiatric follow-up since 2004. The follow-up records were not available. She suffered with low mood and insomnia over several years. She consulted private practitioners for insomnia and was prescribed hypnotics. June bought over-the-counter hypnotics to promote sleep as well. She took up to two tablets of hypnotics every night. She had episodes of irritability and scolding her colleagues and even clients. Despite these episodes, she was able to maintain her job.

June met a client at work in March 2014. He was a married, African American man whose family was abroad. She reported being raped by the client when her colleagues and she were viewing an apartment with him. She dared not tell anyone about the incident because she was afraid that she would be "judged." She was raped again on another occasion when she was getting a document for the client at her office. She later confided in a colleague who was close to her. The client then pursued her, and eventually they developed a romantic relationship. The client borrowed money from her many times, adding up to more than US$10,000. She discovered that by the end of 2015, a sum of US$50,000 had been transferred from her into his account, but still he didn't pay her back. She was disappointed and upset about it. She also found out that he had other girlfriends. She called him repeatedly and confronted him about the money. Eventually, the man blocked her on all the messenger applications.

Her mood deteriorated a lot with frequent crying spells. Her appetite was poor. She had a weight loss of 20 pounds over 3 months. Her sleep was also poor. She used to take three tablets of over-the-counter hypnotics to promote sleep. She lost interest and volition in her daily activities. She felt tired during the day. She was unable to concentrate at work. She did not have feelings of hopelessness and helplessness because her children were supportive. She harbored fleeting suicidal ideas, but no attempts or plans were made. No perceptual disturbances or abnormal beliefs were expressed. She attended the accident and emergency department on February 2017 twice for "unstable emotions". The consultation liaison psychiatrist assessed her. The impression was that she suffered from a mixed anxiety and depressive disorder and from hypnotic abuse. Fluoxetine 20 mg daily was started. Ativan was prescribed on an as needed basis. She was referred to the local psychiatric center. The new case appointment was scheduled for December 2017. June was diagnosed with a moderate depressive episode.

Consultation

JM noted that this was thorough assessment and concise and asked what the doctor's understanding of why June was so unhappy.

The doctor responded that the formulation of this case was discussed with their supervisor. Her broken marriage made her vulnerable to her future relationships because she was afraid of getting disappointment and decided to stay single. Also, she tried to present herself as being tough on the outside while she remained fragile inside. She said she had a poor life and I think she meant that she felt lonely. This broken marriage was later horrible, and this new relationship happened at a time when she felt she should try something new and move on from her past relationship. However, she didn't really work it through but tried to get on by taking on more work. The failure of this new relationship brought on more unhappy feelings.

JM noted that the first point is that June is lonely and asked what are the other things that make her unhappy. The doctor replied that she knows that she cannot find "the man," she is trying to make contact with him, but he never replies. She feels betrayed and angry.

JM responded then the second element of her unhappiness is anger. Has she also lost hope that she will ever have a relationship with the same man? Does she still want a relationship with the man who stole US$ 50,000 from her? The doctor replied that she is unsure on this point because she fears that the man will never treat her right again, but on the other hand, she feels that they may "just be friends."

JM asked so, the same man who stole US$50,000 from her is the man who raped her—is that right? The doctor replied affirmatively.

JM asked how she developed a relationship with the man who raped her? The doctor said that he tried to ask her the same question; she said she tried to keep a distance from him after the rape happened because she was afraid it would happen again, but the man pursued her in an intense way so she felt that someone "is caring about me." She felt this was a good feeling, so she changed her mind.

JM noted that there is a need to understand how June went from being abused to wanting to have a relationship with her abuser. We do know that this happens: Abused women do maintain relationships with their abusive partners, and we do know that many people seek to maintain relationships with people who abuse them and who are even physically violent to them. So there is no doubt that it happened and happened in this case, but it needs to be considered how June feels and why she allowed these painful events to happen. What does she feel about her own worth to allow herself to be abused both sexually and financially?

The doctor responded that this is due to a blow to her self-esteem. So JM inquired what her self-esteem was. She views herself as a substandard person. When she was growing up, she had many difficulties. Her first marriage did not turn out well, but she is grateful that her children are still supportive and loving toward her.

JM observed that somebody who has a solid self-esteem does not allow themselves to be abused sexually and financially and still seek a relationship with that person. If a person values themself and somebody abuses them, they become angry; they take the abuser to court; they seek retribution against the abuser; they seek restoration from and perhaps punishment of the abuser. I expect that if someone does something improper toward you, I expect you would be furious; you would want them to apologize, to make a reparation, and not to repeat the same behavior. Further, you are unlikely to say, "you abused me now let's be friends."

JM suggested is that her self-esteem will need to be reexplored. It is good that you have taken her on for therapy because many things have happened to June without her understanding why they did. She is right to be so unhappy; she is lonely and abused, and unless she changes her tactic, the future does not look good for her. On the other hand, she is an able woman, not at the end of her career, is in her 50s, and can rebuild her life. She is young enough to have a new relationship with another person, and she does have a good relationship with her children. So, there are many positive things about her. But with a person who feels that it's OK to be abused, that it's OK to be taken advantage of, and who does not have a significant sense of worth and self-respect, traumatic events are likely to happen again and again. For example, why does she not take legal action against this man who owes her so much money? She is not owed a negligible amount. The doctor replied that she has been thinking of taking legal action now. It is hard to define whether the money was given to him as a present or as a loan.

JM asked if she does not think she has a legal case or if she had sought legal advice. She discussed it with her children, but she has not taken any action. JM observed that his is a half-hearted approach. It is not a person who feels: "I have been wronged; I do not deserve to be treated like this." June's view of herself is of someone who is at fault and not worth respecting. Perhaps reexploring how that rape happened: was it a violent assault or was it something into which she was pressured or seduced? I don't expect you to know the answer to this now, but it would be useful to explore this further. From the limited information that we have, it seems that pressure was exerted, and she was seduced and pressured into consenting to a sexual act even though it was against her wishes. In this way, you will find that she is vulnerable. If one's starting point is that you do not think of yourself as a worthy woman as a sexual being and you find somebody who does want you sexually, you are more inclined to succumb to this seduction. If, on the other hand, you feel that you are a worthwhile person, you do not allow people to abuse you. If somebody approaches you with a proposal for a sexual relationship, you set the conditions and insist that you form a relationship first and, if this relationship is satisfactory, then you include a sexual aspect to it. You first insist on forming a relationship in which mutual respect is a central point. It is a woman who has damaged self-esteem (for whatever reason, and in this case, we are not sure what caused the damage) who allows damaging events to happen to her.

I would have thought that the first thing one would do in therapy was to help her regain a sense of self-worth. I think it is fortunate that her therapist is a woman because as a woman, you can talk about empowerment of women. I know that there is sometimes a sexist element in the therapeutic relationship and to hear a professional woman tell her that she is also a woman with a profession (she is an estate agent) with the ability to earn money, who can stand on her own two feet, is an intelligent and healthy woman, who has been a good mother, whose children love her, and she can have a full life. There are good things about her that she needs to be mindful of, so she does not feel completely worthless.

If she regained her sense of self-worth she is more likely to become better at protecting herself, and she will be better at managing relationships. It is going to be difficult to help her rebuild her self-esteem because she has made some important mistakes, and these mistakes would understandably undermine her self-esteem. You cannot give her a false reassurance by telling her things like, "you do not need to worry; everyone loses a million in gambling." If you are to maintain credibility as a therapist, you need to help her develop a realistic and balanced view of herself. "Yes, you have made mistakes; let us understand how you allowed yourself to make these mistakes, but the mistakes are not all there is about you. There is another side of you that is both worthy and able." "Worthy" so that she does not feel demoralized and "able" in a realistic way as she does have several abilities both as a person who works but also as a person who relates. For example, if her children have done well, that must be partly a credit to her. If her work has earned her some money, that must also be partly a credit to her. If she has friends, that must be also partly a credit to her because other people must consider her worthwhile to be their friend. One needs to find real things that are solid and positive about her. Then we need to work at understanding her negative aspects.

It would be worthwhile to find out how she managed to gamble away hundreds of thousands of dollars. What was the emotion that was driving her to persevere with the gambling when she was losing this enormous amount of money? We do not know, but I imagine that it is connected with having a massive gain that would give her a sense of significant security and worth. She could be thinking that, "if I am a billionaire, I am somebody." The extra money would be necessary for her to restore her sense of self-worth. We cannot be sure about this now; this is only an idea worth exploring with her. It would be worthwhile exploring the reason why the relationship with her "good husband" broke down. What went wrong?

The doctor replied that it had to do with her gambling. Partly it was the gambling and partly the emotional relationship between them, and this is something I will need to have to go into. JM noted, as you say, it is important to understand better how she handled the relationship with her husband. It is also worth exploring and understanding further how and why they lived together for 2 years while they were divorced. The situation must have been strange for both. Did they have a sexual relationship in these 2 years? Were they sleeping in the same bed even though they were divorced?

The doctor replied that was not asked about. JM said that it would be useful to find out. She said that she was feeling betrayed when, while they were divorced, her husband had a relationship with another woman. It is not really betrayal if two people are divorced and live separate sexual lives. Therefore, they were not properly divorced or at least that she was not emotionally divorced from her husband. She had not clearly separated emotionally from him; she was still attached to her ex-husband.

The doctor noted that even after the divorce she was still treating him as her husband. JM responded, so, psychologically, this was not a divorce. It would be useful to go one step further and explore why she was not psychologically divorced from her husband. What was making it so difficult for her to separate emotionally from the man who did not feel that he should be her husband anymore? We do not know how her husband dealt with what must have been a big problem—her gambling. How did he deal with his wife spending a so much of the family resources? Unless they were multimillionaires, the lost sum is not negligible. One has the impression that the couple did not thoroughly deal with emotional aspects of their actions. Certainly, she does not thoroughly explore her feelings about actions, and, instead, moves on to the next step without exploring or resolving feelings. In this way, she accumulates traumata—one trauma on top of the other. The doctor said that they didn't even touch, but she is still thinking of him a lot.

JM observed that many aspects of this woman's psyche were explored in 20 minutes and that he hoped this discussion has given some direction on which to follow in sessions June. I am warming up to this woman. I am thinking: "poor thing." How come this woman who had everything going for her ended up alone, unmarried, abused, and at risk of ending her life? This is a sad story. The optimistic thing is that she is young, healthy, intelligent, and has a profession. She also has some support from others. The doctor noted that June is trying to find some answers and that is why therapy will help her.

Summary

A middle aged woman with many positive attributes who lived through a vicious spiral of her actions that worsened her predicament and who was subjected to abusive and exploitative relationships (see, Leung, 2019; Wong et al., 2016); a vulnerable sense of self-worth was further undermined, and this weakened her ability to restore her sense of self and her trajectory in life. A psychiatric (multimodal) approach will address not only her illness of "depression" but also give her an opportunity to restore a realistic sense of self-worth, which will give her a better opportunity of restructuring her life.

Since discussing this case, JM searched the literature on intimate partner violence (IPV). Although this woman was not "violated" by a man with whom she had a relationship, she did wish to develop a romantic relationship with her abuser. It is therefore justifiable to consider her as a victim of such violence. There is an excellent review of the literature on the subject (Ades et al., 2019; Dillon et al., 2013). One sees that there is a good description and analysis of consequences but little information about women who engage in such relationships. The present case gives a glimpse of this area, which seems neglected in the scientific literature.

References

Ades, V., Goddard, B., Pearson Ayala, S., & Greene, J. A. (2019). Caring for long term health needs in women with a history of sexual trauma. *British Medical Journal*, *367*, l5825. http://dx.doi.org/10.1136/bmj.l5825

Dillon, G., Hussain, R., Loxton, D., & Rahman, S. (2013). Mental and physical health and intimate partner violence against women: A review of the literature. *International Journal of Family Medicine*, *2013*, 313909. http://dx.doi.org/10.1155/2013/313909

Leung, L. C. (2019). Deconstructing the myths about intimate partner violence: A critical discourse analysis of news reporting in the city. *Journal of Interpersonal Violence*, *34*(11), 2227–2245.

Wong, J. Y., Tiwari, A., Fong, D. Y., & Bullock, L. (2016). A cross-cultural understanding of depression among abused women. *Violence Against Women*, *22*(11), 1371–1396. http://dx.doi.org/10.1177/1077801215624791

Marie

Presenting complaint

Marie is a 55-year-old divorced, unemployed woman who presented with low mood, anxiety, and poor sleep.

History of present condition

Marie attended a follow-up appointment in September 2019. She reported that her condition had been similar to the previous consultation. She had constant right-sided body pain with numbness, weakness, and spasm; this had significantly affected her mood and sleep quality. She felt anxious most of the time in fear that her pain could be exacerbated at any moment. She also reported "flashbacks" of the image of her finger being trapped at the lift door; this was related to an injury she had sustained almost 5 years previously. She would startle when these images appeared. Apart from flashbacks, she also reported nightmares of a similar theme, which make her sleep mostly interrupted and shallow. She mostly stays at home now because she feels the need to take a rest with a hot bath when her pain is intense. Marie is able to attend follow-up, if required to, but tends to avoid the lift door; she either takes the stairs or faces inward if she takes the lift. She showed low mood and hopelessness toward her pain. She felt guilty, blaming herself for the accident. She had poor concentration and most of the time she ruminated on why the accident happened to her. She had vague suicidal thoughts, which are mostly transient when she was in pain. She had no self-harm behavior or a concrete suicidal plan.

Family history

There is no family history of mental illness.

Personal history

Marie was born in the country. She is the eldest of six siblings. Her father died in the 1990s after a cerebrovascular accident. Her mother and siblings currently live in the country. She was educated up to senior secondary school level in the country. She came to the city in 1987 with her grandmother and worked as a factory worker until she got married at the age of 29 in 1991. She had been living with her mother-in-law and her husband. The marriage "went sour" in 2010 when her husband had an extramarital affair. She divorced him and started to live alone in a public housing unit. She worked as a waitress in a restaurant until she suffered an injury on duty in 2014. She is unemployed and relies on social welfare. She is visited and supported by a friend regularly. She has maintained regular contact with her family who also visit her at times. Marie reported that she was an optimistic and cheerful person before the accident. She is not a drinker or a smoker. She had no history of substance abuse or a forensic record.

Past psychiatric history

Marie first presented to mental health service in August 2016. She reported recurrent nightmares, flashbacks, startle response, and anxiety symptoms since suffering an injury at work in November 2014. In that incident, she had her right ring finger trapped at a lift door of a small lift used to transfer dishes within the restaurant. As a result of the accident, she suffered trauma to her right ring finger soft tissue and a muscle tear to her right shoulder. The pain had gradually spread from her right arm toward her whole right side. She also started to feel numbness, weakness, and spasm that had progressed throughout the years. She had seen a pain team about her pain and was prescribed opioid analgesics; these were repeatedly prescribed, and a ganglion block was carried out in 2016. She had been followed-up by physiotherapists, and alternative medicine practitioners had tried some alternative treatment. However, her painful condition had not improved, and most treatments only provided temporary relief.

Marie had regular follow-up by the psychiatric outpatient clinic since her first presentation in 2016; she had been admitted once in April–July 2017 for low mood and vague suicidal thoughts. In addition to medication, she had received follow-up by our clinical psychologist with eye movement desensitization and reprocessing (EMDR) during her inpatient stay. Her symptoms had improved partly when she was discharged, but her condition had never achieved complete remission. Thirty sessions of repetitive transcranial magnetic stimulation (rTMS) were carried out in October–November 2018 on the basis that the symptoms may be related to a depressive illness. This led to a temporary and partial improvement.

Marie had a history of a traumatic right temporal subdural hematoma, which required decompressive craniotomy with clot evacuation and subsequent cranioplasty in 1999. Following this, she developed long-term right-sided hearing impairment and transient left-sided hand spasm with left-sided leg numbness. A magnetic resonance imaging (MRI) of the head and neck region in 2007 showed cervical degenerative changes. She had no known history of allergies.

Present treatment and management   Marie will continue with regular follow-up (appointments every 2 weeks) at the psychiatric clinic and will receive clinical psychologist support. Her pain condition is followed up by the pain team and a physiotherapist.

Consultation JM congratulated the doctor for the thorough assessment. JM then inquired about how Marie acquired the brain injury. The doctor replied that this was caused by an accidental fall not related to work. JM then asked about the recovery following the operation, and the doctor added that she had right-sided hearing loss that was not causing her any difficulties, but she was also left with some left-sided hand spasm, which persisted for several years. Then the doctor added that the cervical spinal changes were not severe. The doctor clarified that there was no association between Marie's current symptoms and the degenerative changes in her cervical spine.

JM then asked for clarification if Marie's main complaints were physical and not related to her emotional state. Marie saw her emotions as consequent to her physical complaints. JM then focused on Marie's function. What impaired her function, according to Marie, were the physical complaints. The doctor added that whenever interventions offered to her, like physiotherapy, she would decline, claiming that her pain and the spasm made it impossible for her to attend, and this was because when the symptoms emerged, she needed to go home and have a warm shower. Marie even found it difficult to attend outpatient appointments, thinking that she would be lost about what to do if the pain emerged because she would not be able to have a hot shower to ease her symptoms. The doctor clarified that a hot shower reduces her pain and numbness. The shower also makes her calmer and less agitated.

JM then asked the doctor to what he attributed the physical symptoms. The doctor replied that the basis of these symptoms was Marie's emotions and not her physical state. JM then introduced the notion of a depressive equivalent (Lesse, 1968; Magni et al., 1983). In certain cases, a depressive illness does not manifest itself in the classical form but, with different symptomatology, such as in this case, physical symptoms. With children, adolescents, and persons with learning difficulties it can manifest itself with behavioral difficulties or other disorders. If this was the case with Marie, she should have shown some greater improvement with the antidepressant treatment such as with the rTMS. Marie had also been treated with antidepressants, but her response was limited and variable. JM then summed up the case as that of a 55-year-old woman who lives alone and has no children to support her. The doctor added that Marie still has connections with her work colleagues who used to visit her when she was in hospital. Marie did have a circle of friends.

JM then asked if Marie is continuously unable to function or if she has only periods of incapacity. The doctor clarified that Marie is not continuously in pain, and she is not continuously unable to function but only has periods of dysfunction and discomfort. The doctor clarified that there is a baseline of discomfort and pain that is low grade but has exacerbations that are incapacitating. Each exacerbation lasts for a few hours. The doctor clarified that Marie suffers these exacerbations daily and sometimes two to three times a day. JM commented that Marie is experiencing almost daily torture and wanted the doctor's view whether Marie appeared to him as if she is a woman who is under constant torture. JM wanted to confirm that Marie's presentation of her situation was exactly or similar to that observed by the nursing staff and asked about the nurses' and other staff observations during the period when Marie was an inpatient. It seemed that when Marie was an inpatient, she suffered less than the picture described by her when she was outside the hospital. The doctor attributed the improved clinical picture during the period of inpatient treatment to adjustment of medication and the EMDR. In response JM asked why, if the improvement was attributed to these therapeutic interventions, the improvement did not last. The safe conclusion would be that there were emotional contributions that led to Marie's improvement during the inpatient stay: the support of the staff and the work with the psychologist. A study of Marie's condition in detail points toward the emotional underpinning of her complaints, and this needs to form the basis of any psychological intervention.

JM pointed out that the psychotherapeutic treatment of psychosomatic symptoms is notoriously resistant to psychotherapeutic interventions. The prognosis of treatment of patients with significant somatic complaints that are of psychological origin is poor indeed. As a result, the therapeutic target with Marie should be support and gentle interventions rather than any deep and heroic attempts aimed at a personality transformation and a cure.

JM then pointed out that the work of the consultation is for the benefit of us gaining a deeper understanding and not for the application of it in any more dynamic sort of psychotherapy in every case. Our dynamic understanding will help us offer the treatment that is most appropriate to Marie, and the treatment most appropriate is the regular and not too frequent but mainly supportive psychotherapy. The fact that when Marie is supported suffers less is both evidence of the cause of her discomfort and, at the same time, a pointer toward the right treatment for her.

JM then explored other factors that may be contributing to Marie's continued suffering. He raised the possibility of compensation. The understanding is that compensation has still not been settled for years after the accident. Resolution of the compensation issue can only remove an uncertainty that is contributing to Marie's unsettled condition. JM clarified that he was not suggesting that Marie was pretending to be suffering to augment her compensation claim but that the uncertainty over the outcome was a contributory factor (Mayou, 1996; Miller, 1961, 1962). The relationship of this to her treatment is that it could be helpful if the psychiatrists or the hospital could intervene to encourage the prompt resolution of the claim. JM presented an overview that Marie had suffered a minor accident—a ring finger been trapped. This by itself would not normally justify incapacity to work, which would last for 4 years nor would it justify an escalation of symptomatology. It is uncertain why this initially limited injury would cause such major incapacity.

The consultation then moved to the matter of psychotherapy of this psychosomatic condition (Shoenberg, 2007). JM suggested that it is likely that Marie would feel resistant to talk about her feelings about the incident, her feelings about her employer, and what relationship she has with a solicitor and the advice that that solicitor is giving. JM pointed out that Marie is a relatively young woman with probably 10 or 15 years of working life ahead of her and that it would be extremely useful to her to have the compensation issue settled so that she can look forward to her life.

JM then addressed the issue of Marie's perception of the origin of her symptoms. He pointed out that it would be helpful to Marie to be reassured that the origin of her symptoms is not an illness that will be getting worse and not even a physical condition. The symptoms are real, but they are not the result of a physical condition that is incurable. That should give her some hope about her own future, which can only improve her mental state.

JM cautioned against challenging Marie's perception because such a challenge would make her see the therapist as somebody who does not understand her, is not sympathetic, and not on her side.

Finally, JM suggested that the appointments are not too frequent because these may encourage dependency of Marie to the doctor, and this dependency may contribute to her presenting with increasing number of complaints aimed, possibly unconsciously, at maintaining this dependent relationship.

As a last advice, JM suggested that the doctor should be mindful that they maintained the relationship at a strictly professional level. He pointed out that dependent patients often aim to change the relationship to a friendly, family, social, or even amorous one and that any shift from the strictly professional is definitely counterproductive for the patient and quite often for the therapist as well. The doctor needs to give the message that he is a person and a caring person but that their relationship can be most useful to her only if it is within the confines of a professional boundary.

References

Lesse, S. (1968). The multivariant masks of depression. *American Journal of Psychiatry*, 124(11S), 35–40.

Magni, G., de Bertolini, C., Aldrich, C. K., Florence, D. W., & Parris, W. C. V. (1983). Chronic pain as a depressive equivalent. *Postgraduate Medicine*, 73(3), 79–90.

Mayou, R. (1996). Accident neurosis revisited. *The British Journal of Psychiatry*, 168(4), 399–403.

Miller, H. (1961). Accident neurosis. *British Medical Journal*, 1(5231), 992–998.

Miller, H. (1962). Accident neurosis. *Proceedings of the Royal Society of Medicine*, 55, 509–511.

Shoenberg, P. (2007). Psychotherapy with psychosomatic patients. In P. Shoenberg (Ed.), *Psychosomatics: The uses of psychotherapy* (pp. 27–54). Palgrave Macmillan.

Cindy

Cindy, a 50-year-old single woman working as a security guard.

Presenting condition

Voluntary admission for unstable emotions and self-harming behavior of drug overdose with six tablets of Panadol and eight tablets of fluoxetine.

History of present illness

Cindy's mood had been mostly stable, and she could maintain her job as a security guard despite long-standing family problems. Her mood worsened late in May 2018 when she was diagnosed with eczema on her periorbital regions and neck. Her sleep and appetite worsened. She had poor concentration. She needed to make a great effort to cope with her job. She complained of easy fatigability. Cindy presented with no negative cognitions or suicidal ideas at that time. Her drug compliance was good.

Cindy's mood further worsened 2 days before the day of admission. She went gambling to relieve stress. She lost about US$3,000. She had no prior debt. Cindy became more agitated after having an overnight shift the following day. She had a temper outburst and threw books, newspapers, and paper boxes out of the corridor. She called her second elder brother and asked him to return home, threatening that she would burn the flat if he did not return home immediately. She also made a verbal threat of suicide. Out of impulse, she took six tablets of Panadol and eight tablets of fluoxetine in her room. Cindy left no suicidal note or plan. She denied informing anyone about the suicidal act beforehand. Her self-harm behavior was stopped by her elder sister, who brought her to the accident and emergency unit. Cindy was seen by the psychiatrist of the consultation liaison team who suggested inpatient management.

Cindy is a middle-aged woman of average build; she makes fair eye contact. Her mood is depressed and her speech is relevant and forthcoming. Cindy expressed negative cognitions of uselessness and hopelessness. There were no psychotic symptoms and no suicidal ideas at the time of admission.

Physical examination revealed an eczematous rash over the periorbital region and neck. She was clinically euthyroid and presented with no focal neurological deficit.

Cindy was thought to be suffering from a recurrent depressive disorder, with the current episode of moderate severity.

Family history

There is a strong family history of psychiatric illness. Her mother suffers from schizophrenia and has had psychiatric treatment; she committed suicide by overdose with Dettol in 2010. Her third elder sister suffers from depression and currently receives psychiatric treatment. Her second elder brother has severe hoarding problems (paper boxes and other objects), but he strongly refuses psychiatric assessment.

Personal history

Cindy was born in the city. She is the youngest of five siblings (one older sister and three older brothers). She described her childhood as unhappy. She had a distant relationship with her father because he spent most of his time working. Her eldest brother took up the parental role in family. He had poor temper control. There is a history of him beating Cindy with sticks when she was young, and it was felt that he was displacing his anger in this way. Cindy had a good relationship with her mother and elder sister, but she found they were too submissive and did not protect her from her brother. Cindy was educated to secondary level 5; her academic results were consistently poor. This was attributed to her lack of interest. Cindy is currently working as a security guard, a job that she has held for 5 years. There is no history of a courtship, and she has no forensic record. She lives with her second older brother and third older sister in a public housing unit. Cindy had longstanding family problems. She had a poor relationship with her second older brother who had severe hoarding problems. He refused to seek psychiatric help despite repeated advice from family members. Cindy and her older sister would avoid staying at home with him to avoid conflicts. In addition, she has recently been the only breadwinner in the family. She found this to be stressful and unfair.

Past psychiatric history

Cindy had been known to the mental health service since 2011. She presented with depressed mood after her mother committed suicide in January 2010. Cindy was then diagnosed with a mild depressive episode. She was well stabilized with fluoxetine 20 mg daily. There is no previous history of suicidal attempt or violence. There are no previous psychiatric admissions.

Cindy suffers from eczema, which is being treated by her general practitioner; the eczema affects her appearance and on her self-esteem; she thinks of herself as "ugly." There is no known drug allergy.

Cindy described herself as hot-tempered and impulsive. She has few friends. She tends to bottle-up her feelings. She observes no religion. She is a nonsmoker, nondrinker, and has no history of substance misuse. There is a history of gambling once in mid-2017 (when she lost US$1,000). Cindy claimed she then wanted to relieve stress arising from conflicts with her second older brother regarding his hoarding.

Present treatment and management   The purpose of admission was to titrate the dosage of fluoxetine to optimize her mental condition; to consult medical physician for treatment of eczema; to refer her to a clinical psychologist for anger management and poor stress coping; and to refer to medical social worker for family therapy.

Consultation   JM thanked the doctor for the thorough presentation who clarified that Cindy had been discharged on medication, that appointments with a psychologist had been set up. but the doctor was not certain whether she had begun attending those. Cindy would be followed-up at the psychiatric clinic.

JM invited participants to explore the reasons why living at home had been stressful for her. The brother's hoarding affects every room of the house and makes life for her unpleasant. JM expressed sympathy for Cindy's predicament who cannot afford to live in a separate flat and does not have any effective means of improving the home situation. The doctor clarified that every shared space in the house is affected by brother's hoarding. JM asked what her brother's likely response would be had she decided to clear the flat of his hoardings. This was not known. JM then asked if social services had been involved in this problem. The social services had been involved in trying to find a public housing unit for her, but this had not been successful. Because there is a great demand for public housing in the city, it had been impossible to provide a flat for her on her own. JM then asked if it would be possible for Cindy to share a flat with another person rather than her brother. The doctor responded that seeking a flat on psychiatric grounds would be "the last resort," and JM suggested that it was time to use this last resort. JM then suggested that it would be impossible to make someone feel contented with words and medication if their living environment is equivalent to a rubbish tip.

JM asked what the therapeutic aim could be and if she could be expected to learn to put up with this situation. Such an aim would be unrealistic in the sense that no person can be expected to be satisfied living in that situation. JM suggested that this was a deserving case for a woman who needs a different living environment, and this could be arranged either through finding a flat for her to share with another person or for the local authority to take legal action against the brother for causing this distress to his sisters. His motive may not be criminal, but his behavior is undoubtedly damaging.

JM then moved to another area of psychiatric concern for Cindy, which was that of her self-esteem. JM invited the doctor to consider her positive aspects, which she could base a healthier self-esteem. JM asked, "what would you say is that of which Cindy could be proud of?" The doctor responded that she could be proud of being the sole breadwinner for the household. JM accepted this was a major issue on which she could realistically be proud. She is supporting not only herself but also her two siblings. JM asked if Cindy was proud of her contribution, and the doctor responded that she was preoccupied with frustration and feeling of unfairness that she would have to do that. She was consumed by feelings of unfairness and that she had not even contemplated that she could be proud of her contribution.

JM stressed that it is useful to concentrate on Cindy's self-psychology separately from her relationship feelings. For example, she needed to give herself credit for her ability to support her brother and sister and to do so separately from the feelings of resentment for having been placed in that position. Cindy could be valued as a person who is able to work and who is able to support her brother and sister.

JM asked if there are other aspects of her life for which Cindy could be proud of, and the doctor responded that she could be proud of her good work record. She had kept the same job for 5 years, that she is appreciated at her work, and that she is a naturally hardworking person. JM highlighted the fact that Cindy could be proud of herself as a worker.

JM then asked about the feelings of her colleagues and seniors toward her. She had good relationships with her colleagues, and she had earned the respect of her seniors. The respect of the colleagues will be reflected in her own self-respect. The respect of the colleagues will enable her to develop he own self-respect.

JM then asked about relationships outside family and work, and it seemed that Cindy has few contacts outside those settings. JM then diverted the consultation to the issue of Cindy's self-view as a woman. The doctor responded that Cindy has not had any romantic relationships since she had been rejected by a boy at high school. Since that episode, Cindy became shy and expressed that she did not deserve to be in a relationship. Cindy based this view on her appearance, which she felt was "ugly" because of her eczema. Cindy had also expressed to the doctor that the eczema is not only on her face and neck but also on other parts of her body and that this was making her unattractive to men. Cindy takes extra care to cover her body even on warm days. It was not made clear whether on examination Cindy did manifest facial eczema, which would make her unattractive to look at.

The consultation then moved on to any possible historical reason why Cindy should feel herself to be so unattractive as to exclude any possible relationship with a man. JM pointed out that the attribution of 40 years of shyness and withdrawal to a single episode needs further understanding because most people experience an episode of rejection in their lives but not all of them develop in the same way that Cindy has and that there must be an additional reason why an event that is almost normal in somebody's life experience should take such deciding dimensions with Cindy. JM then focused on to the more realistic view of how married women look. Cindy thinks of herself as being unattractive, but there are plenty of women (and men) who would be considered unattractive but still enter romantic and even marital relationships. There are factors, other than appearance, that make two people decide to form a relationship.

Cindy had also negative thoughts about her age (she is 50). She believed that men would want only younger women, forgetting that there is not a glut of younger women who would happily pair up with an elderly man. If Cindy restored her self-esteem to a more realistic level (which is that she does have an unattractive facial characteristic—the eczema) and that she also has other characteristics that are she is hardworking, she is respected, she is able to support herself and others, that complete picture would be something attractive to many men, perhaps even of similar age to her.

JM then repeated the question of why her appearance and age are the deciding factors of her view of herself. JM suggested that it would be worthwhile helping her take a more global view of herself and with this to explore why she either did not take up opportunities to form a relationship with other people or why she did not even seek a relationship with another person. The appearance by itself cannot account for this behavior. Simply the appearance does not explain why she does not feel herself worthy to make somebody content to be connected with her or to be in a relationship with her, either in a romantic sense or in a sense of friendship.

JM then also added the impact of her poor educational achievement on her. There was a high possibility that she may think herself not only as unattractive and old but also as not clever enough. JM suggested that in a more careful exploration of her life one would find other realistically positive characteristics of her personality that she could be made more aware of and she could be encouraged to value them. For example, it sounded that she could be quite a caring person. This would be a strong positive realistic attribute. It is quite erroneous that she should write herself off as a potential partner because there must be men in their 50s or 60s who are available and who would benefit from a relationship with her. Unfortunately, she does not think that and she needs help to develop a more realistic view of herself. Cindy needs to be helped to learn to value herself for what she can realistically offer even though she does have eczema, is not young, and is not brilliant.

This case demonstrates the vicious circle in which a poor self-esteem leads to problematic interpersonal relationships and how the latter, in turn, can damage a person's self-esteem.

Mr. K

Mr. K is a 48-year-old, married, government clerical worker, who lives with his family in a self-owned flat.

Presenting condition

Mr. K was admitted from the outpatient clinic because of unstable emotions and the fleeting idea of burning his house.

History of present complaint

Mr. K is married and lives with his wife and two children (14 and 9 years old). He reported that his mood had become increasingly low over the last year when his wife suggested that they get a divorce. They have been married for 20 years and previously had a good relationship, but their relationship progressively deteriorated over the past 10 years due to conflicts over childcare and Mr. K's overspending.

Last year, Mr. K had the opportunity to receive housing allowance from the government because he had been working there for 20 years. They planned to relocate their family into a bigger house. Mr. K's wife went for a financial assessment, only to discover that Mr. K still had a debt of around US$30,000; this made them ineligible for housing allowance. Mr. K's wife subsequently expressed her wish for a divorce, claiming that he "had not done anything for their family over the years" and that she could no longer tolerate his overspending behavior. Since then, they have been sleeping in separate rooms, and their relationship has become distant. Mr. K was worried that he might say something that would further worsen their relationship.

In the past month, Mr. K suspected that his wife may be having an extramarital affair with her senior because he noted that she had started purchasing new clothes and fancy underwear and recently saw her buying a beautifully wrapped present that was not intended for him. He believed this affair was part of the reason why she wanted a divorce. His children had also started talking back to him and often took his wife's side in arguments. His 14-year-old son refused to live in their house and moved in Mr. K's mother-in-law's home because he complained that their home had become a "rubbish dump," cluttered with objects that Mr. K had bought over the years.

Mr. K's mood further worsened. He believed that he could not control his emotions and would cry at one moment, only to feel angry and irritable afterward. He also developed a fleeting idea of burning his house down because he believed this would solve all their problems and clear away all the "rubbish" that he had bought over the years. He denied any planning or acting. He denied having any recent overspending or expansive plans. Mr. K has obstructive sleep apnea but has not been using the machine for this purpose and has fair sleep. He denied hearing nonexistent voices or having other abnormal perceptions. He denied any actual violence toward his wife or children or any self-harm or suicidal behavior. He agreed to inpatient treatment to stabilize his mood.

Family history

Mr. K has no family history of mental illness.

Personal history

Mr. K was born in the city. He was the second of four brothers and reported he had felt inferior to his brothers as a child because they had better academic results. He was educated to Form 5, with below-average academic results. He felt scolded and humiliated by his teachers due to his poor academic performance. He also reported being bullied by classmates in secondary school "as he was quite chubby," and they would call him names and draw on his uniform. He had a good relationship with his parents; his elderly father had died about 10 years previously; his mother, who is Christian, used to take him to church when he was younger.

He had been working as a clerical worker in the government since graduation for about 20 years. He often experienced interpersonal problems at work and felt pinpointed by his supervisors who would ask him to work faster and who would pass uncomplimentary comments about his work.

Mr. K married his wife in 1998 after a courtship of 6 years. They were both Christian, but he reported that a pastor had once told him that they were not suitable for marriage because they had different personalities. They used to have a good relationship. Mr. K believed that his wife was "smarter" than him because she studied further and had completed a university degree. His wife also worked as a supervisor in construction and earned a lot more than him. He felt that since she obtained her degree, she started to spend less time with him and sometimes did not listen to him. Around 10 years ago, he started using a large proportion of his salary to buy things that he liked. He would buy expensive electronic items, cameras, and appliances. He could not control his spending behavior and accumulated debts of more than US$100,000. He was unable to contribute to their mortgage, could not support his own living expenses, and had to ask his wife for help. His wife started paying the mortgage and all the living expenses while he focused on repaying the debt. Their marital relationship worsened since then, and he felt his wife's family of origin also disrespected him and looked down on him. Last year, his wife filed for divorce and their relationship deteriorated further. Mr. K is a non-smoker and a nondrinker. He has no history of substance abuse. He has no forensic record.

Past psychiatric history

Mr. K had been known to the psychiatric service since 2011, when he presented with low mood and anxiety. He was diagnosed with a Mixed Anxiety and Depressive Disorder. He was started on antidepressant treatment. Since 2012, Mr. K was noted to be easily irritable and appeared overtalkative with overspending behavior. He was thought to exhibit risk-taking behavior (he tried to take the subway without purchasing a ticket). His diagnosis was revised to Bipolar Affective Disorder, and he was started on a mood stabilizer. His latest regime includes quetiapine fumarate 400 mg nightly, sodium valproate 1000 mg nightly, and alprazolam 0.25 mg twice daily as needed. He has no past psychiatric admissions.

Present treatment and management of case   Mr. K is thought to suffer from Bipolar Affective Disorder, with the current episode being mixed. Predisposing factors include low self-esteem, starting with a sense of inferiority since childhood when compared to his brothers, being scolded and bullied in school, and later being looked down on by his wife and his wife's maiden family. He also tends to bottle up his thoughts and feelings and did not know how to express his emotions to others. He has maladaptive coping through excessive spending, which led to deterioration of marital and family relationships. This current admission was precipitated by a further deterioration in his marital relationship. Treatment plan includes medication titration, referring to social services for marital and family counseling, and psychological treatment to increase his self-esteem and facilitate development of appropriate coping strategies.

Consultation   JM thanked the doctor for the comprehensive and succinct presentation. He then proceeded to ask why Mr. K and his wife got married. The doctor responded that the couple had met at church, they got on well together, and after 6 years of courtship they decided to marry. Furthermore, at that time, the couple had similar backgrounds and similar salaries. In the later years of their marriage, the wife was promoted to a job that gave her a much higher salary than that of her husband's. JM asked if it was not obvious from the beginning of their relationship that wife's intelligence was higher than that of her husband. It seemed that in the early stages, the couple were not mindful of the difference in their intellectual ability. Although it was obvious that Mr. K had high school results of below average and his then wife-to-be had above average this was not something that they considered in their decision to get married. The doctor pointed out that in the early phases of their relationship Mr. K was proud of his wife's ability but it was in the later stages of their marriage that the discrepancy in earnings and in career progression became an issue. It is relevant that the feelings about the difference in abilities were different at the beginning of the relationship to those of the more recent years. From the husband feeling proud of having a bright wife to then feeling inferior to her. Instead of being a collaborative relationship, it became an antagonistic one. The change was from Mr. K feeling proud and fortunate to have a smart wife to feeling inferior and was possibly envious of her. JM pointed out that there was no change in their respective abilities; the change was in their attitude toward this difference.

JM suggested that the feeling of inferiority and envy may have played a part in his overspending behavior. His overspending could have been a dysfunctional way of bridging the gap that he sensed and the feeling of inferiority that he felt. JM pointed out that it was possible that it was not only Mr. K who was feeling antagonistic to his wife but that his wife may also feel antagonistic toward him. JM suggested that it was possible that his wife may have moved in circles that were appropriate to her career trajectory and not easy to combine with his static and low-level work. The doctor added that she had spoken on the telephone with his wife and that she came across as caring and considerate. The doctor, quite appropriately, did not think it would be right for her to address the issue of her possible extramarital relationship over the telephone. JM asked if a professional had seen the couple. The doctor pointed out that a social worker had invited the wife to a meeting, which she had declined claiming that it was not necessary. His wife felt that it was not appropriate because she had already filed for a divorce and did not feel that working on the marriage was relevant anymore. The couple were still sharing a house, but they were sleeping in different bedrooms.

JM asked about Mr. K's attitude to the divorce. The doctor added that Mr. K felt "heartbroken" and that he wished there was a way to repair the relationship. In fact, he had been thinking of how to clear the house of all the unnecessary items that he had bought and had actually never used. In fact, Mr. K had drawn up a list of a number of actions he could take to improve the relationship, but his wife believed that this was already too late. JM pointed out that Mr. K had not accepted an important fact in his reality, which is that the marriage had ended and is irretrievably broken. Mr. K lives in a fantasy world where he believes that the marriage can be salvaged despite all the evidence pointing to the contrary. This could be one of the central targets of therapy: that he should be helped to accept the reality that his marriage is over. Following this realization, Mr. K needs to think of how he is going to structure his life after the divorce. Mr. K needs to be thinking of how he is going to manage the access and contact with his children and how the relationship with his children will be shaped following the divorce (Sprenkle & Storm, 1983).

JM suggested that a further task for Mr. K would be for him to think more constructively about his work. Although he has not been promoted, neither has he been dismissed from his job, so at some level, he must be offering a useful service. The doctor pointed out that traditionally it is difficult for a person to be dismissed from a government post. The doctor accepted that Mr. K could derive some sense of pride in keeping a job and keeping it for such a long time (20 years). JM pointed out that there are two steps for Mr. K: The first is for him to *realize* what his job reality is, and the second step would be to emotionally *accept* it. If he really accepts this, he will spare himself the distress that he feels every time a younger colleague passes him in a promotion.

JM continued that more importantly, Mr. K needs to realize and then accept that he is only of average intelligence and that he needs to rate his performance in relation to his innate ability and not in relation to what other people achieve or to what his wife had achieved. Failure to accept the level of his ability will lead him to feel miserable for a long time because he is likely to encounter the divergence between his current trajectory and that of other people who are more fortunate. JM pointed out that Mr. K would be helped to accept this if he knew that he is not in a minority and that, by definition, half the population has the intellectual potential lower than average. Despite millions of people being in that intelligence bracket, this does not stop them from performing a function in society that is extremely useful. JM gave the example of the street cleaners, who, although they do not have high qualifications, still perform an enormously useful function in society. Mr. K does not need to be given this example but other examples that would help him see himself as a valuable member of society even though he is not as bright as his wife or others. He could be reminded that people who have below-average intelligence can still manage not only to provide a useful function for society but also to organize a reasonable or even good life for themselves, their marriage, and their children. Mr. K can be helped to accept that he has the potential to offer a useful function and to be a good family man if he does not ruin his chances by adopting dysfunctional behavior such as that of wasting the family resources on purchasing unnecessary objects. Mr. K can be relieved of any sense of shame for not being able to earn as much as his wife if he realized that he is not responsible for the kind of brain that his DNA endowed him with. On the contrary, Mr. K is responsible for the way in which he manages his abilities and for wasting his earnings; this is something that he can manage differently.

JM then pointed out that the *level of discourse* with Mr. K should be at a level on which he could comprehend. JM gave an example of statements like, "it is not your fault that you are not born with an IQ of 140; you have a potential like millions of other people, but you can either live a good life having accepted that or you can use measures that are counterproductive such as overspending, and ruin your life." It is possible for him to feel proud that he has managed to obtain a job that gives him security and a regular income, something that many people with much higher ability than his have not been able to achieve.

JM then pointed out that the role of the therapist is emotionally to show to him that he is accepted and valued for what he can offer. JM referred to the link between how he feels emotionally with what he thinks cognitively. The emotional acceptance by the therapist can be a different experience for him from the emotional experience that he has with his wife (and possibly had with his siblings in his family of origin). JM repeated the link between the cognitive realization of reality and the emotional acceptance of it. He will then be able to value his reality, to value that he has certain ability that can be useful and can lead to a good life as it does to millions of other people. The doctor pointed out that Mr. K does have a positive relationship with his siblings and with his mother. This is something that could sustain him because Mr. K does have some friends—though not many—he does have relationships with some people who value him for who he is. Having accepted these aspects of his reality, he may begin to see his divorce as a natural development and possibly a positive one in the sense that it will save him from the constant comparison with his wife and her friends—a comparison that makes him continuously feel inferior. Mr. K may be helped to accept that his wife and his paths have been divergent.

JM then shifted the attention to Mr. K's role as a father. The children have sensed the *antagonism* between the parents and have been under some pressure to take sides. One can understand that the children would be more attracted to his wife's higher trajectory than his static trajectory. The doctor pointed out that although the son has taken sides and had removed himself from the home (to live with his maternal grandmother) the daughter is still young and has not rejected him. JM then suggested that some attention could be paid in therapy to the relationship of Mr. K with his wife as parents and not only as a couple (Lebow & Newcombe Recart, 2007). The parents have a shared interest in the children's welfare. This shared interest could reduce the antagonism between them. Both parents could be made more aware of the impact of their antagonism on the children's development. It has been well-established that a parental conflictual relationship has a damaging effect of the children's development. JM pointed out that although the children are young, this is the time when they form the models on which they may expect their own relationships to take shape when they grow up. The parents need to be more mindful that they sort out their own antagonism so that it does not adversely affect their children's development. What would be helpful to all of them is if they accept that the divorce is a reality but that a damaging consequence to the children is not inevitable. They need to accept that though in the past their differences were indeed compatible with having children and bringing the children up together, the way the relationship has developed, it has become of a kind that is not compatible with bringing the children up together as a couple. Mr. K could be helped to accept that he is a valuable person in society and that he has achieved his potential in relation to his innate ability by not comparing himself with those who are more fortunate than he is. This may go some way toward relieving him of any shame or guilt that he may feel because of this difference.

JM then added that the emotional acceptance that he will experience through his sessions with his therapist will enable him to accept himself with the qualities that he has been born with. This is the emotional role in developing some cognitions that are positive. The doctor added that the hospital admission has been helpful to Mr. K because he came across other patients who are as able as he is or even less able than him. The doctor also pointed out that Mr. K shows his caring for the children by buying objects for them instead of accepting what he can offer as a father in a relationship kind of way to them. Mr. K can be guided to accept that his concern for his children is worthwhile and that it cannot be substituted by buying trinkets for them. Mr. K can also be helped to be mindful that his children's needs will be changing with their growth. His 10-year-old daughter will have different needs when she becomes 14.

This case demonstrates several points of interest. For example, how different intellectual abilities of spouses or partners of a couple can be handled constructively (as they were originally when husband felt pride in his wife's ability) or destructively when the same difference later became a source of family conflict when addressed antagonistically. Similarly with the overspending, he used that as a compensatory mechanism for his nonacceptance that his ability was lower than that of his wife and the possible envy of her. The case also points to the stages of realizing, accepting, and valuing ability. Furthermore, highlights the role of a therapist is in such cases to provide emotional support so that these things can be achieved. A separate issue is that the difference between marital and parental relationship of the couple can be addressed helpfully in divorcing couples.

References

Lebow, J., & Newcombe Recart, K. (2007). Integrative family therapy for high-conflict divorce with disputes over child custody and visitation. *Family Process*, 46(1), 79–91.

Sprenkle, D. H., & Storm, C. L. (1983). Divorce therapy outcome research: A substantive and methodological review. *Journal of Marital and Family Therapy*, 9(3), 239–258.

10
Adjustment Disorder

Jo

Jo, a 39-year-old married housewife, who was referred from general outpatient clinic for low mood and suicidal ideation after her husband's injury while on duty.

Historyv of present complaint

Jo was functioning well mentally until August 2017 when her husband suffered a brain injury. He was treated by neurosurgeons and was eventually discharged from hospital in July 2018. He remained mostly bedbound and needed assistance to move and could only walk with a "rollator" (a walking frame on wheels) and the assistance of one or two people.

Since her husband's accident, Jo became depressed and irritable. She frequently had unprovoked crying spells and had difficulties in coping with household chores. Her concentration and memory also worsened. She frequently forgot what she needed to buy when she was in a supermarket and even needed to jot down reminders to herself of things to do, which she regarded as a sign of worthlessness. She attended church activities because she felt that these lifted her mood. Her sleep was reduced to only 1 to 3 hours a night. Her appetite was reduced, and she had unintentional weight loss of 10 pounds in 1 year.

Jo became pessimistic, felt helpless and directionless. She did not know how to help her husband or her son. She believed that she should provide the best care to her son. She felt guilty for being more emotional and scolding her son when she was upset. She also blamed herself for spending insufficient time with her son after he voiced his need for more attention from her. She had no sense of hopelessness. For the most recent 6 months, she slapped and pinched herself out of anger or frustration, and she banged her head against a wall to calm herself down. She also harbored fleeting suicidal ideation of jumping from a height or dashing into traffic. Once she looked down from a window and thought about a suicidal attempt but she had no concrete plan to act. She further did not write a suicide note. She abandoned this idea because she felt responsible for her son.

Dynamic Consultations with Psychiatrists: Understanding Severely Troubled Patients, First Edition. Jason Maratos.
© 2022 John Wiley & Sons Ltd. Published 2022 by John Wiley & Sons Ltd.

Jo was first seen at general outpatient clinic in September 2018 and was started on fluoxetine 20 mg daily, after which her mood remained unchanged, but her sleep improved to 4 to 5 hours a night. She was followed up at the general outpatient clinic 2 weeks later and was referred to psychiatric outpatient clinic for further management.

There was no history of manic symptoms, abnormal perceptions or beliefs, or of substance misuse. Jo was tidy-looking with dyed hair. She was forthcoming, friendly with social smiles, and had good eye contact. She had normal psychomotor pace. Her mood was slightly depressed, and her affect was reactive and appropriate. Her speech was coherent, relevant, and spontaneous. Her volume of speech was appropriate. She had no hallucinations or delusions and had no active suicidal ideation. She did not have any active negative cognitions. Her insight was fair. She was motivated to seek medical help and agreed with medication titration and follow-ups.

Family history

There was no family history of mental illness or suicide.

Personal history

Jo was born in the country. She was the youngest of four siblings. There were two elder sisters (ages 53 and 47) and one elder brother (age 46). She reported an uneventful childhood. There was no history of childhood trauma. She had good relationships with her parents and siblings since childhood. Her father is 80 years old and her mother is 76. Her parents, together with other siblings, were residing in the country. She maintained a good relationship with her family members despite not seeing them often.

She completed secondary school in the country and then earned a diploma in business administration. After her diploma study, she worked in sales in the country and then in the electronics company owned by her father-in-law.

She was introduced to her husband by her father-in-law, and they dated for few years before getting married in 2006. Jo's family initially objected to the marriage, but Jo insisted and her family, eventually, agreed to the marriage. Her husband declared bankruptcy in the same year. They sold all five flats that they owned to repay the debts. In addition, Jo's family subsidized them to overcome the financial difficulty. She immigrated to the city in 2011. They have a 6-year-old son. Jo's relationship with her son had been consistently good and she cared for him. Her son had fair performance and no behavioral problems in kindergarten. This was the second marriage for her husband (age 42). Her husband had a daughter from his first marriage.

Jo had recently transferred to another public housing unit; her husband was living with his parents since his discharge from hospital and it was intended that he would return home at a later date. The family was sustained on her husband's disability allowance, her husband's salary, and loans from her elder sister.

Jo lives with her 6-year-old son, who is a Primary 1 pupil, in a public housing unit. Jo is a nonsmoker and a nondrinker. She has no history of substance abuse and no forensic record.

Jo described herself as a good-tempered and optimistic person. She is a Christian and enjoys attending church activities to meet up with fellow church members.

Past psychiatric history

Jo was new to mental health service. She has had no history of suicidal attempt or violence. She enjoyed good physical health.

Present management

Jo was thought to be suffering from an adjustment disorder with the ongoing stressor of her husband's physical condition and incapacity to work. Differential diagnosis included depression.

She continued on fluoxetine, which was initiated at the general outpatient clinic. She had good adherence to medication. However, she reported to have slowness in thinking and tiredness after taking fluoxetine, so it was switched to sertraline in a subsequent follow-up session. Her son started voicing his need to have more attention from his mother. She experienced more self-blame because she spent most of her time and attention on her husband, but she perceived there was limited progress in her husband's recovery. She felt that taking care of her husband and her son at the same time was stressful to her. She remained depressed and irritable. She still managed to cope with household chores and enjoyed attending church activities. Sleep improved to 5 to 6 hours a night. She was eager to have a medication adjustment for improving her mood.

Recently, Jo became more positive because she was hoping that additional neurosurgery would bring some improvement to her husband's condition. She had less frequent acts of self-harm because she was afraid that continuing such acts might make her out of control and that she would no longer be able to take care of her son. She tried to cope with her emotional distress by looking at old photographs of her husband and her son to remind her of happier times. Eventually, she decided to seek medical help because she believed that helping her emotional problem could improve the whole family's situation.

Consultation   JM thanked the doctor for the thorough presentation. The doctor then clarified that the objective of psychiatric contact would be to understand more about Jo's early childhood experience so to understand better the guilt that Jo feels for not spending enough time with her son, which makes her feel that she is not a good mother. JM then asked the doctor to clarify what was the implicit treatment contract. The doctor explained that he would be able to see this patient about once a month for a few appointments until the medication was stabilized and then he would then refer her to a psychologist for therapy.

JM then asked the doctor what he thought Jo's suffering was that was beyond the acceptable and understandable distress that a woman in her situation would experience. She was married to a competent husband, and they were jointly looking after their son; however, now she was left to care for a seriously incapacitated man who lived in another house (with his parents) and was finding herself traveling between households to care for two people who were highly dependent on her, her husband and her son. As psychiatrists, sympathy is important, but something beyond sympathy must be offered to address the symptoms that are beyond the natural and understandable. The doctor responded that Jo's suicidal ideation and her activities of self-harm were indeed in the sphere of dysfunctional responses. JM then asked about the duration within which an adjustment reaction would be considered normal. The husband's accident took place in August 2017 and asked if the present reaction still qualified as an "adjustment reaction." The doctor clarified that the first adjustment was with the accident in August 2017 and the second adjustment was her husband's discharge from the hospital in July 2018. Additionally, there was the threat of additional stress if the husband moved to live with his wife and son.

JM suggested that it would be useful if Jo's workload was looked into in some detail so that the burden that she carries was understood more comprehensively. A detailed history of her daytime activities, which would involve all the time it takes for her to prepare her son for nursery; the time to travel; the time she spends with her husband, the activities that she carries out there, and the activities that she helps her husband with; the time she takes traveling; the time she takes to prepare food for herself and her son; and the time it takes for her to attend church and other activities. Understanding her workload will help in having a more accurate picture of the stress that she experiences. In particular, an opinion could be formed as to whether the stress is purely because of the workload or if there are other emotional factors complicating the picture. The doctor thought that there was no additional help at Jo's husband's home such as help from community physiotherapy or from district nurses. It did not seem that Jo's husband was in an active rehabilitation program.

There was no fixed date for his return to live with his son and wife, nor was there any plan for what sort of help would be offered him and her after his return. There was uncertainty whether there would be an occupational therapy assessment of the home so that appropriate appliances could be fitted, which would improve his mobility and reduce his reliance on other people. An occupational therapy assessment, for example, could even recommend a different flat for him and include things such as moving to a ground-floor flat or a flat in which there is easy access to a wheelchair (and possibility getting him a wheelchair) to move from one room to another as well as an appropriate and well-equipped bathroom. Greater clarity on how Jo will cope with her husband would help her in adjusting psychologically to the new situation.

JM posed the question why this manifestly intelligent woman had not mobilized the services that already existed in the city for cases similar to her husband's. The two hypotheses that came to mind were: She may not be familiar with the services in the city because she is a migrant, and as a migrant, her expectation of what services are available may be based on her memories of what services used to be available in the country when she lived there. In other words, her expectations may be outdated for the city and for the country. If this is the case, a social worker would be able to inform her what services are presently available in the city.

The second factor maybe that she is troubled by conflicting feelings that reduce her effectiveness in seeking help, including feelings of guilt and of ambivalence and frustration or anger for what has befallen her.

One of these factors was the guilt that she was feeling in failing to provide her son the attention for which he was asking. JM pointed out that it could be useful for Jo to be reminded that intentionally causing harm to someone else is a cause for guilt and that she should work on not feeling guilty for everything that happens because it is disadvantageous or hurtful. If she is pulled in all directions by conflicting demands that cannot be realistically met, then she can be helped to be relieved of the unjustified guilt. She cannot do more than her best, and she is doing her best anyway. She is dealing with pathological guilt, which is not a healthy feeling that results from awareness of culpability.

Pathological guilt can be part of an adjustment reaction. It is common, for example, for mothers of children who have been struck by an illness (e.g., leukemia) in which they feel that the illness is a punishment from God because they had not been good at observing the demands of their religion. Mothers are vulnerable to such feelings when things go wrong with their children. For some psychoanalytic views of guilt, see Winnicott (1958).

JM then expanded on the relationship between workload and perceived stress. He used the example of junior doctors who are often faced with long hours and intensive demands on their time. Some doctors perceive this stress only negatively (and elaborate on negative thoughts and feelings about it), whereas others suffer the stress but also see it as part of gaining experience that enriches their understanding of illness and that will make them doctors who are more competent in treating a wider variety of conditions in future. The latter doctors experience the same stress but are less likely to develop dysfunctional symptomatology and are more likely to benefit from the same stressful experience. The relevance of this to Jo is that there is a possibility that complex negative emotions and cognitions make the stress, which is there, much more destructive than it needs be.

JM then pointed out how a mother's guilt can affect a child's expectations and a child's relationship with her. For example, a mother who explains pragmatically that she will now be able to give a lot less to her child because this major catastrophe has hit their household will help the child accept the situation and draw more on their own resources instead of increasing their demands on their mother and making the family situation more problematic. The child may even experience by learning to cope with difficult situations and feeling that they are helping in the difficult family situation. It is not a mother's fault that she is not able to provide a family environment for the child that is like that of their friends.

As the child grows up, they may be able to see their life in a greater perspective and even consider themself to be a little more fortunate than children of parents who abuse them or who have serious behavior problems (like drug addiction), which causes even greater distress. There are children who grow up in a family environment with hate and aggression who are much more unfortunate than this child is. It is important not to patronize the child and give the impression that the doctor believes that the child should feel lucky to have had a father with serious brain damage. That would be a seriously unsympathetic approach and will reduce the doctor's credibility and may even cause the doctor-patient relationship to cease. Nevertheless, it would help the child appreciate that reality is rarely perfect and that many families must cope with various degrees of misfortunes.

A solid introduction to the psychoanalytical understanding of guilt can be found in Winnicott (1965). In those articles, Winnicott addresses the issue of guilt developmentally (the development of the capacity to feel guilt and the pathological absence of guilt) and also addresses situations like Jo's when he refers to "the absurdities of guilt feelings" (Winnicott, 1958, p. 18).

References

Winnicott, D. W. (1958). Psycho-analysis and the sense of guilt. In J. D. Sutherland (Ed.), *Psychoanalysis and contemporary thought* (Vol. 1, pp. 15–32). Hogarth Press Ltd.

Winnicott, D. W. (1965). *The maturational processes and the facilitating environment*. Hogarth Press.

Section III

Eating Disorders

11
Bulimia

Catherine

Catherine is an 18-year-old, single, unemployed woman, living with her parents and a domestic helper in a private flat. She was admitted voluntarily at the hospital in October 2017 following a paracetamol overdose; she had been suffering from bulimia for a few weeks.

History of presenting complaint

Since September 2017, Catherine suffered with recurrent binge eating. She described the bingeing episodes as impulsive acts that were triggered by thoughts of her broken love affairs and her unhappy family. She reported bingeing up to 10 cakes a day. Such binge-eating episodes were followed by subsequent starving and self-induced vomiting. She had a weight loss of 10 pounds within a month. She was reported to be highly preoccupied with food craving and with her self-image. She had a fear of gaining weight and expressed guilt about her binge eating.

On the day of admission, she had attempted to contact her former boyfriend. After she failed to reach him, she developed suicidal ideation. She purchased ant poison from a local store and left a suicidal note on the internet. Her family discovered this before she attempted suicide. She was brought to the emergency department to seek medical attention. She threw a temper tantrum and impulsively overdosed with 12 tablets of paracetamol during her wait at the observation room but denied actual suicidal intent. Catherine expressed no remorse afterward. Subsequent psychiatric admission to the hospital was arranged in view of her unstable emotions and the abnormal eating pattern.

Catherine appeared with dyed purple hair, thin body build, multiple tattoos over hand and forearm, and old slash scars over wrist and forearm. Her mood was low, and her affect was reactive and congruent. She had vague suicidal ideas but no definite plan. Insight was limited, and she showed minimal remorse about her self-harm or maladaptive behavior. Her body mass index was 16.2.

Family history

There is no family history of mental illness or suicide.

Dynamic Consultations with Psychiatrists: Understanding Severely Troubled Patients, First Edition. Jason Maratos.
© 2022 John Wiley & Sons Ltd. Published 2022 by John Wiley & Sons Ltd.

Personal history

Catherine was born in the city and is the youngest of her siblings. She perceived her childhood as unhappy and was raised up by two domestic helpers hired by her parents because her parents were busy with their jobs. She had a distant relationship with her parents and felt that there was a lack of emotional flow within the family. Catherine perceived her parents to be emotionally unavailable. Her parents tended to invalidate her emotions at an early age; for example, when she cried, her parents would demand her to stop immediately, and when she failed to comply with their instructions, they would further scold and physically punish her. There was a history of corporal punishment by her mother when she failed to meet academic expectations. Her relationship with her family became more distant with the start of her parents' business. They had increased conflicts and arguments. High intrafamilial tension was reported. She recalled seeing her parents fighting, and in some episodes, her father held her mother's neck and threatened to kill her. When she turned 16, the family discovered that her father had an extramarital affair. Mother decided to file for divorce.

There was no history of sexual abuse.

Her father is a 60-year-old, businessman; he is the owner of a seafood shop. Catherine felt more emotionally attached to her father when she was young because he tended to spoil her. Their relationship gradually became more distant as she grew up and as her father seldom stayed at home.

Her mother is a 44-year-old, business partner of her father. She was described as stubborn, hot-tempered, dominant, strict, and overprotective. Her mother tended to take control of various aspects of family and business life. She adopted harsh scolding and hitting as punishment. Catherine disliked her mother and described their relationship as stormy.

Her elder sister is a 31-year-old, married housewife; they live separately. She was described as caring and supportive. She shared a confiding relationship with Catherine; however, she failed to provide regular support to Catherine because she was busy with the childcare of her two young children. Her elder brother is 21 years old; he has lived separately from the family following recurrent conflicts with parents. They have maintained minimal interaction.

Catherine received education in local schools. Her mother set high academic expectations from an early age. Catherine scored above average academic results in primary school; however, her academic performance deteriorated in secondary school. This was attributed to a lack of motivation in learning and to being subjected to bullying by peers.

Catherine considers herself to be bisexual. Her first courtship was when she was 13. Her longest courtship lasted for 3 years. She had unstable and intense interpersonal relationships. Catherine used to alternate between extremes of idealizing her partners (when they showed care toward her) and devaluing them (when they did not meet her needs). She was described to be emotionally overdependent to her partners and highly devoted to her relationships. She claimed that she was prepared to "give up everything" for her partner. She described her previous relationships as "stormy." She was easily prompted to get involved in conflicts. She had a strong sense of insecurity, with a tendency to polarize to extreme emotions when she anticipated abandonment. Catherine adopted frantic efforts to avoid abandonment. For example, she would make repeated telephone calls, would threaten suicide, and would attempt to overcompensate by repeatedly apologizing. She would impulsively self-harm when she was faced with separation. She would quickly establish new relationships after separation to seek for a new attachment figure to meet her need for security.

Catherine had worked as a receptionist and in sales in the past. The longest employment was for 1 year. She has currently been unemployed for a year.

She is impulsive, overdependent, has excessive fear of being abandoned, feels insecure, and has low self-esteem. She has adopted self-harm and the seeking of new relationships as a coping strategy.

Catherine considers spending time with her partners and shopping as her hobbies. She is a social drinker and a chronic smoker but has no history of substance abuse. She has no forensic record.

Past psychiatric history

Catherine suffered with chronic affective instability and low mood since her teenage years; this had been related to her unhappy childhood and to dysfunctional family dynamics. She was described to have low self-esteem with unstable self-image.

Catherine was first known to a child psychiatric service in 2015 at age 16. She had presented with low mood and suicidal ideation, which she attributed to her father's extramarital affair and to her parents' divorce. She experienced the divorce as a form of abandonment. She had repeated episodes of deliberate self-harm by slashing her wrists; these were triggered by thoughts of family conflict and relationship crises. Catherine was diagnosed with adjustment disorder, with a suspected underlying personality disorder. She was treated with antidepressants and a mood stabilizer. Minimal clinical improvement was noted.

Her mental condition further deteriorated in June 2017 following a broken love affair with her female partner. After their separation, she quickly started a new relationship with a male friend who was in a relationship with another girl. She described their relationship as "stormy and turbulent" with multiple arguments and fights. She feared abandonment by her partner and made repeated suicidal threats aimed at gaining her partner's care and attention. Eventually, the relationship with her male friend ended because he decided to return to his girlfriend. She was markedly distressed about her loss, which she perceived as a form of betrayal. Catherine made excessive efforts to avoid the abandonment, including making multiple phone calls and stalking. Her mood was depressed, and she exhibited increased crying spells, loss of interest, and social withdrawal. She perceived herself as worthless and viewed her future as hopeless. Her mode of "coping" was to slash her wrists with a cutter; her intention was to inflict physical pain.

There were no previous psychiatric admissions. Catherine had many episodes of low mood since her teenage years; these were associated with social withdrawal, anhedonia, reduced motivation, disturbed sleep, poor appetite, pessimistic thoughts, and suicidal ideation.

Catherine took an overdose of antidepressants in 2015. This was precipitated by a broken love affair. As a teenager, she had multiple episodes of deliberate self-harm by slashing her wrists; these were triggered by conflict with family and by broken love affairs. Catherine fought with former boyfriends during heated arguments.

She has been treated with venlafaxine, bupropion, valproate, Lyrica, quetiapine, clonazepam, diazepam, and zolpidem. She has been diagnosed as having an emotionally unstable personality disorder, borderline type; recurrent depressive disorder, and Bulimia Nervosa.

It was considered that her condition was caused by the following predisposing factors: a dysfunctional family dynamic marked by intrafamilial conflict, dysfunctional communication pattern; tendency of her parents to devalue her while they remained emotionally unavailable to her; the influence of inconsistent parenting with a distant father and a controlling mother; an insecure attachment; a personality with low self-esteem and a tendency to be impulsive and insecure; and an unclear self-image.

The following were thought to have been precipitating factors: her father's extramarital affair—from idealization to denigration; parental pending divorce; and anticipatory fear of loss and a broken love affair.

The following were thought to be perpetuating factors: maladaptive behavior, such as deliberate self-harm; unstable relationships—lack of a stable and confiding attachment figure; intrafamilial discord, invalidating environment; and uncertain life goals and internal preferences.

Present treatment and management of case   A multidisciplinary management approach was adopted, with the active involvement of clinical psychologist, occupational therapist, social worker, and dietician. The focus was the exploration and reflection on cognitive errors, dysfunctional core beliefs (self-worth versus body image) and cyclical maladaptive behavior (e.g., acting out, suicidal threat, self-harm). Components from dialectical behavioral therapy were implemented. Coaching was conducted on distress tolerance skills, emotional regulation, interpersonal skills, and relaxation skills. Catherine was encouraged to discuss and establish life goals, to strengthen self-worth, and to facilitate individuation.

Catherine was observed to have marked discord with difficulty in collaborating in the care for herself. A dysfunctional communication pattern was noted with her parents who refused to communicate with each other, who lapsed into arguments easily, and dominated conversations. Coaching on effective communication skills was conducted. Catherine was advised to validate others' thoughts while voicing her own feelings. Her parents were encouraged to validate Catherine's emotions. She was treated with mirtazapine, venlafaxine, quetiapine XR, and diazepam.

Consultation   JM thanked the doctor for making such a thorough presentation. He then asked the doctor to specify what the issue was that they would like to address. The doctor enumerated the difficulties in proceeding with treatment and these were the lack of motivation, the patient's refusal to leave the hospital (because she did not wish to return home), and that medication had not proved to be useful in the past. JM stated that he appreciated that these were the difficulties in treatment but the group still needed to specify what the issue to be discussed at the present consultation was. The doctor responded by explaining an additional difficulty to progress, which was the lack of insight on the part of the patient's parents. JM advised that the issue to be addressed had not yet been clarified. The doctor explained that they would wish to clarify if there was any direction in which the psychological interventions could move that would be effective for Catherine. JM restated the question as a need to base the psychological intervention on understanding what was pathological in this patient's psychological structure. JM then added that to work on the pathological we needed to be aware of what is healthy within her psychological structure.

JM proceeded to ask if the doctors considered that there was anything positive or healthy in this patient's psychological structure, and the response was an unequivocal "no." This was said with some obvious discomfort by those present. JM then responded: "Well, she is not dead" because he wished to build an image of a healthy aspect and second was that she was in hospital (implying that she was at some level accepting treatment). Then JM added that Catherine had the capacity to argue, that she had the volition to cut herself, she had the mental capacity to almost plan a suicide, and she could write suicidal notes. JM pointed out that all these aspects implied some degree of ability on Catherine's part. Furthermore, she was thought to be of at least average intelligence. JM pointed out that the presence of intelligence is an asset (something healthy) even though she uses it in the wrong way.

Additionally, Catherine was, except for the weight loss, physically healthy. For example, her body mass index was almost within an acceptable range and so she was a young lady who was slim but physically healthy. Furthermore, she was a young woman of only 18 years of age and as such, she had the future ahead of her.

The doctor confirmed that Catherine had completed her secondary education. She had the potential to build a life based on her youth, health, intelligence, and education.

JM then introduced the notion of countertransference (Heimann, 1950; Kernberg, 1965; Winnicott, 1960). The doctors' feelings of hopelessness about this case reflected Catherine's own hopelessness about herself. She did not see anything healthy or strong within herself despite that there were the positives that were highlighted: health, youth, intelligence, and education. Catherine felt that there was nothing positive about her. She was a desperate young woman. JM then pointed out that the emotional and geographical distance of the consultant from the doctors, who were in face-to-face contact with her, enabled him to have a more detached and more objective view and, as a result, a more balanced and realistic view of her.

JM pointed out that Catherine gave a convincing account that her emotions were never healthily contained and responded to; they have been consistently denied or devalued by her parents. Catherine's parents did not have the capacity to show sympathy, to accept her emotions, and to support her. JM then asked the doctors about the role of the other carers in the house, such as the maids who sometimes become emotionally important figures. The doctor responded that the maids frequently changed and so there was no constant figure to whom Catherine could attach herself. JM then continued the exploration for other possible caring figures within the family by asking about the elder siblings, but this seemed also not to be the case because the older sister was distant and had moved early out of the family to build her own family. JM pointed out that there may be more to this relationship rather than just the age gap because in other situations even when there is an age gap the older siblings play a complementary parental role. JM pointed out that emotionally this girl did not have any support from parents, elder siblings, or nannies. She was "dropped" in an emotional vacuum. As a result, Catherine was desperate to meet somebody who would understand, support, and contain her.

Catherine tended to form new relationships from a starting point of despair. There are few people who are keen to form a relationship with somebody who is desperate. As a result, her relationships were either based on a wrong choice of partner, or they were poorly managed because of the despair that she was experiencing.

A relationship stands a better chance of being successful if it is based on mutuality and equivalence of input and gain derived from it. A relationship based on one partner's despair is unlikely to prove successful for either party. In this way, the deprived person enters a vicious circle through which they come out as not only deprived but also additionally traumatized. A trauma is a confirmation of prior feeling that indeed they are not worth loving.

JM then pointed to the more complicated dynamic of being "spoiled" by her father and denigrated by her mother. The doctor clarified that the spoiling had gone on until she was 13 when the demands of the business took father away from her. From the age of 13 onward, she needed to contend with the loss of father's attention, even though the attention was not the most developmentally positive. JM added that spoiling is a form of neglect, and spoiling or indulgence does not promote an ability in a child to cope with frustration neither does it promote a sense of self-reliance. Spoiling is neglect even though the external appearance is that of extreme care. It is not accidental that this kind of care—noncare—is considered "spoiling," which means destroying.

JM then proceeded to give another example of spoiling only at the emotional level. He gave the example of a child going to a parent distressed because of a conflict in school. The neglectful/spoiling parent will collude with the child and simply place the blame on the other people. A properly caring parent would first acknowledge the child's distress and support them but would not stop there. A caring parent will then explore with the child the process of interaction that led to the distressing incident, help the child understand the whole process, and enable the child to interact next time in a different way so that the outcome is positive and not distressing. One aspect of this proper care is to help the child to see the incident in a wider perspective because the child most likely will be distressed because that incident has taken their mind dimensions well beyond that the incident merits. Through this exploration of the interaction, the caring parent can prevent the incident of becoming damaging to the child's self-esteem. This outcome is more likely to give the child hope for the future and empower them to return in this situation at school and try to reshape the relationship in a constructive way.

Having received this overview of this young person, JM suggested that Catherine will require the service of an environment that will provide for her what her natural life was not able. The environment will need to provide validation and containment of her feelings. The same professionals in that environment would enable her to have a realistic (balanced) view of herself and a realistic evaluation of her qualities.

This means that she will be able to have a realistic view of her potential, which would include the positive aspects of her potential. The professionals will recognize (and not dismiss) her difficulties but will not see the difficulties as the whole of her existence. The professionals will need to particularly acknowledge her loneliness and how painful this must be for her but will not stop there and will help her develop a sense that there is a realistic hope for her because she has a realistic potential. This potential is enough for her to make a good life for herself.

The context that can provide these services has, for the moment, been dictated by her threat of suicide and her dangerous eating pattern. JM pointed out that people who hold a borderline personality structure are more likely to receive benefit if they are treated in the context of a therapeutic community (Main, 1977; Pearce et al., 2017). The elements that will make the setting therapeutic would be the ability of the environment to contain her and the ability to promote her psychological growth. Such a setting would help her to develop a more constructive way of relating with other people. The cognitive input is essential, but it is rarely enough if it is not coupled with the emotional support. Catherine needs to feel that she is accepted and welcomed by the caring staff.

It was pointed out that the service of a therapeutic community does not exist in the city, and JM suggested that perhaps, in due course, the doctors could develop such a service. In the absence of such a community, these points could be the therapeutic elements of an already existing therapeutic structure in the city. JM pointed out that it is difficult for people with borderline personality structures to respond to occasional (even regular) outpatient appointments. Borderline personality requires a more comprehensive approach. JM pointed out that it is not only the input from the therapists that is therapeutic in the context of a therapeutic community but also the input from the other clients of the service. JM suggested that the young doctors consider the creation of a therapeutic community in the city future.

References

Heimann, P. (1950). On countertransference. *The International Journal of Psycho-Analysis*, *31*, 81–84.

Kernberg, O. F. (1965). Notes on countertransference. *Journal of American Psychoanalysis Assessment*, *13*, 38–56.

Main, T. F. (1977). The concept of the therapeutic community: Variations and vicissitudes, 1st S. H.Foulkes annual lecture. *Group Analysis*, *10*(2 Suppl), 2–16.

Pearce, S., Scott, L., Attwood, G., Saunders, K., Dean, M., De Ridder, R., Galea, D., Konstantinidou, H., & Crawford, M. (2017). Democratic therapeutic community treatment for personality disorder: Randomised controlled trial. *The British Journal of Psychiatry*, *210*(2), 149–156.

Winnicott, D. W. (1960). Countertransference. *The British Journal of Medical Psychology*, *33*, 17–21.

12
Deliberate Self-Harm; Self-Neglect

Jane

Presenting condition

Jane, is a 59-year-old single, unemployed woman, living alone in a public housing unit, and financially dependent on social security. The present admission was compulsory; she was transferred from the medical ward on account of self-neglect and abnormal experiences.

History of present complaint

Jane was suspicious and reported that workers threatened to kill her with a meat chopper and tried to push her into busy traffic during an escort service. She also accused male social workers of sexually harassing her by staring at her chest. She believed that poison was being added to the meals that she had bought from restaurants, and she henceforth kept the receipts as proof of the (imagined) persecution. She experienced no auditory hallucinations or other psychotic phenomena. During home visits, her house was found to be "in a mess" with dangerous disregard for hygiene. Her belongings were put in plastic bags stacked to a height greater than an average adult, leaving only a narrow passage for daily activities. She put everything, including electrical appliances, into plastic bags for no apparent reason and wore gloves whenever she touched anything. She was observed to be washing her hands a lot. Her bed was stained with excreta. The toilet was covered with fungus. Her mood was on the low side, and she expressed that she would kill herself after she finished launching all the complaints. No suicidal note was left, and there was no actual attempt.

Family history

There was no family history of mental illness or suicide.

Dynamic Consultations with Psychiatrists: Understanding Severely Troubled Patients, First Edition. Jason Maratos.
© 2022 John Wiley & Sons Ltd. Published 2022 by John Wiley & Sons Ltd.

Personal history

Jane was born in the city. She was the youngest of three children. She felt that her father favored her elder brother but that her mother treated the children equally. Her family of origin was well off. She studied in a prestigious secondary school in the city and achieved good academic results.

Jane emigrated to the US with her family. She completed bachelor's and master's degrees in Business administration in the US. She aspired to become a successful businesswoman. She sprained her back in a gym, and this resulted in low back pain. She returned to the city after her master's degree because her father was physically unwell. She found out that her family business had been closed and that the family was in debt. She blamed her family for not being supportive and for ignoring her concerns regarding her low back pain, when in fact, her mother financially covered her medical expenses. Jane returned to the city to work as secondary school teacher for a few years. She worked as a clerk and as a secondary school teacher only briefly because she felt that that was not what she wanted to do.

Jane had been unemployed for several years and relied on her savings and, later, on support from the Social Welfare Department and nongovernmental organizations (NGOs). She has no relatives in the city and no visitors except staff from the welfare services.

Jane has limited social support. Her parents are deceased. All her siblings live in the US. She has had accommodation problems for years before moving to the current public housing unit. Previously, she had stayed at budget guest houses and temporary shelters. Jane is a nonsmoker and a nondrinker; she has no history of substance misuse and does not have a forensic record.

Past psychiatric history

Jane had been known to various psychiatric outpatient clinics since the mid-1990s and had been under the care of both psychiatrists and psychologists. She discontinued attending after she was last seen by a psychiatrist in 2008. Various diagnoses have been given, including Generalized Anxiety Disorder, Dysthymia, Neurotic Depression, Somatisation disorder, and others.

Jane suffered from progressive physical deterioration in the last 5 years. She complained of back pain and inability to walk, becoming homebound. She was reported to be selective toward services she received and often launched complaints against hospitals and NGOs. She was "picky" in choosing meals delivered to her and made demands that the services could not meet. She would then phone various workers, whom she had known in the past, to ask them for help in buying food and necessities. However, often, she launched complaints against these services and as a result, would be left out of supply of food. She was reported to have starved herself on and off over many years, surviving on just drinking water; this resulted in hyponatraemia and hospitalization. She hadn't taken a bath for years and attributed this to her back pain.

Present treatment and management of case   The doctor has been her case officer since July 1, 2017. At first, her speech was overinclusive, and she spoke in fast pace because she was worried that she would not have enough time to tell the whole story to the doctor. In the subsequent sessions, she was given 20-minute sessions. She felt more comfortable with this arrangement. She was put on fluoxetine 50 mg and risperidone 4 mg. There was limited improvement. She complained of generalized discomfort and urinary urgency that was attributed to risperidone. She was found to have hyponatraemia with sodium down to 120 (normal blood sodium level is between 135 and 145 mEq/l). Fluoxetine was discontinued. She is currently on risperidone 2 mg. She received input from a clinical psychologist.

Consultation   The first issue that was addressed was the current understanding of the reason for Jane's present deterioration. This was thought to be partly due to her physical complains (the back pain). JM questioned whether the back pain was of a severity that would justify the degree of incapacity and disability. The doctor explained that the back pain had been extensively investigated and that there were no physical abnormalities identified. JM returned to the issue of whether the existing back pain could justify the degree of neglect and the squalor within which she lived. Would the back pain justify the degree of undernutrition to the degree that it caused electrolyte imbalance? The doctor added that a further factor was the family's deterioration in financial situation. She had been brought up by an affluent family that was now bankrupt.

JM persisted in the exploration of how back pain and family bankruptcy could justify life in squalor and serious undernourishment. JM questioned how a woman, who was not dementing and not suffering from a neurological or an orthopedic condition, could arrive at this state of serious neglect, squalor, and risk to her life through an electrolyte imbalance. JM stated that it was important to accept that the attribution of her situation to back pain was Jane's explanation of her predicament and that this was not supported by objective evidence. JM pointed out that if the physical complaints were the cause of this serious incapacity, they would have been detected in some of the numerous examinations and tests that she had undergone. This discrepancy between her perception and of the objective reality, leads one to wish to explore the sphere of her emotions and her cognitions. For a review of literature regarding the difference among illness, disability, and handicap, see Susser (1990).

The doctor added that Jane feels that she is a failure in life because she has not been able to achieve goals that she feels she should have been able. JM then proceeded to address the expectations that Jane had when she returned to the city about her own life and achievements. One needed to be mindful that Jane returned from the US having achieved good secondary school grades and university degrees. This indicated that she had the capacity of a person with above-average intelligence. JM then inquired what would be an appropriate expectation for Jane and asked about Jane's expectations of her parents on her return to the city. The doctor responded that this was not an area that had been considered jointly with Jane. JM suggested that this phase in her life when she graduated successfully from a US university but then failed to remain on this positive trajectory and instead expected important people in her environment (her family initially and services later) to make it possible for her to have the life that she expected.

JM pointed out that Jane had been able to address constructively the demands of her previous phases of life. She had managed both high school and university positively. JM felt that on return to the city, she stopped addressing her issues herself and instead expected other people to do that for her. Jane did not think that with the tools and experience that she had she could make a better life for herself. The reason why this competent young woman did not mobilize her resources for her own benefit is obscure.

JM then addressed Jane's current expectations for her own future. The doctor responded that her current expectations were unrealistic. For example, Jane insisted that she should be allowed to return to her flat and claimed that she would be able to look after herself. When Jane was asked to explain how she will be looked after, she claimed that social services and the NGOs would provide for her. JM interpreted that Jane is currently using a primitive defense mechanism—that of denial (see Laplanche & Pontalis, 1983).

JM asked about the current understanding professionals have of why Jane would resort to the unhelpful and dysfunctional defense of denial. It is possible that she resorted to denial because the prospect that she imagined for her was unthinkable, totally unacceptable to her, or too painful. JM suggested that in her mind, Jane felt desperate and that she had "written herself off." Rather than feel the pain of despair, she resorted to denial. It is possible that Jane thought that she was unlikely to ever have a partner, unlikely ever to have a job, would never recover from her chronic physical symptoms, and would always depend on agencies for her survival.

JM proposed that it was this despair that needed to be addressed. She needed to be helped to develop and accept a more realistic and positive perspective for her life.

JM proposed that Jane would need to accept that she has both limitations and a problematic history, that she is unlikely to realize her dream of starting a business, and that she is unlikely to find a partner now or to find a proper employment. It is unlikely that when she is at this stage, a potential employer would give her a job. But Jane is not demented, and she does have some residual thinking ability that she could use. It is possible that her intellectual ability remained above average. Jane's intellectual ability is something real and something substantial on which she can found a realistic prospect for her life even at the age of 59.

Then JM pointed out that in 21st century, there are indeed agencies the city that can help her, but the help needs to be appropriate in a developmental way. By developmental support, it is understood that she is being helped to develop her abilities and is helped to adopt more healthy practices; it is not a support to sustain her in her present position or, worse, to aggravate her present helplessness. JM expanded on the nature of developmental support in contrast with growth inhibiting support. JM used examples from the area of bringing children up. In the simplest way, a parent who helps a child who has a difficulty with eating would help the child to overcome that difficulty and develop in a way that they can eat on their own, properly. An anxious or unhelpful parent would do for the child what the child cannot do; in the case of eating, they would spoon-feed the child, thus depriving the child of the opportunity to develop their own skill of feeding themselves. JM pointed out the difference between developmental and dysfunctional support. Jane requires developmental support that will help her develop the residual capacities that she realistically has. JM proposed that, in the beginning, the support Jane required was to begin to socialize and to do something constructive with her time. The doctor responded that Jane had already been referred to the occupational therapy department but that she was resistant to the help they provide. Jane tended to denigrate the service offered and commented that the service was too simple and below her ability.

JM suggested that the occupational therapy service perseveres and that she be encouraged that there is progress possible beyond the initial stages, which seem too easy and "silly." JM suggested that she could be shown that even the silly tasks or, the tasks that she considered silly, do have aspects that are not negligible; for example, the task of turning up on time for a particular activity, the task of learning to be with other people, the task of listening (obeying) to instructors, and the task of finishing a task that has been allocated to her. Jane could be encouraged to undertake these simple tasks because they are the door for her better life in the future. Jane could be given hope (something that she lacks at present), that if she achieves these easy early steps, there are better, more significant steps that she can take at a later stage in her life. JM pointed out, that in her case, one would not offer her analytical psychotherapy in the traditional sense but would use the psychoanalytical concepts in formulating her treatment. The package of treatment that she will receive needs to include psychiatric supervision, psychotherapeutic support, and occupational therapy that would aim at restoring some realistic hope for some realistic (achievable) plan for her own life. It may not be realistic to encourage her to aim toward employment, but it would be realistic for her to aim toward some creative activity, some life that is better than living in a flat of this state and with this degree of self-neglect. The transitional period of occupational therapy could be extremely useful to her, beginning with the overcoming the difficulty of being with others.

JM then suggested that Jane's tendency to nag and demand excessively is managed therapeutically. JM suggested that it is pointed out that professionals who are employed to help her will put up with her tendency to be overdemanding and nagging but that people in her natural environment are not likely to accept this and are more likely to distance themselves from her. By being overly demanding, Jane is undermining her own chances of receiving appropriate help. It was suggested that this be pointed out to Jane that the way she treats people influences their relationship in such way that her needs are not net. In this way, she is placing herself in a vicious cycle where her needs are made even worse by her tendency to alienate the people that can be of use to her. The doctor pointed out that when this is being tried with Jane, she tends to respond by continuing to blame other people. JM then suggested that the therapist returns to Jane and points out that people do want to help her, but by alienating them, she ends up with less help than she can get.

JM then suggested that although the process is not going to be easy or quick, that this is the direction that stands the best chance of effecting a change in Jane's approach. JM further added that although, in a consultation session the process is concentrated and appears simple and quick, in real therapy time, this is the line that is standing a better chance of having results in the long run. JM suggested that this is a process that will take many months before any substantial change takes place. It is for the therapist to maintain the therapeutic objective in mind and persevere along this line, accepting that the changes are going to be in small increments over repeated sessions.

JM returned to the issue of instilling realistic hope. JM then proceeded to point out that the trauma of losing her father and the trauma of the family bankruptcy obviously contributed to her deterioration and suggested that this series of events is acknowledged with sympathy but that it is also coupled with an instillation of realistic hope.

JM then proceeded to address the need for the therapist to have realistic expectations. A patient who has been in that pattern for more than 30 years is unlikely to be able to make this dramatic change in personality easily. The therapist runs the risk of being either demoralized by having high expectations and passing on this demoralization back to the patient who already feels without hope. The issue of returning to Jane and pointing out that her explanation that back pain and inadequacy of others justify her present state is just not helpful. The treating psychiatrist needs to (a) maintain a realistic hope and (b) try to convey this realistic functional attitude, what is likely to work for her and trying to get her to think in a functional realistic and constructive way. The psychiatrist needs to be mindful that the dynamic that fuels this functional approach is her own sense of hopelessness.

JM repeated the issue that by attributing her misfortune to her family, to her physical complains, and to the (perceived inadequacy of the) helping services is not an approach that will ever improve her own predicament. JM asked if Jane is dextrous at engaging other agents (services) in giving help for her. The doctor pointed out that Jane does do that. JM suggested that this capacity of hers should be used therapeutically in the sense that it is pointed out that she does have the ability to engage other people and that she could use this capacity in a more constructive way—in a way that she is reminded that she is not without ability and not without capacity. Some effort could be made to point out that she does demonstrate a certain capacity to engage other people, and if she used that to get a constructive help to develop her own abilities further, she would benefit a lot more then she benefits, or does not, in this case.

JM then gave an example. Instead of using the services to buy food for her, she could use the services to help her go and buy the food herself, and the same could be done with the state of her flat. Instead of using other agents to make her flat more habitable she could use the service so that she herself could play a part in making her flat more habitable. It could be pointed out that she does have the capacity to do these simple tasks if her emotions were directing her in the right way.

The doctor then suggested that the efforts of the therapists should be toward empowering her, and JM reinforced this. JM then added that although it is unlikely at the age of 59, and after more than 30 years unemployment, that she is likely to get employed work but that did not mean that it was necessary for her to live in squalor and to undernourish herself to a degree that she puts her life at risk through an electrolyte imbalance. JM suggested that examples of people who are more incapacitated than she was could be used. For example, the case of people without legs and of people who are blind who are still able to look after themselves much better than she does, and she could be reminded that she still has a mind with above-average intelligence.

JM asked if this Jane could walk. This was confirmed. Because Jane could walk she could certainly be escorted to the shops and helped so that she herself could do some of her shopping. If Jane argues that she is unable to carry any shopping, it could be pointed out that she is able to carry some, if not all, her shopping. The doctor pointed out that Jane was not able to carry more than 5 pounds in weight. JM responded that could be seen in a positive way in the sense that she was able to carry up to 5 pounds in weight, so there was indeed something that she could do for herself. Also, in relation to her back pain, it could be pointed out to her that walking is a good exercise for it.

The doctor expressed the concern that she will be institutionalized. JM confirmed this concern and added that this is what the rehabilitation ward will have as a task. The rehabilitation ward will have to instil hope, that she is still a bright woman, that she can do better for herself, that this is a step toward something realistically better for her, and that she needs to be kept there to achieve improvement. If she complains, the complaint needs to be seen as part of her pathology and not as a genuine complaint. The ward staff may need to be protected from her complaints, which should not be escalated to the management. Because she is a clever woman and may manipulate the environment by escalating her complaints, it would be useful if there was good networking among the treating psychiatrist, the staff, the nurses of the ward, and the administration; the senior staff of the hospital need to be prepared about what to expect of this woman who has difficulties in adjusting and her response of having the difficulties is to regress and to retire to where she feels comfortable, instead of moving on toward being discharged and coping in real life. This is indeed a difficult case.

References

Laplanche, J., & Pontalis, J.-B. (1983). *The language of psycho-analysis*. Hogarth Press and the Institute of Psycho-Analysis.

Susser, M. (1990). Disease, illness, sickness; impairment, disability and handicap. *Psychological Medicine*, 20(3), 471–473.

Section IV

Addictions

13
Alcoholism

Peter

Peter is a 40-year-old married man who is unemployed and lives in a public housing unit with his wife, two daughters, and a son. He was admitted to the hospital 1 week ago after threatening to kill himself and his family when he was under the influence of alcohol.

History of present complaint

Peter drank 9–10 cans of beer every day, starting with an "eye opener" (the early morning drink to cope with symptoms). He drank 'round the clock to relieve withdrawal symptoms such as tremor and restlessness. There had been craving, difficulty to control use, and continued use of alcohol despite the harmful effect on his liver. There had been no periods of abstinence in the community. There had been multiple psychosocial and forensic complications. While intoxicated, he had history of punching his wife and of causing lacerations that required suturing; this resulted in 18 months of probation. He had a history of abusing his daughter by scratching her hand with a beer lid opener. His relationship with his wife and children had been poor "due to his drinking." He denied a history of confusion or seizures. He denied recent use of illicit substances.

His mental state deteriorated in the previous 2 to 3 weeks. He became easily irritable. He slept for 3 hours only and experienced increased energy level. He made excessive planning to earn money by trading expensive watches. He asked his younger sister to give him back his credit cards and US$4,000, which she kept for him. He became agitated when she refused. He planned to spend US$40,000 to purchase a flat in the country as an investment. He overspent US$500 in a supermarket to buy food and cash coupons and spent US$900 to buy a new television. He went fishing overnight and got injured after slipping on a rock 2 days before admission. He denied any abnormal perceptions or beliefs.

On the day of admission, he called the police because his younger sister refused to give him back his credit cards and money. Police arrived and found a fruit knife on a table. He threatened to harm himself with a small knife placed near his forearm. He locked himself at home. He took off the

Dynamic Consultations with Psychiatrists: Understanding Severely Troubled Patients, First Edition. Jason Maratos.
© 2022 John Wiley & Sons Ltd. Published 2022 by John Wiley & Sons Ltd.

window frame and sat next to the open window. He claimed that he wanted to threaten the police only and denied true suicidal ideas. He later calmed down, and the police left. He went fishing alone and sent voice messages to his younger sister. He threatened to burn her flat and asked her to be careful of losing her children. He mentioned that he would not suffer any legal consequences after killing people because he was a mental patient. He also threatened to burn his wife and asked her to move out with their two daughters. He denied any true intention of harming them. He showed no remorse about his behavior. He believed that his younger sister should bear all the responsibility because she refused to give him back his money. His younger sister called police to bring him to hospital.

Family history

There is no known family history of mental illness.

Personal history

Peter was born in the city. His parents favored him because he was the oldest son. His father was strict and used physical punishment. His mother was submissive in parenting. He was the eldest of five siblings. He has two younger sisters and two younger brothers. The family relationship was not close. He was educated up to Form three with below-average performance and poor conduct. He dropped out of school to earn for the family. He worked as a construction site worker. He was unemployed in the last year after he got injured in a traffic accident. He relied on government allowances.

Peter got married in his 20s. His wife is a 31-year-old housewife; she is a quick-tempered person. They had frequent conflicts because of his drinking. His wife wanted to divorce him but did not proceed for financial reasons. He has two daughters, aged 8 and 9, and a 2-year-old son. He has a history of child abuse by scratching his daughter's hand with a beer lid opener.

He is a quick-tempered person. He enjoys fishing. He was a smoker and regular drinker. He had no suicidal history. He was given 18 months of probation for punching his wife 3 years ago. He is currently under police investigation for a suspected case of criminal intimidation.

Past psychiatric history

Peter has a longstanding history of alcohol misuse as well as cannabis and ketamine abuse since his teenage years. He had been known to mental health services in 2002, when he was admitted to a psychiatric hospital for irritability, irrelevant speech, and abnormal belief about black magic. He was diagnosed with a Delusional Disorder and Harmful Use of Alcohol. He was treated with risperidone and thiamine. He only attended follow-up once and later did not attend any further because he felt that he had no mental illness. He denied illicit drug use in the last 10 years. He had another psychiatric admission from June to August 2018 for irritability, overspending, increased planning, and child abuse. He was diagnosed with Bipolar Affective Disorder, Manic Episode, and Alcohol Dependence Syndrome. He was treated with olanzapine 10 mg nightly and valproate sodium 400 mg every morning and 800 mg nightly. He attended psychiatric follow-ups regularly, but he had poor drug compliance.

Present treatment   The provisional diagnosis is Bipolar Affective Disorder, Manic Episode, and Alcohol Dependence Syndrome. Olanzapine 10 mg nightly and valproate sodium 800 mg were resumed after admission. He was given diazepam 5 mg twice daily. He was referred to medical social worker for family relationship problems and to occupational therapy for vocational assessment.

Consultation   JM thanked the doctor for her thorough presentation and then asked about Peter's spending of excessive amounts and questioned whether this was part of him being in a hypomanic phase. JM also asked if Peter tended to have overvalued ideas about his wealth and his position as a man who can invest thousands of US dollars in various property schemes. These were factors that needed to be considered in relation to Peter's diagnosis.

JM then asked about Peter's relationship with his sister and, in particular, the way through which his sister gained control of some of his money and of his credit cards. Was this arrangement one in which Peter engaged willingly as a way of protecting some of his money? JM then asked why it was the younger sister who helped in this way rather than his wife. The doctor explained that at the time, his wife was in the country where she stayed for 2 to 3 months. The doctor suggested that because he had a history of being violent and hitting his wife, his sister would be in a better position to control his money. In clarifying the relationship between sister and Peter, it was pointed out that sister has been quite responsible and protective of Peter, and there was no question of her exploiting him or profiting from controlling his money.

JM asked how Peter managed to have control of such big sums, and the doctor clarified that at that time Peter was working in the construction industry where his wages were good. The relationship between Peter and this sister required a different understanding because his sister was being helpful to him by protecting his finances.

JM then focused on the reasons why Peter remained unemployed after his accident. The doctor pointed out that Peter suffered an accident a year previously when he was driving a motorbike. The doctor noted that the accident did not cause any serious physical injury and that after the accident Peter was given a government allowance, which made it unnecessary for him to earn a living. (About a pathological reaction to accidents, see Miller [1961, 1962]). JM questioned whether the allowance for an accident that did not cause serious injury could be so generous as to support him and his family and make it unnecessary for him to ever work again. The doctor confirmed that this was indeed the case. JM questioned whether 40-year-old ever wanted to return to work, and the doctor responded that he did not. There did not seem to be a long-term plan for Peter in his life, and he simply makes excuses whenever a doctor suggests returning to work to him. JM asked if Peter was at all troubled by the prospect of a life without work, and the doctor responded that he did not seem concerned. This was thought to be related to the possibility of him being in a hypomanic phase. Furthermore, Peter used to justify his earnings by selling luxury watches, and he felt that he did not need to earn any more. His concept of his earnings was not in keeping with reality and was a pathological defense, thinking of himself as a rich financier when he is an unemployed laborer living in a public housing unit. The doctor added that the situation was also difficult for Peter's wife. JM asked about Peter's view of himself as a father: Was he concerned about what sort of model he would present to his children and was he concerned to be a provider for them? The doctor added that it was his wife that had most of the concern and who carried out most of the caring for the children. The doctor mentioned that Peter claimed that he cared about his children, but JM commented that his behavior did not indicate this because he used to start his days by drinking alcohol and remained inebriated throughout the day.

JM asked if the current mental state represented a significant change in Peter and if in the past Peter had a good track record regarding work and in his function as a family man. The doctor pointed out that Peter had a good work record, but his relationship with his wife had been marred by his alcoholism, which had been longstanding. JM asked if Peter had any insight on his alcohol problem. The doctor stated that Peter lacked insight completely because he did not think that he has an alcohol problem. JM pointed out that it would be difficult to establish a therapeutic contract with Peter. JM asked if the doctor knew what Peter's hopes were about the purpose of the psychiatric treatment. The doctor responded that Peter's wish was that the psychiatrist would support his application for greater financial assistance from the government. JM pointed out that such an attitude was a difficult position for doctors because, on the one hand, a doctor wants to be helpful but, on the other, they do not wish to be exploited or used for the wrong purpose. If one simply refused to support Peter's application, that would lead to the end of the therapeutic contact. On the other hand, if one simply supported his unjustified claims, one would be colluding in a possibly illegal and most likely antitherapeutic process.

JM suggested that Peter was likely to continue his search until he found a psychiatrist who would be prepared to support his application for further funds. JM elaborated on the difficulty of maintaining the therapeutic relationship while avoiding any collusion or participating in a marginally illegal activity. The doctor could suggest that Peter could make a better life for himself if, as a first measure, he stopped drinking altogether. JM pointed out that it is unlikely that a target of measured or only sociable drinking would be realistic for Peter. For him, the most appropriate target regarding his alcoholism would be total abstinence.

The second difficulty in Peter's case is the possible double pathology of alcoholism and bipolar disorder. There is a possibility that one exacerbates the other. For example, the idea that he can cope with any amount of alcohol and his dismissive attitude about the difficulties that alcohol brings may be an expression of a hypomanic phase. Any therapeutic contract needs to make clear that defrauding the state is not only illegal, but it is also not the best plan for him and not in his best interests. He can be helped to have a more realistic view of himself as a young able man who has responsibilities (i.e., wife and three children) and who can make himself a much better role model for his children. Also, Peter can acquire a better status in his community, as that of a working man rather than that of an alcoholic who lives off the state.

JM then suggested the possibility that Peter is at the beginning of a career as a vexatious litigant (Mullen & Lester, 2006). JM referred to a small group of people who make a living out of relentless pursuing of compensation through litigation. Quite often, this group of people rely on the understanding that many individuals or companies would rather concede to their demands instead of being embroiled in a time-consuming and expensive litigation process. Some people sue the doctors or the hospital for failing to treat them or by making their case worse by failing to support their application for funds. Some litigants show themselves to be adept at finding weak points in the system on which they base their claims. Litigation becomes their primary concern, and it is like a "job" for them. JM concluded by stating that the most helpful approach is one of firmness, in the sense that one is willing to help their patient but only in their capacity as a doctor and not as party to a dubious scheme of enrichment.

References

Miller, H. (1961). Accident neurosis. *British Medical Journal, 1*(5231), 992–998.

Miller, H. (1962). Accident neurosis. *Proceedings of the Royal Society of Medicine, 55*, 509–511.

Mullen, P. E., & Lester, G. (2006). Vexatious litigants and unusually persistent complainants and petitioners: From querulous paranoia to querulous behaviour. *Behavioral Sciences & the Law, 24*(3), 333–349.

14
Cocaine Addiction

Ms. T

Presenting condition

Ms. T is a 35-year-old, single, hairstylist who was voluntarily admitted from the general hospital.

History of presenting illness

Ms. T had been known to the mental health service since 2015 when she presented with low mood and cocaine abuse. She was last seen in clinic in December 2018 with fair mood and increased use of cocaine to daily consumption. Since the last follow-up, she continued her daily use of inhaled cocaine. She often asked her mother for money to purchase illicit drugs. When her mother refused, she would get agitated and frustrated. She carried out many self-harm gestures, including slashing her left arm whenever she felt frustrated. In addition, there were many violent gestures demonstrated to obtain money from her mother. She once attempted to lock the gate of the flat with an iron chain to stop her mother from leaving. She also pointed a pen knife at her mother while requesting money to purchase cocaine.

On the day of admission, Ms. T again requested money for cocaine. Her mother refused, and she felt frustrated. She drank 500 mL of apple cider after her mother left the house. Afterward, she went downstairs and purchased a packet of charcoal. She also took a belt and fixed it at the upper deck of her bed. She then took the photo of the charcoal and of the belt and sent it to her social worker. Then, when she noticed that her mother had returned to the house, she began to burn the charcoal. Her mother immediately detected smoke, so she went into the room and discovered the fire. Her mother then informed the police and took Ms. T to the hospital for medical management. When these events were further explored, Ms. T claimed that this was a way of gaining her mother's attention.

Family history

No family history of mental illness was found.

Dynamic Consultations with Psychiatrists: Understanding Severely Troubled Patients, First Edition. Jason Maratos.
© 2022 John Wiley & Sons Ltd. Published 2022 by John Wiley & Sons Ltd.

Personal history

Ms. T was born in the city; she has a young sister. Her parents divorced when she was in primary school, and her father was heavily engaged in gambling. Her mother took care of both daughters, and they have had no contact with their father. Ms. T felt that she had a distant relationship with her mother because she felt that her mother preferred her younger sister over her. This is because her younger sister was more obedient r and had better academic results. She also felt that her mother was not caring enough and tended to leave Ms. T alone whenever Ms. T faced difficulties.

Regarding the relationship with her younger sister, Ms. T described that she felt jealous of her because she had most of their mother's attention. She admitted she would frequently scold her young sister over trivial matters as a way of releasing her jealousy. Later, her sister continued her studies and life in the US. After her departure, there was an improvement in their relationship and the relationship with her mother. Ms. T was able to finish secondary school with fair academic results. She made many friends during study, yet she felt that each friendship did not last long and has few contacts with her classmates now. After completing her studies, Ms. T worked as a hairstylist. Apart from working as a hairstylist, she currently also holds classes teaching hairstyling.

Ms. T has had many romantic relationships; the longest one was in her 20s. She met her boyfriend at work, and they fell in love after knowing each other for 2 weeks. After being in the relationship for 3 months, Ms. T decided to move into his apartment. This relationship lasted for 5 years, but they broke up many times. Ms. T was also engaged in other brief relationships, which lasted for a few weeks during this relationship. Ms. T claimed that the reason behind that was that her boyfriend was busy working, so she felt lonely and would go to bars when she was off work.

For the premorbid personality, she described herself as an "extrovert mixed with introvert." She would be able to make friends easily if she wanted to, but she somehow believed that those friends didn't truly know her. Her interests are drawing pictures and listening to music.

Past psychiatric history

Since adolescence, Ms. T has a history of self-harm with many occasions of arm slashing. She would slash her arm when experiencing low mood. Ms. T used cocaine initially 5 years ago under peer influence and following conflict with her family. Initially she consumed cocaine 3 to 4 days per week. There was a noted increase to daily cocaine consumption since December 2018. This followed the imminent return of her sister from the US. She was worried that her mother would focus her attention on her sister again.

At that time, she presented with 3 months' history of low mood with insomnia and negative cognitions. She was diagnosed with a moderate depressive episode and was treated with fluoxetine. She also had a history of cocaine use. She consumed cocaine when she felt low, especially after conflict with family.

Treatment　Ms. T was treated with antidepressants (Remeron 30 mg nightly) to which she responded well. She was given the opportunity to explore the cognitive distortions, and she was more able to recognize that she jumps to conclusions, such as that her younger sister's return to the city meant that her mother would abandon her. She was also able to consider more possibilities when her young sister returned. There could be improvement in the relationship between them and with their mother. Stress coping methods were discussed with her. She was encouraged to develop further her own personal interests, such as painting, after discharge from the hospital instead of relying on cocaine. Further treatment plan includes exploration of the family dynamics with her mother. In addition, Ms. T was offered motivational interviewing. She showed more determination in discontinuing the use of cocaine. A joint interview with her mother was conducted. They showed more understanding toward the diagnosis. Her mother agreed to further supervise Ms. T's medication compliance and monitor Ms. T's mental state on discharge.

Consultation   JM thanked the doctor for the thorough presentation and then shared his impression that this was a case of a 35-year-old woman and not that of a younger child. Ms. T was still preoccupied, as it would have been appropriate for a young child, with who her mother loves most. The significant matter in this case is that she is not only mindful that she is not the favorite child but that she is made sick by the perception that she is not. This is a pathological preoccupation. A better adjusted person would be aware that she is not the favorite child and at the same time get on with her life. This is not the case with Ms. T. By age 35, most people would divert their attention to finding other sources through which their legitimate emotional needs could be met.

JM then pointed out that any mother is more likely to feel closer to a child who is not manipulative, who is addressing her own needs such as her studies, and who manages to leave home to study abroad (like her sister) than to somebody who is making incessant demands and pressures her for money to buy cocaine. It would not be helpful to try to convince her that her mother loves both children equally. It may be more constructive if Ms. T was helped to appreciate the role that she is playing in turning her mother away from her or in making her mother like her and love her less. It would be more helpful if Ms. T was made more aware of the role that she is playing in shaping the relationship with her mother and that if she wants a better relationship with her mother she should stop manipulating her, stop harassing her for money for cocaine, and concentrate on addressing the real issues of her 35-year-old life, which are to build her career, build a romantic relationship, and build a circle of good friends. In summary, Ms. T needs to be made aware that she plays a part in bringing about the thing that causes her so much pain.

In therapy, it would help if the therapist acknowledged that Ms. T's need for love and some admiration from her mother are legitimate. Both love and admiration are interconnected, but it is useful to think of them separately to start with. JM then offered examples of parents who love their children even if they have major difficulties. A parent can feel (and show) a sense of pride in the child if their achievements are of a level appropriate to their abilities. Some parents have arbitrary expectations of their children without taking account of their children's potential. For example, a parent of a child with average potential may have expectations that they would go to university and have a professional career. Such an approach is going to make the parent feel that the child is failing, and as a result, they are going to convey this feeling of failure and undermine the child's self-esteem. The child is going to feel a like failure. That is why, in psychiatry for children, one often helps parents develop realistic expectations of their children. For example, if a child has below-average potential, this needs to be recognized, the expectations adjusted to that level, and the child can be made to feel proud of achieving results in accordance with their potential. This is how a child will learn to value their own self and to develop a positive attitude toward themselves. Arbitrary expectations and arbitrary comparisons with other siblings are counterproductive. It is possible that in this family there was an expectation that Ms. T performed as well as her sister and that this expectation was not only mother's but also Ms. T's.

Obviously, being a hairstylist is not considered as highly as being a university graduate, but nevertheless, it sounds that Ms. T has good reasons to feel proud of being a good hairstylist and of being good enough to be asked to teach others.

Ms. T would be helped if in therapy she accepted that she is not as academically bright as her sister and that her career is not going to be as highly regarded as that of a university graduate. "Accepted" implies also that she grew to value her skills and her career.

Another objective in therapy would be for Ms. T to accept that, for whatever reason, she is not her mother's favorite child and that her relationship with her mother is not going to be as good as that of her sister and her mother. This is a process akin to mourning because Ms. T will need to mourn the loss of the hoped-for close relationship with her mother. Having accepted this bitter reality, Ms. T can divert her attentions to have her legitimate needs being met in other ways. She can divert her attention to developing a relationship with a good man, she can develop good relationships with her work colleagues, and she can develop friendships which are supportive; she needs to find people who will love her and look up to her (or simply value her for who she is) instead of people who are collusive with her, agree with everything she says, and then supply her or even pressurize her to take cocaine. Ms. T needs to be more careful who she chooses as friends.

One objective of therapy is for Ms. T to accept that she may not be the brightest and she may not be the most attractive person, but she can still make a good life for herself, she can still form relationships that give her love, and she can still perform work that makes her feel proud.

It is understandable that Ms. T finds the feelings of not being loved and not being admired unbearable; having acknowledged that, we can then try to understand what is it that makes it impossible for Ms. T to cope with such feelings. We know that she finds it impossible to cope with it because she resorts to self-harming and to taking drugs instead of working through these feelings. As this had not been explored with Ms. T, JM invited the doctor to reflect on occasions when he had to cope with the disappointment of originally high expectations and how he had to readjust these personal expectations. Such an experience of being disappointed and making readjustment is common and has happened to most people. JM then invited the exploration of the process. The doctor suggested that one coping technique is distracting oneself to other matters. The other suggestion was that time sometime helps. JM accepted this but also pointed out that with time, certain problems become more entrenched and certain feelings become even more painful. It is not time in itself that is therapeutic, but the way in which one addresses the issues during time that brings about improvement. The case of Ms. T is an example in which things have become worse with time.

There are several factors that help one cope with such disappointments. The first is the presence of people who you feel are on your side, like friends or family. These people will show you that the reality is that you did not achieve your goal, but that is not a disaster because you can still have a good job and can still be a valuable person in society. You can still be a good friend and you can still be, say, a good hairstylist; therefore, you can still be loved and can still be admired despite the disappointment.

In the case of Ms. T, she needs to be helped to develop the ability to form relationships with friends who are supportive and more long lasting. Ms. T clearly has difficulties with relationships, and these difficulties need to be identified and worked through. The context of this process cannot be effective if it is only in the form of education (i.e., if she is only informed that she is playing a part in destroying the relationships). Ms. T needs to feel safe in the relationship with the therapist who will be helping her to come to terms with certain difficult truths while the therapist shows her acceptance, human concern, and appropriate appreciation.

JM then pointed out that Ms. T needs to be clear that people who push drugs on her are not a good influence, are not people who have her best interest at heart, and are not people who she should consider friends. There is no uncertainty about the effect of cocaine; it is a toxic drug that does not resolve anything and that also stores troubles for the future. She clearly needs to distance herself from drug pushers.

The therapeutic task for Ms. T is to mourn the negative experiences in her life and to concentrate on the positive aspects of it. Ms. T can begin to feel proud for her job and the appreciation she must derive from her clients and her pupils. This is a solid achievement on which she can begin to build a positive value of herself. Furthermore, she has maintained the working relationships with the same company for many years, so she is appreciated by them. The doctor added that she was also popular at work and with her pupils. These are solid and realistic foundations of a good self-esteem. JM asked the doctor of the reason why Ms. T had not been sacked from her work. As this was not known, JM suggested that certain positive aspects of her behavior at work may be ignored when in fact it would be useful for her to be reminded of them so that they can form solid building blocks of a realistic and positive sense of self. JM pointed out that she may not value the many positive things in her life because she only judges them in comparison with those of her sister. A therapist may be able to help her move her comparisons from the sister and the family of origin to her present and her future life in the community.

Based on this, the therapist can help Ms. T see the future with some greater hope. Knowing that she can work, that her work is valued, and that she can earn a living and support herself she can look at the future as a more positive experience than her recent past has been.

JM then pointed out that another counterproductive source of counseling is that of simple support in the form of collusion. Sympathy that comes across as "poor you, you have been so unlucky, you have a mother who does not prefer you" will only confirm her worse feelings of herself. Sympathy is a necessary step in developing a therapeutic relationship but becomes toxic if the therapeutic relationship stays at that level. Sympathy is essential so that the patient can feel appreciated and cared for so that they can effect change necessary for them. Collusion is as toxic as cocaine.

Flores and Mahon (1993) highlight the issues referred to in this consultation and is not only useful for those interested in providing group therapy for their patients.

Reference

Flores, P. J., & Mahon, L. (1993). The treatment of addiction in group psychotherapy. *International Journal of Group Psychotherapy*, 43(2), 143–156.

Section V

Psychosomatic Presentations

15
Fatigue

Paul

Presenting complaint

Paul is an 18-year-old student attending Form 4 presenting with fatigue and a wish to die.

History of present illness

Paul's mental condition was stable until August 2016 when he was abroad and hit by a vehicle while riding a motorcycle. He suffered from lower limb injuries and was unable to work. This loss of income brought about financial stress. His mother stopped contacting him, and his father became more dependent on him as his mental illness deteriorated. He felt lonely because he had no one to depend on anymore. His mood became low most of the time despite being able to cope with routines during the day. His sleep and appetite were maintained. He felt anxious about his future because he was uncertain what options remained available to him. He made an impulsive attempt of overdosing with 30 tablets of amisulpride, which had been prescribed for his father. He fell asleep and did not seek medical attention after waking up the following day. He made no other self-harm gestures.

Paul felt that he was unable to cope and returned to the city to live with his paternal grandmother in 2016. He soon heard that his mother took the compensation from his road traffic accident and sold his motor bike. He felt disappointed about the past and wanted to start over in the city and started repeating Form 2. At first, his mood improved because he performed well at school and had good relationships with classmates and teachers. He tried to sustain these relationships by doing what he felt they liked him to do. However, he felt that he was being pretentious, and he tired of behaving so. He started skipping school and stopped talking to his classmates because he felt uninterested. He felt that he was treated differently by teachers and classmates and that he was disappointing them. He became more worried about his interpersonal relationships and was uncertain about his own image. He felt that he had been living for the sake of others and felt empty at times. He described that

Dynamic Consultations with Psychiatrists: Understanding Severely Troubled Patients, First Edition. Jason Maratos.

his mood had been low most of the time during the last 2 years despite coping well at school. He was able to concentrate at school. His sleep was fair. His appetite was good. He felt lonely and worthless at times. He was pessimistic about the future.

Paul suffers an intermittent obsession on symmetry, which was not affecting his daily function. He had no history of overspending or elated mood. He had no perceptual disturbances. He had no abnormal beliefs. He had no violent ideas. One or 2 weeks before admission, he had repeatedly refused going to school and spent most of his time at home. He didn't take a bath, and he locked himself in his room and started drinking red wine and smoking. His grandmother was worried and advised him, but he felt irritable and had similar behavior. On the day before admission, he felt tired and did not want to attend school. His grandmother criticized him for skipping school and told him that he might as well go abroad if he was not trying hard in the city. He felt that his grandmother, who was his only family member, was giving up on him too. He felt abandoned because there was no one who cared about him anymore. He went back to his room and took 50 tabs of Bromazepam and swallowed them in front of his grandmother, after telling her that he loved her. He believed that this method was lethal. He then became unconscious. His grandmother was worried and called an ambulance. Paul denied any preparation before this attempt. No suicidal note was written. At the emergency medical ward, friends and family visited him. He felt that he was not lonely, and his mood improved. He strongly requested discharge because he believed that he was well and had to prepare for a concert in March. He covered his face with a pillow when his application for discharge was turned down. He alleged that he was only trying to rest his neck, and he was misunderstood. The consultation liaison team saw him, and he eventually agreed to inpatient observation and management. Voluntary admission to the psychiatric hospital was arranged.

Family history

His mother and paternal grandmother suffer from depression. His father has psychosis and is followed abroad. A paternal uncle has psychosis and depression and is followed up in the country. There is no family history of suicide.

Personal history

Paul was born in the country. He is an only child, who had an unhappy childhood. His mother was demanding of him and repeatedly physically punished him. His parents divorced when he was 10, and he lived with his father since then. He met his mother once a month after the divorce and their relationship became distant. His father's mental condition gradually deteriorated, and he was not able work. Paul started working when he was 12–13 years old. He worked as toilet cleaner, labor worker, delivery worker, and waiter and attended school irregularly since then. He started to use alcohol about 1 year ago "to cope with study stress." Paul started drinking half a bottle of red wine daily. Gradually, his consumption increased over the year. He is currently drinking 3 cans of beer every night on weekdays and 3 bottles of red wine until getting drunk on weekends. He denied withdrawal symptoms or drinking in daytime on weekdays.

Paul studied up to Form 4 abroad and had not skipped school since Primary 5 when he was no longer supervised by his mother. Paul came to the city in 2016 and started school in the city from Form 4; he had good academic performance. He presented with no conduct problems. He had a girlfriend in abroad for many years and broke up in 2017 after coming to the city. He is a smoker (one pack every weekend). He has no history of substance abuse and has no forensic record.

Past psychiatric history

Paul attended a psychiatrist abroad in 2016 (after the injury) and was diagnosed with Obsessive-Compulsive Disorder because he had repeated intrusive thoughts about symmetry and ritualistic behavior. He was prescribed sulpiride, later switching to amisulpride, but there was no major improvement. Paul became known to mental health service in the city via the child team in 2017; he was diagnosed with depression with Obsessive-Compulsive Disorder symptoms and was given escitalopram, which was gradually titrated up. Bromazepam was added due to on and off low mood, anxiety, and stress from studies.

Present treatment and management   Escitalopram was resumed after hospital admission; it was tolerated with no reported side effects. Detox for alcohol was completed. Valium was gradually tailed off with no withdrawal symptoms. Paul was referred to a clinical psychologist for personality assessment and to learn coping strategies. He was referred to an occupational therapist for a rehabilitation program. His mood remained stable since admission. He had no prominent negative cognitions. His sleep and appetite were normal. His energy level was normal. He enjoyed playing guitar and chatting with other patients. He made no self-harm gestures and had no suicidal ideas. He was regularly visited by a social worker and his grandmother during admission. Paul and his family requested an early discharge so that he could perform in a concert. A contingency plan was discussed and explained. Paul agreed to stop using alcohol after discharge. He was referred to a community psychiatric nurse. He attended regular follow-up at clinic and was seen by clinical psychologist at an outpatient department.

Consultation   JM thanked the doctor for the thorough presentation and then asked why Paul had not been able to work after his accident, especially because he had suffered only lower limb injuries that were reparable. The doctor responded that he was no longer able to ride his motorcycle. JM returned to the question of why he did not return to riding his motorcycle after his legs were restored. The doctor then added that Paul had a low mood after the accident. JM then suggested that it seemed that the physical sequelae of the accident would not justify Paul being out of work for 2 years. The doctor confirmed that Paul was able to ride his motorcycle. It, therefore, was clear that the injury to his legs was not enough to justify absence from work for 2 years. JM stressed that the matter of injury to his legs and his inability to work is a matter that was a lot more complex than the way it was presented. Paul had not returned to work even though he had recovered from the physical consequences of the accident and that a 3-month absence from work could be justified but not 2 years. On the matter of illness and disability, see Susser (1990).

It seemed that it would be helpful, in considering Paul's emotions, if reality, as it can be independently assessed, was taken account of, rather than only according to Paul's narrative. The doctor then pointed out that following the accident, the Paul's father became more dependent on him. The doctor explained that Paul's father suffered from psychosis. His father started having persecutory ideation and refused to leave the home. His father also refused medical help. Paul undertook more responsibilities in running the home. There was no other adult who could undertake these functions because his parents were divorced. His father expected Paul to do these things because he had no other activity to demand on his time. JM suggested that it was reasonable of Paul's father to expect Paul to do a bit more at home now that he was not at work but also pointed out that it is not stressful for an unemployed man to do a bit of shopping and a bit of cooking. The fact that Paul found these simple chores stressful needs to be understood in psychological terms. The doctor added that it was not only the additional chores but also the lack of a functioning father that affected Paul. JM added that Paul may have resented doing household duties when he was not at work.

JM then asked the doctor to expand on the nature of Paul's obsessions about symmetry. The doctor explained that the obsessions did not seem to be causing Paul a lot of trouble; he was only preoccupied that things should be symmetrical. JM then clarified that Paul did not seem to be suffering from Obsessive-Compulsive Disorder but that he may simply have a trait of obsessiveness in his personality. Paul may also have some personality trait of rigidity, which is not a disability in itself.

JM then asked that Paul's sense that he had been abandoned by his grandmother to be reexamined. The question was raised because his grandmother was actually looking after him; the grandmother's attitude could be stated as: "you are welcome to come to the city to live with me as long as you study but if you do not study then you should go abroad to live with your father." His grandmother seemed to expect of Paul (or even encourage him) to attend school. This did not seem an attitude of abandoning. Despite this approach, Paul saw his grandmother's attitude as a rejection. The doctor explained that Paul tended to experience a rejection any challenge to his own narrative. JM added that this approach would make it difficult for any health professional to help him adopt a more constructive narrative. Paul is likely to perceive any advice as hostility. This approach indicates that the health professional who will undertake his treatment will need to proceed slowly to avoid developing a negative relationship with Paul.

JM then focused on the overdose Paul took in front of his grandmother. The doctor explained that Paul took the tablets, went to his room, and started swallowing mouthfuls of them. He was doing that while he was telling his grandmother that he loved her. JM then asked if it was known what sense Paul made of this behavior. JM pointed out that if one intends to kill themselves that is not the way they would try to do it. Although this was obviously a gesture, Paul claimed he intended on ending his life. This assertion obviously lacks credibility.

JM then asked the doctor if he knew what Paul's plan was for his life after his discharged from hospital. The doctor added that Paul intended to return to his studies and to attend psychiatric follow-up. His school attendance was not regular. The reason for this erratic attendance was, according to Paul, that he had problems with the attitudes of his classmates. He found it difficult to be 2 years older than his peers. Paul saw himself as a man who had experience in working, while his peers were "childish" because they had only been school pupils in their life. Paul had found the interaction with his classmates to be stressful and tiring.

JM asked if Paul's motivation for returning to school had been explored. The doctor explained that Paul had expressed "high expectations" of himself; he wanted to do well in public examinations and that he intended to study at university to work in the "professional sector." JM asked if the doctor thought that this was a realistic objective. The doctor felt that this was because Paul had consistently been in the top 10% of his class when he was a pupil. Paul had good grades when he was attending school, and it was realistic of him to expect to cope with state exams. It, therefore, became clear that the reason for him not being likely to perform well in state exams was his poor school attendance. The doctor added that it was not certain that Paul was doing homework. JM pointed out that his actions (not doing homework and not attending regularly) were not consistent with somebody who wants to achieve well at school and go to university. The doctor pointed out that Paul had an unrealistic attitude that he could pass the exams without necessarily attending school or doing homework.

The doctor then expressed a different view, which was that he believed that Paul was studying hard at home and that, therefore, it would not be unrealistic to expect of him to pass the state exams. JM was concerned that this was not exactly the case. JM expressed the view that Paul may have had an immature approach toward work, particularly that he could get by, by not doing the whole range of activities that work expected of him, and further, that Paul's approach was not that of a mature person who appreciates that work is a form of a package of enjoyable activities but also of other but not attractive engagements. Work is not entertainment in which people do only what they enjoy;

work is doing what is expected irrespective of whether it is considered enjoyable. JM pointed out that attending school prepares a person for work in the sense that it trains them to do all that is required even if it is difficult or not entirely pleasant and not only the parts that they find enjoyable. Work, like school, expects of a person to attend regularly, to get along with peers, and to do things that are difficult and maybe not to their liking. JM pointed out that if Paul is to make a good life for himself, he needs to develop a more mature approach to work, including schoolwork. He needs to be helped to approach difficulties as something to overcome and not something to avoid, as is his present practice.

JM repeated the point that Paul's approach was to avoid when things were unpleasant or difficult and that is where his alcoholism fits in. When he encounters difficulties, he resorts to alcohol instead of addressing the difficulties. It is his systematic and persistent avoidance of problems that is driving him further away even from his own objectives and not only his family's objectives but of his own. Even if he passes the exams, nobody will hire somebody who consumes several bottles of wine per week. JM pointed out that one could have sympathy with him because of his early history (his mother being negative toward him, his parents divorcing, and his father suffering from a psychosis), but at the same time, he is no longer a child and has a greater part to play in shaping his own life.

JM also added that it was extraordinary and indicative that his mother took the money from the compensation from his accident. It justifies his ambivalent feelings about his parents. The doctor reinforced this issue by pointing out that when he was much younger, Paul was afraid of his mother who had high expectations of him and who would physically chastise him if he did not do what he was required. Although his father was more supportive up to the age of 10, he was not an effective father after that because of his severe mental illness.

JM then asked why Paul was sent to work at the young age of 13, which was a young age even for the cultural context in which he was growing up. The doctor explained that after his parents divorced, he was left as being the only person who could support his severely ill father. JM pointed out that Paul became a parental child (Jurkovic et al., 1991), a father figure to his father at the age of 13. The doctor explained that Paul thought that he had no choice but to go to work and provide for his father. JM pointed out that whoever worked with him therapeutically needed first to acknowledge the deprivation and psychological maltreatment that he suffered when he was much younger. He had been deprived of a proper adolescence when he was entitled to have his needs looked after by his parents. It is understandable that he would have ambivalent feelings about his parents, some of which would be a degree of resentment, sadness, and anger at them depriving him and at not meeting his justifiable needs. Although it is a fact that he experienced a less than ideal childhood, it is also a fact that he is currently no longer a young child and that he can do better for himself. Paul is still uncertain whether, for example, he attends school to achieve his own aims or to meet parental expectations. JM clarified that Paul was in two minds: the part of him the brings him to school is the part where he wishes to achieve well for himself and the other that takes him away from these tasks when he thinks he is doing these activities to meet parental expectations. He rebels against meeting the expectations of his mother, father, and grandmother even though these coincide with his own.

Therapy will need to help him disentangle what his aspirations are from those of his family. It could be pointed out, or he could be helped to appreciate, that he is still young, able, and has appropriate expectations, in the sense that he could achieve those if he tackles them in a more functional way. Furthermore, his grandmother is not only somebody who may have unrealistic expectations of him but also somebody who does provide a home and the support that is inherent in this. His grandmother does not seem to be making any demands on him for her own sake; her demands are for his sake. He could be helped to realize that at present he is in a much better position than he was when he was 13. Paul could be given the realistic hope that he can achieve a lot more for himself if he were to adopt a more age-appropriate and functional approach to his life tasks. Paul needs to develop a view of himself as somebody who is young, healthy, and intellectually capable. Paul could be helped to disengage and distance himself from his past to build his present and his future.

References

Jurkovic, G. J., Jessee, E. H., & Goglia, L. R. (1991). Treatment of parental children and their families: Conceptual and technical issues. *The American Journal of Family Therapy, 19*(4), 302–314.

Susser, M. (1990). Disease, illness, sickness; impairment, disability and handicap. *Psychological Medicine, 20*(3), 471–473.

16

Sleeping Disorders

Wendy

Presenting complaint

Wendy is a 45-year-old divorced woman who presented with initial insomnia.

History of the present condition

Wendy's mood started to deteriorate as a result of multiple stressors. She had a decreased wish to carry out housework and had reduced motivation during the rehabilitation program that had been arranged by the department of orthopedics and trauma. Her sleep became fragmented but her appetite remained fair. She was able to cope with activities of daily living and housework but at times would throw a tantrum with her mother when she was distressed. She had episodes of ignoring requests from her mother. Wendy felt guilty for not being able to take care of her mother and felt that she was useless. She had fleeting ideas of killing her mother with a knife and of committing suicide afterward by burning charcoal. She also had ideas of jumping from heights. She had an episode of standing next to a window and looking down, but otherwise she did not act on any of these intentions. There was no history of suicidal attempts or of violent acts. No definite preparation for suicide was undertaken.

Wendy repeatedly ruminated about how she showed her temper at her mother and had not been able to take care of her. She thinks that she is responsible for her mother's death and that her mother would have lived longer if she took better care of her. She also regretted that she did not spend time listening to her mother and acknowledging her emotional needs. She felt that her mother was "pathetic" during her final days because of her ignorance.

Wendy had difficulty initiating sleep and was easily woken. She sleeps for 2 hours each night. Her appetite had recently been poor. She lost interest in meeting with friends. She was not keen to resume work despite being assessed fit to drive small vehicles. She is tired during the day and is unable to concentrate. She feels hopeless at times. She resorted to drinking in the last 2 weeks, drinking up to

Dynamic Consultations with Psychiatrists: Understanding Severely Troubled Patients, First Edition. Jason Maratos.

six cans of king-size beer a day. She denied substance abuse. She has had no previous episodes of elated mood or overspending. Wendy suffered no perceptual disturbance and held no irrational beliefs. There are no anxiety symptoms. There were no flashbacks. She has no active suicidal or aggressive ideas.

Family history

There is no family history of mental illness.

Personal history

Wendy was born in the city in 1973. She is the second child and has one older brother with whom she has a distant relationship. She described the history of her childhood as "unremarkable." Wendy described her mother as demanding of her since her childhood. Wendy studied up to Form 5. She worked as a receptionist at a driving school for about 20 years and gave up her job when its nature was changed. Wendy worked as a clerk briefly, then worked as a bus driver, and then started working as a driver in government.

Wendy's father died from cholangiocarcinoma more than 10 years ago. In August 2018, her mother's condition deteriorated and she was admitted for oncological care; her mother eventually died in August 2018. Her funeral took place in September of the same year.

Wendy married at 22 and had a daughter who is now 23 years old with whom she has infrequent contact. Wendy divorced her husband after suffering domestic violence; he repeatedly hit her, even when she was pregnant. Her ex-husband experienced marital problems in his second marriage and died by suicide about 10 years ago.

Wendy stopped smoking about 1 year ago, following the recommendation of an orthopedic surgeon (for better bone growth). She was a social drinker; stopped drinking for the same reason; however, she started drinking six cans of 500 mL of beer daily since her mother's death. There is no history of substance abuse or forensic history. She has hobbies of badminton, hiking, and traveling.

Since her divorce, Wendy had lived with her mother for more than 10 years. She had been her mother's main carer. Wendy returned home to live with mother after discharge and is currently living with her paternal grandmother.

Past medical and psychiatric history

Wendy had been mentally stable until 2017. Wendy was hit by private car when she was riding a motorcycle in January 2017; this resulted in a fracture of her left foot that required surgical repair. She stayed in the hospital for rehabilitation for 2 months. At that time, she was motivated to engage in physiotherapy and occupational therapy as part of her rehabilitation. Her mood was stable, and she was looking forward to resuming work.

On discharge, Wendy still had to walk with a walking aid and required help in preparing meals. Her mother had been able to help at first but was later found to have relapse of breast cancer with lymph node metastases. Her arm was swollen and was unable to cope with some household chores. Wendy was unable to help much due to her persistent and disabling foot injury.

In July 2017, Wendy had used up her fully paid sick leave and was started on low-pay sick leave. She sought help from her elder bother but was not supported by him emotionally or financially. Her mother's physical condition deteriorated, and she spent most of the time indoors or in bed requiring help in activities of daily living. Wendy was not able to help at that time because of her walking difficulty. Later, Wendy attended driver training assessment and training and was deemed not fit to resume work.

Present treatment and management   Wendy had been attending a clinical psychologist since early 2017 for cognitive behavioral therapy (CBT), which had limited effect. It was suggested that she attend a psychiatric service for her persistent low mood. She had not attended previously because she thought she could cope with the stress on her own. However, she felt that her sleep remained poor recently and started attending psychiatric clinic for hypnotics. Organic workup was performed and was unremarkable. She was started on mirtazapine in September 2018 and was gradually titrated up to 30 mg nightly. She was given promethazine to take when necessary to promote her sleep. She continues to attend a clinical psychologist for CBT. She will be seeing a new therapist at her next appointment because her current therapist is being transferred to another hospital.

Consultation   JM thanked the doctor for the thorough preparation of this case. The doctor continued that Wendy had set her heart on returning to a driving job because she was hoping that her foot would be restored to normal functioning. Wendy had not explored alternative solutions or alternative occupations. "All she wanted to do was to continue driving after her foot got better." JM pointed out that this was a year prior and that she had at least 1 year in which to reconsider her future. JM pointed out that in the last year instead of recovering and becoming increasingly capable, she became increasingly incapacitated with the clinical picture being more complicated. In fact even though her physical condition (the foot) was improving, her overall adjustment was deteriorating. The doctor confirmed that from the beginning of 2018, Wendy was thought fit to undertake driving, but at that time, she felt too fatigued and did not have the "volition" to start work. JM pointed out that at present Wendy is physically fit to undertake a job as a driver. The doctor added that Wendy had not driven her motorcycle since her injury because she felt it is too dangerous. Wendy was fit to drive a commercial vehicle.

JM asked the doctor to clarify that the only reason Wendy was not at work presently is her emotional state. This was confirmed. JM then addressed the issue of the lack of motivation for work especially because work would have improved Wendy's quality of life enormously. The doctor pointed out that since her mother's death in August 2018 Wendy was troubled by feelings about her mother's death. Wendy was always feeling tired and was ruminating about the recent past, and more particularly, she was troubled with feelings of guilt about how she had neglected her mother. JM then summarized the case as one in which during the last year, up to her mother's death, Wendy had been affected by two major events (the foot injury and mother's illness and death), and after her mother's death she was troubled by a prolonged and complicated grief reaction. What was incapacitating her since her mother's death were her ambivalent feelings about her mother and her sense of guilt.

JM then suggested that this formulation would be a useful guide in directing the type of therapy that was likely to help Wendy. The target would need to be appropriate grief processing, resolving ambivalent feelings, accepting failings in a realistic way, and being able to put that behind her so that she can reconstruct her life toward her future.

The doctor then pointed out that Wendy had expressed to him feelings of guilt for "not being able" to look after her mother better in the last days of her life. JM picked out the sense of guilt and suggested that one cannot realistically feel guilty for something that they are unable to do. She would be entitled to feel guilty if she was able to do something and did not do it. The nature of Wendy's guilt could further be explored along those lines and be resolved.

The doctor added that Wendy failed to care for her mother in things that she could have carried out. In trying to understand Wendy's sense of guilt, JM asked the doctor if he had taken a detailed history of the way in which Wendy had failed to look after her mother. The doctor added that when things worked "normal," it was Wendy's mother who was preparing the meals. When mother became unwell, it was up to Wendy to prepare the meals. Wendy felt that she was not preparing meals that could have been as elaborate as her mother would have done and that she was only preparing the bare essentials. The doctor added that although she prepared meals and also looked after mother's physical and hygienic well-being, Wendy felt that she did not do it to a good enough standard.

JM then suggested that a psychiatrist who is acting a little like a priest and who gives absolution would not hold great credibility with Wendy. JM pointed out that one should accept that the care that Wendy gave to her mother was less than optimal and that it reflected her mixed feelings toward her mother. JM then proposed that once the mixed feelings had been identified, then the source of these feelings could be explored and be traced to previous experiences of a mother who was overly demanding or, perhaps, controlling. Although a psychiatrist could not offer "absolution of sins," they could work with her to reach a more thorough understanding of the origin of her feelings across time.

JM then returned to the issue of Wendy being a young woman who has the full capacity of her mind, who regained her physical fitness but who has adopted the identity and the existence of an invalid. JM suggested that Wendy could think of herself as somebody who had a really traumatic recent past (from the divorce, the noncommunication with her daughter, the cancer and the incapacity of her mother and her own accident, pain and incapacity immediately after) but who is still relatively young and able to build a good life for herself. JM added the importance of giving Wendy realistic hope for her future because hope is the basis of good motivation. High motivation can be based on hope and a realistic perspective.

Wendy's reality is that she has the ability to hold a job, has the ability to make a better life for herself, and so she is entitled to have a realistic hope for her own future. Although she has had difficulties with other people, she has had a few friends and she could reignite those friendships with professional support. One can give Wendy considerable sympathy for all the unfortunate events and difficulties that she experienced, but the support needs to be in the service of giving her realistic hope, a realistic perspective, and the impetus to start building her life.

This case highlights several important issues among which:

The pathology of guilt, for which see Winnicott (1958);
The pathology of mourning and grief, for which see Freud (1917), Boelen and Smid (2017), and Parkes and Markus (1998);
The pathology of response to trauma and illness, for which see Susser (1990); and
The pathology of intimate partner (or domestic) violence, for which see Dillon et al. (2013) and Leung (2019).

References

Boelen, P. A., & Smid, G. E. (2017). Disturbed grief: Prolonged grief disorder and persistent complex bereavement disorder. *British Medical Journal*, *357*, j2016.

Dillon, G., Hussain, R., Loxton, D., & Rahman, S. (2013). Mental and physical health and intimate partner violence against women: A review of the literature. *International Journal of Family Medicine*, *2013*, 313909.

Freud, S. (1917). Mourning and melancholia. In *The Standard Edition of the Complete Psychological Works of Sigmund Freud* (Vol. XIV, pp. 243–258). Hogarth Press.

Leung, L. C. (2019). Deconstructing the myths about intimate partner violence: A critical discourse analysis of news reporting in the city. *Journal of Interpersonal Violence*, *34*(11), 2227–2245.

Parkes, C. M., & Markus, A. C. (1998). Coping with loss: Helping patients and their families. *BMJ Clinical Research*, *316*(7143), 1521–1524.

Susser, M. (1990). Disease, illness, sickness; impairment, disability and handicap. *Psychological Medicine*, *20*(3), 471–473.

Winnicott, D. W. (1958). Psycho-analysis and the sense of guilt. In J. D. Sutherland (Ed.), *Psychoanalysis and contemporary thought* (Vol. (Vol. 1, pp. 15–32). Hogarth Press.

Ben

Ben is a single, 37-year-old unemployed man who previously worked as part-time private English tutor and who lives with his mother in a public housing unit.

Presenting condition

He was voluntarily admitted from the accident and emergency department due to insomnia.

History of present complaint

Since his last discharge in June 2018, Ben reported that he had followed up with different private psychiatrists. He refused to disclose to the hospital psychiatrist any details, including his usual medications because he claimed that this information was "confidential." The hospital psychiatrist explained the importance of continuing his usual dose of medication and the risk of changing the usual dose, especially for long-acting benzodiazepines, but he still withheld permission to the hospital psychiatrist to contact the private psychiatrist. The hospital psychiatrist tried to contact his mother, but he reported his mother was not familiar with his medications and follow-up. He reported he was on Stilnox 10 mg at bedtime, clonazepam 0.5 mg three times a day, Artane 4 mg twice daily, Quetiapine XR 300 mg nightly, and paroxetine.

Ben had been settled in the community despite his difficult adjustment until 2 weeks prior to admission when he caught the "flu." He visited a private general practitioner, but he had difficulty in initiating sleep despite taking Stilnox. He attributed this difficulty to his flu symptoms. He found this distressing because he was tired during the day, and he became more forgetful and ruminated about the numbers 7, 8, and 9. He was checking the closed door after he left his home. He was more anxious, and the obsessive thoughts disrupted his daily activities. He wanted to take a break and get a good rest in the hospital and strongly requested admission at the emergency unit on the day of admission. He denied any intention to self-harm or any suicidal or violent ideation. He reported no low mood and no perceptual disturbance.

Ben is an average built man with fair self-care and poor eye contact. He appeared not interested in the consultation and was difficult to engage. Ben's attitude was self-righteous, carefree, and guarded. His speech was coherent, relevant, and spontaneous. There was no formal thought disorder. He speaks using English but in the syntax of the native language. Ben readily talked about his previous experiences in other psychiatric units and mentioned that his requests were always fulfilled. Ben repeatedly tested boundaries with many requests (e.g., hospital psychiatrist must grant day leave with mother to visit dentist and a transfer to a ward for chronic patients). Ben appeared less challenging when his requests were granted. Ben stated that the hospital psychiatrist's attitude was "disrespectful" when he inquired about medication history.

Ben's mood was euthymic, and his affect was congruent but also exaggerated. He manifested no psychotic symptoms. Ben complained of a similar rumination about numbers 7, 8, and 9. Ben was not suicidal or violent. He was oriented in time, place, and person. Insight: Ben knew the diagnosis of Obsessive-Compulsive Disorder (OCD). He had his own plan for admission and discharge (e.g., he intended to tail off all benzodiazepines and hypnotics and requested to be transferred to the ward for chronic patients "ASAP"). He threatened the hospital psychiatrist that he would file complaints against him to the CEO if his requests were not fulfilled because he had stayed in psychiatric hospitals since he was 20. Ben requested clinical psychology service to be offered to him as his "life coach" during his inpatient stay. He was given the diagnosis of OCD and dissocial personality disorder.

Family history

There was no family history of mental illness, sexual abuse, or suicide.

Personal history

Ben was born in the city and was the eldest of three siblings. He was educated up to Form 5 and worked in various jobs. He is a smoker and a nondrinker and has no history of abuse.

He started working as a private English tutor (teaching another foreign language and basic English vocabulary to survive in the city) and was able to earn US$2,000 a month (when the average monthly income was in the region of US$1,700). He could not elaborate on the working pattern and the number of students he had and later revealed that he idled at home and enjoyed a listless lifestyle. He found it difficult to cope with housework because he spent most of his life in a psychiatric unit and found it exhausting to take public transport, especially on a hot summer's day. He complained of the size of his flat, which, he felt, was not spacious enough for himself and his mother.

Attempts to inquire about developmental history were not fruitful because his mother could not recall much information; she claimed she had been busy with work. She recalled that he was a difficult child who had frequent conflicts with his father.

Past psychiatric history

Ben has been known to the psychiatric service since 1994 when he was 14. He presented to a private psychiatrist with fear of contamination and compulsive handwashing and rechecking behavior; the diagnosis at the time was Obsessive-Compulsive Disorder. He became known to the public psychiatric service in 2003. Ben has had 35 psychiatric admissions to different psychiatric units mainly due to increased obsessive preoccupations with certain numbers and anxiety. Ben mostly requested admission himself, claiming that he could not cope with living in community.

Ben was last admitted to in 2018 (for 6 months). He was then reported to have playful, challenging, and demonstrated disturbing behavior that required frequent reporting to the police. He threw chairs, splashed water, and spat at a nurse. He was charged with common assault and was sentenced to the psychiatric center (Forensic Unit) for a week. He had declined the offer of a halfway house placement in 2015 and had turned down an offer for a public housing unit in 2016. He also repeatedly wrote letters to the CEO or the local authority applying for a larger flat. He had frequent day leaves with his mother to renovate their flat and to visit a private dentist. He was discharged when he did not return after day leave because he went to another city to see his friends.

Compassionate rehousing was offered in a public housing unit and follow-up was arranged later in the same year, but he did not attend. It was later discovered that he had been admitted to another hospital due to increase in obsessive-compulsive features and harmful use of medication. At that time, following conflict with the ward staff, he was discharged on clonazepam 0.5 mg three times daily, 1 mg nightly Stilnox 10 mg nightly, Quetiapine 300 mg nightly, Artane 4 mg twice daily, and paroxetine 60 mg nightly. Follow-up was arranged, but he did not attend. Since 2003, Ben has had a total of 43 hospital admissions. There are repeated documented episodes of self-harm by cutting or hurting his head. There is an extensive history of violent attacks on staff and family members. Ben frequently absconded from the ward and failed to show up for follow-up appointments.

Ben had been seeing a private psychiatrist for 8 years until 2003. In 2005–2006, Ben underwent plastic surgery and had changed his name.

In 2014 Ben was convicted of common assault; he was imprisoned for 2 weeks and received an additional 18 months suspended sentence. In 2017, he was fined US$50 for threatening behavior in the ward.

Ben is allergic to seafood, beef, pineapple, and alcohol. He enjoyed good past health.

Present treatment   Since admission, Ben agreed, after a lengthy discussion, to switch to mirtazapine for sleep and OCD symptoms. Clonazepam was titrated up, and his sleep improved. He agreed to titrate down benzodiazepines during the day. He was rigid in his medication regimen and treatment goal and requested to be transferred to a chronic ward for further rehabilitation for 2 months. He expected to have quiet time for reading an English dictionary before discharge. When other treatment options were discussed with him (e.g., private hostel or halfway house for independent living training), he refused almost all options.

Ben had regular meetings with a clinical psychologist, and he was also noted to be rigid and stubborn in thinking and to lack "parallel" thinking. He was challenging in the ward; he would provoke fellow patients and made different complaints toward other patients. He also requested to have shower time alone and complained about the ward environment. He refused to try any other treatment change in rituals unless he was transferred to the rehabilitation ward. He spent his time sitting in a corner of the bedroom and did not engage in ward activities. He liked staying in a quiet environment but refused to be discharged home or to a supervised setting. He spent a lot of time speaking with the manager in the ward, up to an hour a day and made complaints to other nurses (and spat at them).

His mother visited him regularly and complied with his requests such as for her to write letters of complaint against the hospital.

Consultation   JM thanked the doctor for the thorough presentation and congratulated her on persevering with this difficult patient. The first point that was raised was in relation to Ben's tendency to control the information relating to his other psychiatric contacts and treatments. Under the premise of "confidentiality," he refused to allow the present hospital psychiatrists to have any contact with his previous private psychiatrists. This was clearly a manipulative and unhelpful act, which was not conducive to a more effective treatment for him. Neither, of course, was it conducive to a trusting relationship with his present psychiatrist.

JM pointed out that this kind of behavior must have made him one of the least likable patients in the ward. At this stage, JM introduced the notions of disease, illness, and sickness and the parallel notions of disease, disability, and handicap (Hofmann, 2002; Susser, 1990).

JM gave the example of the disease diabetes, which sometimes causes blindness that then limits a person's ability to function. Although many people have the same *illness*, they do not become equally *incapacitated* by it. For example there are many blind people who are gainfully employed and who live a well-functioning life. The relevance of these notions to somebody who attributes their dysfunction to a mental illness (Obsessive-Compulsive Disorder or personality disorder) is that one needs to look into additional factors to justify the person's poor adjustment in life. The diagnosis of the disease in itself does not complete the full picture.

In trying to understand how Ben developed these conditions, JM suggested that his early life history be explored. The doctor responded that she had attempted to do that but the mother found it difficult to divulge useful information. Having this limitation in mind, we are restricted in focusing on the few facts that have been divulged. One such fact was that his parents divorced because his father was visiting prostitutes.

The second element in his upbringing is that he was the only son and the first child of his family. We also know that his mother is colluding with him in making complaints to various authorities. We can guess that this may well be a repetition of a previous pattern in which his mother colluded with him against his father and that she was extremely keen to please her treasured only son. JM asked the doctor if Ben had been "spoiled" as the only son and if this was something to be expected in some parts of that city's culture. JM linked this upbringing with his current demands for preferential treatment and for an advantageous abode with luxuries within. This may also be related with his excessive demands for personal privileges when he is in the hospital.

JM also posed to this that there is another part of him that enabled him in the recent past to earn a living as a language teacher. According to his story, he was able to earn something that approximated the average income in the city (between US$500 and US$2000).

JM then moved on to the treatment plan that would be dynamically informed. The first measure would be one of containment, which would be applied in the form of restriction of hospital admissions. Ben has had numerous (more than 40) admissions, and it is questionable whether he emerged any better adjusted on discharge from any of them. On the basis that admissions have not helped him in the past and are unlikely to help him in the near future, admissions should be restricted as far as possible. A man as dexterous as Ben in manipulating services is likely to engineer admissions, but these should be restricted and be left only for true emergencies and not for capricious demands for care. When he is admitted, the admission needs to be as brief as possible. Another reason for limiting admissions is that these are costly and should only be used when there is a strong indication that they are necessary and are likely to be helpful. It is wasteful to use an admission, an expensive resource, when it has not been and it is unlikely to be helpful.

JM then considered the possibility of influencing Ben's immediate caring environment, which is his mother. JM asked if there was any possibility of informing his mother that colluding with Ben's often capricious wishes does not help Ben make a better use of his life. The potential of the mother to make this change needs to be separately assessed. One always tries to rely on mother's natural love for her son to point out to her that some refusal to collude with his wishes gives the parent an opportunity to direct their child to a way of personal development, personal growth, and better personal adjustment.

JM then pointed out that Ben does have some forcefulness, which he unfortunately misdirects at getting other people to do various jobs for him. The same forcefulness could be used for his own benefit. This is something that can be considered with him. For example, if instead of complaining to the hospital and getting other people to fit in with his withes, if he could use the same energy to look for a job, to search for pupils, and structure his teaching practice, he would have two important benefits. The first would be an income on which to improve his standard of living and the second a sense of pride for his achievements.

JM then turned the attention into the treatment of his Obsessive-Compulsive Disorder. JM expressed his doubts whether he suffered from a genuine OCD, but even so, measures that are employed in the hospital treatment of OCD could be usefully employed with him. For example, one of the measures is curtailing or interrupting compulsive activities. If he were handwashing, a nurse in an OCD unit would be stopping this handwashing. In his case, he should not be allowed to have a shower for longer than it is reasonable and would allow its use for other patients. There are also techniques for interrupting obsessive thinking that would be in a domain of treatment by a psychologist.

Finally, because it seems inevitable that there will be further appointments for him within the health service, consideration should be given to planning these appointments, knowing full well that the likelihood of his attending would be uncertain, but at least, when he turns up unannounced he could be told to address the issues that he brings at the appointment that has been reserved for him in the near future. His mother could also be informed of the appointments so that she can support the hospital process to the extent that she can.

Finally, the aspect of his life that has to do with the opposite sex was briefly considered. Ben did have a girlfriend, and it can be a motivating factor for him to know that if he made a better adjustment for himself, he may improve his chances of forming a good relationship with a woman.

References

Hofmann, B. (2002). On the triad disease, illness and sickness. *The Journal of Medicine and Philosophy*, 27(6), 651–673.

Susser, M. (1990). Disease, illness, sickness; impairment, disability and handicap. *Psychological Medicine*, 20(3), 471–473.

Dorothy

Presenting condition

Dorothy, is a 46-year-old married, unemployed woman, who lives alone while her husband lives in the country. She was admitted voluntarily because of low mood and insomnia.

History of present complaint

Dorothy's 26-year-old daughter broke off contact with her in January 2018, leaving a 5-year-old son under the care of a nanny. Dorothy felt increasingly stressed and developed low mood, insomnia, and fleeting suicidal ideas in October 2018, during which she sought help from the accident and emergency department. She was referred to the psychiatric outpatient clinic and was diagnosed with an adjustment disorder, with mixed anxiety and depressive features. She was commenced on antidepressant medication.

One week before admission, Dorothy was contacted by the police who told her that her daughter had reported to the police station and was no longer a "missing person." However, the police reported that they could not reveal her daughter's contact information because she was already 26 years old and was an adult with the right of privacy. As for her grandson, because he was well cared for by a nanny, the police had no power to intervene. The police asked her to wait for news from her daughter directly and seek help from the social welfare department.

On the day before admission, Dorothy's daughter finally contacted her via WhatsApp, saying that she would deposit US$300 into Dorothy's account, and asked Dorothy to keep taking care of her son. She refused to reveal details of her location and also said she was unable to meet up with Dorothy in the meantime. Dorothy also noticed that her daughter's WhatsApp profile picture was that of a newborn baby. She suspected that her daughter had again given birth to yet another baby despite never having been married. She felt highly distressed by what she thought to be her daughter's irresponsible behavior and refusal to meet her. She cried throughout the night. She could not sleep despite taking two tablets of promethazine 25 mg. She had a fleeting idea to take all the tablets for sleep but did not enact it. Her neighbor heard her crying and advised her to seek medical attention. Her outpatient appointment was moved forward, and she opted for inpatient treatment in view of the limited social support available to her and her unstable emotions.

Family history

Dorothy has no family history of mental illness.

Personal history

Dorothy was born in the country and is the fifth of seven siblings. Her mother is currently in her 80s and healthy. Her father died of a medical illness in 1997. She reported having a good relationship with her siblings and her parents but that they all currently live the country. She described her childhood to be happy, and she studied for around 6 years before starting to work as a factory worker. She met her first husband and was married from 1990 to 1999. The marriage ended in a divorce because her husband was a gambler. She had two children in her first marriage, a son (born in 1991, currently aged 27, previously under her ex-husband's care) and a daughter (born in 1992, currently aged 26).

Dorothy's daughter was put under Dorothy's care but was looked after by Dorothy's relatives during her entire childhood and had later attended boarding school. Her daughter has had complicated romantic relationships, had never been married, and had given birth to a son in 2013. Dorothy used to see her grandson once or twice a year. Her daughter broke off contact with Dorothy from January to November 2018, leaving her 5-year-old son under care of a nanny to be looked after in her daughter's flat. Her daughter may have also recently given birth to another child.

Dorothy started working on a cruise ship in the city in 2000; she met her second husband on the ship. They were married from 2006 to 2012, but the marriage ended in divorce because her second husband was a gambler and a substance abuser. She had no children from her second marriage.

Dorothy met her present husband, who was introduced by a friend, in 2013. They have been married since 2014, and she reports her current marriage to be harmonious, although her husband usually stays in the country where he runs a small diesel business. Her husband is intending to come to live in the city. They have no children.

Dorothy lives alone in a rented subdivided room. She has limited social support because her relatives and current husband are all in the country most of the time. Dorothy has one close friend, her neighbor, who has recently been diagnosed with cancer. Her limited social support is likely to decrease further. She has no history of substance use. She is a nonsmoker and a nondrinker. She has no forensic record. She describes herself as optimistic, with many friends, and extroverted.

Past psychiatric history

Dorothy had been known to mental health services since October 2018, presenting with a 1-month history of low mood, difficulty initiating sleep, and anxiety as well as symptoms of hand tremor, numbness, and nausea. All these symptoms were precipitated by her daughter breaking off contact with her in January 2018 and leaving her grandson under the care of a nanny. She had increasing financial stress from paying the fees for her grandson's nanny and concurrent illnesses and was worried that her daughter was dead. She developed fleeting suicidal ideas of jumping from height, with no actual plan or attempt. She attended the accident and emergency department and was seen by the psychiatric consultation liaison team. She was thought to be suffering from adjustment disorder with mixed anxiety and depressive symptoms. She was referred to the psychiatric outpatient department and prescribed sertraline 50 mg nightly, with promethazine 25 mg nightly as needed. She reported improvement of mood and anxiety symptoms after starting antidepressant treatment but deteriorated when she was informed that her daughter may be pregnant again.

Present treatment and management of case   Dorothy suffers from adjustment disorder with mixed anxiety and depressive features. She had a difficult romantic history, with two past marriages ending in divorce. She has limited social support because her current husband and family members all live in the country. She has limited stress coping skills. Her current treatment plan includes medication titration for better control of her symptoms. She has also been referred to the clinical psychology department for counseling for coping with stress. She is also seeking help from the social welfare department regarding a long-term care plan for her grandson. She will be supported by a community psychiatric nurse on discharge in view of limited social support in the city.

Consultation   JM thanked the doctor for the thorough and succinct presentation. JM then asked the doctor to clarify the treatment plan. The doctor said that Dorothy had already been discharged from the ward and that she was going to be followed up at fortnightly intervals. The doctor then informed of certain positive developments such as that the daughter established contact and that the financial situation had been eased up by contribution from social services. Dorothy had already started feeling better and sleeping better. The doctor added that during the first contact with the psychologist, Dorothy's relationship with her daughter had been broached. Dorothy was concerned about the nature of her daughter's romantic relationships, and she wished she could find a way of controlling what she saw as her daughter's precipitous relationships. Dorothy appreciates that as she has not had a relationship with her daughter throughout her childhood, adolescence, and early adult life, it would be difficult to establish this relationship when her daughter is 26 years old. Therefore, the focus of psychotherapy was helping Dorothy accept the reality instead of aiming to develop a new relationship with her daughter.

JM then commented that at 46 Dorothy was still a young woman and was able to work. The doctor added that Dorothy had not worked since early 2018 "because of stress." JM asked about the origin of stress, and the doctor clarified that although the symptoms were manifest when she was at work the source of stress was the relationship with her daughter and concern about her grandson. The doctor added that Dorothy was previously working as a part-time waitress. Dorothy felt that she was working long hours and found that stressful. Currently, even the thought of returning to work brought on symptoms of anxiety. JM asked if there was a connection between starting work and the onset of the symptoms other than the time relationship. JM asked how Dorothy working part-time reconciled with long working hours. The doctor pointed out that her part-time shifts were 12 hours each. The total hours that Dorothy worked per week was not known. JM suggested that the relationship between symptoms and source of stress needed a little further exploration because, although it was recognized that the source of stress was outside work, the symptoms appeared in relation to work.

JM then pointed out that her own history of looking after her own children was complicated. One wondered how Dorothy understood being looked after or looking after people. The doctor added that even the first marriage was with a man who lived in the country. As for the second husband, there was a suspicion that it was for the purposes of facilitating his move from the country to the city. During the time when she met her second husband, Dorothy was working on a cruise ship and did not have a stable abode in the city. The second husband was a substance abuser. Dorothy tended to be evasive when asked about the relationship with her husbands.

The doctor explained that the immediate future was uncertain for Dorothy. On the one hand she was planning to go and live in the country while she was unwell so that she could receive the support of her husband and the social setting there, but a long-term plan was for her husband to move and live in the city with her. It was not clear how this would fit with him running a diesel business in the country.

JM commented on the doctor's referral to a "mental illness." He pointed out that Dorothy was suffering from "an adjustment reaction," which is not an illness and is a condition dependent on life's stresses. The reason for her suffering was that her approach to these stresses had not been constructive. JM suggested that Dorothy tends to act precipitously without thinking the consequences of her actions thoroughly. JM suggested that this precipitous way may have been responsible for her engaging with three husbands who were in different ways unavailable to her.

JM pointed out that there was an incongruity in her funding a nanny for her grandson, something that should be the expense of her daughter and that it is not as if she has unlimited funds as she herself was on support from a state. How could she afford to give the nanny equivalent of a monthly salary when she herself is dependent on benefits? JM then pointed out that Dorothy had not negotiated with her daughter the conditions under which she would support her daughter (through funding the nanny for the daughter's child) but somehow accepts a decision that had been made for her by the daughter without any conditions. For example it would have been reasonable to negotiate that she has contact with her grandson's mother (her daughter) and with her son. The doctor clarified that Dorothy had access to her grandson who she was seeing at least once a week. The doctor pointed out that when Dorothy had lost contact with her daughter and funding the nanny was difficult, she had considered with social services that her daughter would give up her son for adoption. JM pointed out that the parental authority issue was uncertain here because if grandmother had not been granted legal guardianship she would not be in a position to authorize the adoption of her grandchild because this would have been under the authority of the child's mother. The doctor clarified that Dorothy's daughter is the legal parent of the grandchild.

JM suggested that the overall impression is that Dorothy is repeatedly taken advantage of. When this was confirmed, JM posed a further question which was, "Why does Dorothy allow herself to be taken for granted?" Dorothy had been taken advantage of at first by her husbands, then by her daughter, and possibly by her employers. Why does Dorothy find it difficult to claim her rights and defend herself?

The doctor referred to certain cultural factors. The first was that she had seven siblings, which was unusual in the country. The second is that she was female—a gender that has lower status in certain traditional families. JM tried to separate Dorothy's childhood experience as a female child in the country to her adult experience of a woman who is earning, supporting herself, and is being taken advantage of by the first two husbands who used her earnings for their own habits of either gambling or drug abuse. JM suggested that the main focus in therapy, or one of the early targets of therapy, should be the building her self-esteem in a sense that she develops the right to protect herself and to safeguard her own interests. Dorothy needs to be helped to build her self-respect so that, based on that, she can expect other people to respect her and her work.

JM recommended that Dorothy's immediate future seems uncertain and almost chaotic. For example, the way in which the needs of her grandson and her own needs, in relation to being looked after by her husband who lives in the country, had not been sorted out in a way that is satisfactory to all. JM also pointed out that it is fortuitous that the professionals involved with her are women and, therefore, are in an excellent position to point out to her that she is entitled to be empowered to protect her own interest. A woman is better placed to broach the issue of empowerment of women. The doctor stressed that the cultural discrimination against women is still prevalent in the country, but JM counterposed that there were plenty of empowered women in the country at present and that in the city there is a great shift toward equality of respect for the sexes. JM then asked if Dorothy was overestimating the cultural discriminatory attitude of the culture in the country. JM asked if it is possible that women now have greater empowerment than previously and whether her perception is marked by her own family experience rather than of the culture in general. The doctor pointed out that it was common for women, a quarter of a century ago, to see marriage as a situation through which they could rely on their husbands for life.

JM expressed the concern that treating Dorothy as mentally ill may not be constructive when the effort of therapy is to consider her as a woman who finds herself in an adjustment difficulty, which will not be improved without the adjustment stresses being constructively addressed. The problematic issues were not only because of the stresses arising from the environment but also because of the way she addressed them. The doctor added that she was concerned that the husband may change his attitude toward his wife because he is currently expected to contribute financially for Dorothy's daughter and grandson's expenses. There was a concern that he may begin to find Dorothy a "burden."

JM suggested that there are several issues that need to be settled following respective negotiations. The relationship between Dorothy and her daughter, between Dorothy and her husband, and the respective financial burden that each one is going to carry within the context of precisely what kind of relationship.

JM made a point that if her attitude was changed, Dorothy could even find work as a source of support instead of work being only a source of symptoms of anxiety. Work could give her a near equal standing to that of her husband or to other people, but only if she negotiated her working conditions so that she was not exploited at work.

The particular interest of this case is that it demonstrates the interaction between elements from the personal history and of the cultural environment, including the transition from the country to the city and the change of culture within this setting over time (from traditional to modern). The cultural improvement of the woman's position in society has the potential of improving Dorothy's mental health. It seemed that overwhelming anxiety was making Dorothy unable to sort out each issue separately and lived in a confusion of unresolved problems. These problems were in the relationships with her daughter, with her husband, and with her work.

Margaret

Presenting complaint

Margaret is a 43-year-old single woman who presented with difficulty falling asleep and ideas of self-harm.

History of the present condition

Margaret has a longstanding history of substance abuse. She was last discharged to a detox hostel half a year ago but left the hostel to live with a friend 2 weeks prior to admission. She believed that she could not get along with the other residents and staff of the hostel. She felt that she was being unfairly treated by the hostel staff and attributed this to her being a lesbian. She also believed that the rules were too strict and it was difficult for her to abide by the rules. She found a job as a salon assistant and moved in to live with a colleague from the salon. After leaving the detox hostel, she reinstated on heroin "out of boredom." She abused heroin by "chasing the dragon" daily, using around US$15-US$20 each time. She denied other illicit drug use, other than heroin or intravenous drug use.

Her mood became more irritable since then, and she had difficulty falling asleep. She could only sleep for 3 to 4 hours each night. She felt frustrated when she had difficulty initiating sleep and resorted to self-harm behaviors of slashing her arms and legs with sharp pens. She had an increasingly fleeting urge to slash her arms and legs with sharps for a few weeks prior to admission. She was able to cope with activities of daily living and continued to work as a salon assistant. Margaret denied any perceptual disturbance and held no irrational beliefs. There was no history of suicidal attempts or violent acts.

Family history

Her mother was a substance abuser, who died by suicide by jumping from height when Margaret was 13 years old.

Personal history

Margaret was born in the city in 1976 and had a complicated childhood and upbringing. She has one younger brother who is deaf and dumb. Her father died of cancer when she was an infant. She was brought up by her mother who also abused illicit drugs. Her mother remarried soon after her father died. She was severely abused by her stepfather and was punished heavily for expressing her emotions. When she was 5 years old, her mother once got beaten up for protecting her against her stepfather. She never spoke about her abuse again, and her mother would sometimes wrongly scold her as a result when her clothing or belongings were damaged. Her mother tried to suffocate her two younger stepsisters when she was 9 years old. When she was 13, her mother committed suicide by jumping from height. She believed it was due to her own misconduct problems and felt guilty. She and her younger brother were under her stepfather's care since then. She was also molested once by him in her 20s. She recalled that her stepfather never hit her biological younger brother and treated her two younger stepsisters well. She moved out to live with friends in her 20s and has not contacted her stepfather or younger brother since then.

Margaret was educated up to secondary Form 1 and had worked as a toilet cleaner and salon assistant. She is lesbian and has had a close relationship with a girlfriend for 3 years. Her girlfriend is also a substance abuser. They had been cohabiting on and off. Margaret is a smoker but a nondrinker. She has a longstanding history of substance abuse. She has a forensic record for a number of incidents of theft and possession of dangerous drugs (PODD).

Past medical and psychiatric history

Margaret has a history of polysubstance abuse since 8 years of age; she has used heroin, methamphetamine, cannabis, cough mixture, and nitrazepam. She first started cannabis when she was 8 years old. She experienced euphoria after use and tended to use it for up to 3 times per week. She also used methamphetamine when she was 19 years old with a peak use of 45 grams per day. Previously, she had been using methamphetamine on alternate days (20–25 grams); she last used it a few years ago. She used heroin in recent years. She started heroin abuse by smoking "chasing the dragon" since the age of 11 under peer influence. There was no intravenous use. She used heroin regularly and developed tolerance and craving.

Margaret had two compulsory detoxification periods in her teenage years when she was charged with PODD. She also tried two voluntary detoxification admissions in 2013 and 2015. There were also multiple abstinence periods by herself, with the longest abstinence being for 3 years, when she had a stable job.

She has been known to the psychiatric service since 2011. The diagnoses included polysubstance abuse, drug-induced psychosis, and history of Posttraumatic Stress Disorder (PTSD) from childhood sexual and physical abuse with current mixed anxiety depressive features mixed anxiety/depressive disorder. There were five past psychiatric admissions, due to psychotic relapse and mood symptoms with suicidal/self-harm ideas after increased heroin use. After substance use, she presented with second- and third-person auditory hallucinations and persecutory beliefs. She has had frequent ruminations of past experiences of abuse with flashbacks and somatic hallucinations of her private parts being touched.

In between admissions to hospital and compulsory detox centers, Margaret had regular follow-ups at the substance abuse clinic. She was initially started on risperidone and chlorpromazine in 2011 for control of psychotic symptoms; fluoxetine was prescribed in 2013; Quetiapine was added in 2017; and Remeron was started in 2018. Beside titration of psychiatric medications for control of her mood and psychotic symptoms, she was also offered psychological treatment, including cognitive behavioral therapy (CBT) for PTSD from childhood sexual and physical abuse and was helped to develop coping methods for anger management.

Margaret was sent to a detox center by a court order for 1 year in 2018. Afterward, she was admitted to the current detox center. She absconded from the hostel in May 2019, and she slept on the streets. She reinstated into heroin and was subsequently admitted to another psychiatric unit due to residual auditory hallucinations and harboring fleeting suicidal ideas. It was documented that she suffered from withdrawal symptoms of restlessness and irritability after admission. She was given methadone tablets for a short period, and her mood gradually stabilized. During her admission, she was also seen by a clinical psychologist with psychological treatment given for PTSD and anger management. Admission was then arranged for her into the same detox center, under a probation order.

Present treatment and management   Margaret had been seen by different clinical psychologists (including an in-house clinical psychologists in detox centers) since 2016 for CBT, which had limited effect. She still had periods of the urge to self-harm deliberately. She was occasionally slashing her arms with sewing needles or pen caps. She claimed that she had to "use physical pain to cover her psychological pain" even though there were other coping methods taught to her by the clinical psychologist.

There has been no active psychotic experience since March 2019 after Quetiapine was titrated up. However, Margaret reported there were some second-person internal voices with derogatory comments. She displayed these pseudo-hallucinations to other residents, thus causing her to harbor paranoid feelings toward them.

After admission, in view of her persistent mood symptoms, her medications were further titrated. In September, Margaret was referred to a clinical psychologist and she has had four to five sessions of dialectical behavior therapy (DBT) so far. She was taught methods of understanding and expressing different emotions, as well as methods of coping when facing frustration. Schema Modes Monitoring was introduced to her.

In the DBT sessions, Margaret expressed that she had intense distress with frequent urge to self-harm. She also harbored suicidal ideas with a plan (such as strangling herself with a towel while covering herself with a blanket in bed at night). She was worried that she might not be able to restrain herself from suicidal behaviors.

In the ward, she was noted to be irritable at times, with occasional conflicts with fellow patients. She hid pen caps and slashed her legs in the showers once in September. She alleged that this was triggered by her reading a book about sexual abuse and feeling distressed afterward. In view of her unstable emotions and the risk of self-harm, Ativan 1 mg twice daily was given. She was also put under close observation as a precaution against suicide. Her towel, toothbrush, and pen were removed to prevent further self-harm. She also smoked in the toilet once in October and became sullen and agitated when being told off by ward staff. Restraint was required. In the recent few weeks, her mood had been stable, with a decreased urge to perform acts of self-harm. Her sleep improved with no excessive daytime drowsiness. Her current regime is Remeron 45 mg nightly, Quetiapine 400 mg night, Ativan 1 mg daily as needed. Further DBT sessions with the clinical psychologist before discharge are planned and would continue the sessions in outpatient setting after discharge.

Consultation   JM thanked the doctor for the comprehensive presentation. JM then asked to clarify why the auditory phenomena were called "pseudo-hallucinations." The doctor explained that Margaret was aware that these voices were coming from within her own head. JM then asked the doctor to clarify the "contract" (meaning the understanding) on which therapy was based. The doctor clarified that Margaret was still an inpatient and that she is likely to be so for the next 2 or 3 weeks. After her discharge, Margaret will be cared for by other doctors. JM then expressed the view that the prominent problem is how the transition from one department to another will be managed. JM pointed out that this woman had experienced so many losses in her life that the loss of the treatment team of the ward is going to affect her already vulnerable self in this respect. There is already a social worker who will continue being her key person after discharge from hospital. It was also pointed out that the doctor has a good relationship with the social worker and has confidence in her. JM then asked what sense Margaret made of being transferred from the inpatient unit to the detox center. The doctor was aware that in previous occasions of move, Margaret responded with self-harming behavior. The doctor pointed out that Margaret was not yet thinking of this move. JM suggested that for this reason, the remaining 3 weeks in the ward would be a good time to prepare her for this transition. JM then asked the doctor to consider ways through which Margaret could view the transition in a positive way as a caring step for her. The doctor suggested that Margaret keeps a record of her feelings when distressed and she writes them down instead of cutting herself.

JM then asked what was understood about what Margaret found distressing about the transfer to the detox center. The doctor pointed out that Margaret would be concerned that she may be victimized because she is lesbian. She was also anxious that she would be unfairly treated. JM pointed out that the therapeutic issue ahead is how the present treatment team would prepare Margaret so that she is less anxious about the transfer. The doctor pointed out that Margaret was also concerned that the rules would be too strict and that she would be "compelled" to transgress them. JM asked in what way did she mean that the rules were "too strict." The doctor explained that she had discussed this issue with Margaret, and the rules were not really that strict. As an example of "strictness" Margaret gave that having sharp objects removed from her environment. JM then asked why Margaret considers these measures to protect her as unreasonable or excessive. The doctor pointed out that Margaret felt that slashing her arms was normal for her and that she is different from other people. JM then suggested that this attitude implies that Margaret is determined to continue self-harming and pointed out that exploring this attitude until it is made consciously clear in Margaret's mind would help her appreciate that what she sees as coping mechanisms (cutting herself) are in fact not coping but repeating a previous and unhelpful pattern. A significant issue in Margaret's treatment is to consider with her if she wishes to continue repeating the old pattern of cutting herself when distressed or if she wants to develop a new one where distress is actually resolved and solutions are really found.

Wishing to repeat the old patterns is antitherapeutic; it is incompatible with therapy. The old patterns are self-harm and drug abuse; if she is determined to continue with these patterns, then she does not wish to have any therapy. JM suggested that one major move that needs to be achieved in Margaret's mind is to accept that she is taking on professional help to develop better ways of coping with the demands of her life, better than taking drugs or cutting herself (Gratz et al., 2002; Hawton et al., 2002; Sinclair & Hawton, 2002; King et al., 2008).

JM then asked what the origin of her current distress is. The doctor pointed out that she is still troubled by memories of her childhood physical and sexual abuse by her stepfather. JM pointed out that this is a reasonable therapeutic target: to resolve the feelings about these traumatic experiences so that they do not traumatize the rest of her life. This area was yet to be explored. The first step in resolving such traumatic experiences is to explore them and to reexamine them in realistic detail. Avoidance of painful memories is understandable but is also unhelpful if avoidance perseveres in therapy because it prevents any resolution. This is where the support of the therapist becomes crucial. The patient can feel supported and accepted in the therapeutic relationship so that she can explore the traumatic experience and resolve the hurtful (depressing and angry) feelings that that awful experience must have given rise to (Ingrassia, 2018; Kendall-Tackett et al., 1993).

JM then pointed out that it is fortunate that her treating doctor was female because in the exploration of these experiences with a male therapist the patient may feel that she is giving the male therapist vicarious sexual gratification, and in that way, the therapeutic attempt may in her mind become a repetition of the abusive experience of the past. JM pointed out that delicacy of the approach and that every step should be taken with the expressed permission of the patient to proceed in this way.

The doctor pointed out that because Margaret is lesbian, there is a risk that she may feel that she is being asked to give vicarious sexual pleasure to the female therapist. JM explained that he has been fortunate to have gained the trust of sexually abused women and young girls and that his experience has been of proceeding always with care and always with the patient's permission. Furthermore, if in the process the therapist finds that the patient becomes particularly uneasy or anxious, he stops and invites the patient to explore what the anxiety is about. If the problem is workable with, then the therapy proceeds, but if it is not then JM refers the patient to a female therapist. The psychiatric consultation carries a power imbalance that may lead to the patient feeling intimidated and in that way feel exposed to the same abuse that they suffered as children.

JM advised that in the process of hearing the patient's abusive story, the therapist should not be overwhelmed by the events, even though they may be horrific. Giving the patient the sense that the therapist is overwhelmed is going to inhibit the patient from exploring the experience further. The therapist must not appear too critical or too moralistic because this will also be inhibiting. The therapist needs to remain sympathetic without expressing any extreme emotions or views. The tone of the session needs to remain at a "workable" level (Jones, 2013).

The next issue that needs to be clarified was if the abuse was a violent intrusion or a seduction. This is particularly important because the patient was then 20 years old. To put it simply, the question is if she was seduced or if she was raped. As matters are rarely black and white in human interaction, it would be useful to find out to what extent each parameter was exercised—the parameter of seduction and the parameter of violence. Was the violence in the form of physical violence, was it in the form of threats, or of other forms of psychological violence?

The doctor pointed out that her understanding was that Margaret was raped with penetrative sex once only. JM then asked if there was any behavior prior to the rape that would show stepfather's sexual interest in her. For example, if he made intrusions that he wanted to appear as accidental, such as walking into the bathroom when she was using it or "catching her" partly dressed when she was changing clothes. JM then pointed out that more damage is often inflicted by the abuser making the victim feel as if it was she who instigated the whole action. The statement "look what you made me do" is often used by offenders, and it causes additional harm if the naïve victim believes that she brought this on herself. Accusing a girl of causing her own rape by wearing a short skirt wounds her self- esteem for a long time (Calhoun & Atkeson, 1991).

When during the consultation it becomes apparent that a patient feels guilty for what was done to her, then the therapist can bring in the issues of the power differential and particularly the differential that comes with a 10-year gap in age.

The doctor added that the abuser had a more powerful position because he was in the role of the stepfather and that was in addition to his muscular strength, which made it harder for her to resist. Margaret needs to be helped to realize that she cannot be held responsible for something that was done to her and that she has no reason to feel guilty for the abuse that she suffered.

The next step is to discover if there were any threats made after the abuse to stop the girl from disclosing what happened to her to other persons within the family or in society who were there to support her and protect her. Did the abuser use any means to stop her from reporting him to the police? It needs to be understood why this particular crime of rape was not reported to the police. Particularly, she could be asked if she felt that the police would not be sympathetic to her because, sadly, it often happens that victims of abuse are treated as if they are promiscuous women or wishing to exploit a situation.

JM then pointed out that in some cultures rape carries a stigma on the victim. In the Victorian era, a raped woman was considered "damaged goods," and the attitude is not different in some cultures today. In these cultures, the opportunity for these women to marry and have families is gradually wiped out. JM asked what the attitude would be within the subculture to which she belongs in the city.

The next phase of treatment would be to address the value that she puts on herself. The doctor confirmed that Margaret tends to belittle herself and JM responded that this is the next therapeutic task: To restore in Margaret a realistic sense of self-worth. JM then asked what is there for Margaret to value herself. The doctor responded that she takes pride in her work as a hairdresser and that she is good at dyeing the clients' hair. This seemed a solid and realistic pillar of one aspect of her self-esteem, that she is a valued worker. A second aspect is that she has some level of ability and some level of intelligence. The next area of self-worth is herself as a lover who would make her loved one feel that she is gaining something by being in the relationship with her. In summary, she can value herself because of her work, because of her intellectual ability, because of being valued by friends, and by being valued by an intimate lover.

Finally, Margaret is also young and healthy and is able to earn a living, which are significant pillars on which to base a healthy and realistic sense of self-worth. It would be useful for her to be reminded of these positive aspects so that she does not identify herself only through cutting and taking drugs. Building on these aspects a self with hope for the future, she will need to resort to cutting and drug taking far less that she did previously.

References

Calhoun, K. S., & Atkeson, B. M. (1991). *Treatment of rape victims: Facilitating psychosocial adjustment.* Pergamon Press.

Gratz, K. L., Conrad, S. D., & Roemer, L. (2002). Risk factors for deliberate self-harm among college students. *The American Journal of Orthopsychiatry, 72*(1), 128–140.

Hawton, K., Haw, C., Houston, K., & Townsend, E. (2002). Family history of suicidal behaviour: Prevalence and significance in deliberate self-harm patients. *Acta Psychiatrica Scandinavica, 106*(5), 387–393.

Ingrassia, A. (2018). The independent inquiry into child sexual abuse in the UK: Reflecting on the mental health needs of victims and survivors. *The British Journal of Psychiatry, 213*(4), 571–573.

Jones, D. P. H. (2013). *Interviewing the sexually abused child.* Gaskell/Royal College of Psychiatrists.

Kendall-Tackett, K. A., Williams, L. M., & Finkelhor, D. (1993). Impact of sexual abuse on children: A review and synthesis of recent empirical studies. *Psychological Bulletin, 113*(1), 164–180.

King, M., Semlyen, J., Tai, S. S., Killaspy, H., Osborn, D., Popelyuk, D., & Nazareth, I. (2008). A systematic review of mental disorder, suicide, and deliberate self harm in lesbian, gay and bisexual people. *BMC Psychiatry, 8,* 70.

Sinclair, J. M., & Hawton, K. (2002). Reducing repeated deliberate self-harm. *Practitioner, 246*(1632), 164–166, 169–172

Section VI

Quasi-Psychotic Phenomena

17
Ideas of Persecution

Connie

Presenting complaint

Connie complained of being stared at in public and being the target of persecution for 2 years.

History of presenting illness

Connie is a 56-year-old unemployed woman living with her boyfriend and her 30-year-old son in a public housing unit.

Connie was mentally well until mid-2017 when her nephew's godfather died. She suddenly developed a resurgence of persecutory and referential ideas that her former coworkers were monitoring her. She believed that a former coworker was the mastermind behind a large organization that employed strangers to play tricks on her and to stare at her on the street for the purpose of making her feel like "a target." She had immense distress with emotional reactivity (anxiety and depressive symptoms) and could only go out by wearing sunglasses and a surgical mask so others would not recognize her.

Her symptoms became more severe in September 2018 when she complained of increased feelings of being monitored. She formed the opinion that passers-by were looking at her in an unfriendly manner and believed that they were sent by two former female coworkers whom she worked with in a game arcade. She repeatedly looked behind her to see if others were monitoring her, but this did not give her relief, instead, it increased her tension. She had slept poorly at times when she thought about the persecution and only managed to sleep 2 to 3 hours per night. Her appetite was maintained. She denied any other abnormal perceptions. She had fleeting ideas of committing suicide, such as by hanging from a rope or by jumping from height, but never developed the determination to do so. On the day of admission (October 2018), she attended clinic, and alleged that after thorough discussion with her boyfriend and son, she agreed for psychiatric inpatient treatment for titration of medication and the provision of adjunctive psychotherapy.

Dynamic Consultations with Psychiatrists: Understanding Severely Troubled Patients, First Edition. Jason Maratos.

Family history

Connie has no family history of mental illness.

Personal history

Connie was born in the city. She is the youngest of three siblings, with one brother and one sister. Her father died after an asthmatic attack when she was 4 months old. She lived with her mother and two siblings as a child. She recalls occasionally going to the country to visit her father's first wife and her five older half-brothers. She studied until Form 1 (age 13). She had her first job at the age of 14 when she worked in a garments company, helping her family with sewing. She met her ex-husband when she was a teenager (ex-husband was a family friend) and felt mistreated by him. He was a flirty, masculine figure, and Connie had suspected on many occasions that he had an extramarital affair. She overdosed on medication when she was 20 years old following this romantic crisis. The couple still eventually had two children, a son who works as a registered nurse and a daughter who is a free-lance designer who lives abroad. She eventually divorced him in 2006 when she discovered that he had had an extramarital affair for more than 10 years. Connie met her current boyfriend 10 years ago at a New Life Association (a nongovernmental organization that helps persons with mental health problems). He has been diagnosed with schizophrenia. Her boyfriend, son, and daughter were all supportive of her.

Connie was described as introverted and timid. She is a nonsmoker and nondrinker. She has no history of substance abuse or forensic record.

Past medical and psychiatric history

Connie had taken an overdose in 1982 following a "romantic crisis" but no medical attention was sought then. Since 1991, Connie presented with referential delusions that her neighbors and passers-by looked at her when she spent money buying useless supplies as part of a pyramid scheme. She was known to psychiatric services when she was brought to the accident and emergency department when she felt she was stared at while at the market. Her diagnosis was paranoid schizophrenia. Her course of illness deteriorated since 1994 when she started to work as a cashier in a game arcade. When two colleagues tried to steal money from the cash register, she reported this to the manager, and since then, she harbored paranoid ideas that these two colleagues sent others to monitor her. This necessitated admissions to a psychiatric hospital in 2003 and 2004. She was treated with chlorpromazine, but she developed eczema. She was then tried on trifluoperazine, but she developed a rash. She eventually settled on quetiapine, which she took from 2004 to 2017.

Connie has hypertension, which is managed with diet control. She has chronic low back pain and bilateral osteoarthritis of the knee with pending right total knee replacement in 2022. She has Vogt-Koyanagi-Harada disease with a follow-up with ophthalmology. She has pelvic floor disorders but is not on treatment. She is allergic to trifluoperazine and chlorpromazine. She has adverse drug reactions to enalapril (cough) and atenolol (nausea).

Present treatment and management   Connie has been seen by the doctor for cognitive behavior therapy (CBT) for psychosis. She has completed 26 sessions. She has been taught some CBT principles to manage and amend her thoughts, feelings, and her behavior. Some of her beliefs are being challenged, and additional work is being carried out aimed at reducing the behavior that arises from paranoid beliefs (such as the belief that she is being followed). Connie has been found to be lacking in confidence and has expressed feelings that she is not being liked by other people. Therapy is about to be concluded because she has shown some improvement.

Consultation JM thanked the doctor for the thorough presentation and proceeded to ask some further information about Connie's history and early life. Although aware that her father died when she was young, it would be helpful to know a little bit more about how Connie felt growing up in her family. The doctor responded that early life was difficult because the family was poor. Connie did not have to do the household chores that traditionally are the duty of the eldest child. She had good relationships with her siblings and with her mother until she reached her teenage years.

Connie was hospitalized as a teenager, and following that, she was put on a strict diet because of renal difficulties. The first source of friction between her and her mother was around her mother's insistence that she stuck to a strict diet. The second area of friction was mother's pressure on Connie to get married as soon as possible and to do so with her first boyfriend. Connie suspected that her mother was conveying the pressure that she herself was receiving from peers and extended family. Connie felt that her relationship with her mother continued to deteriorate ever since.

JM then asked the doctor to clarify in what way was Connie's family different from other poor families of the city at the time. It was not possible to identify any characteristics of family life that differentiated Connie's family from that of other poor families. It is true that she had lost her father at a young age, but the pressure about getting married was not too great because Connie did not get married until she was in her mid-20s. This case is not of Connie becoming a "child bride." Connie started dating her husband when she was about 14 and the period of courtship lasted for 10 years. JM pointed out that it is unlikely that she was dating her boyfriend for 10 years because of pressure from her mother; nevertheless, it is significant that this is the picture that she presented.

The doctor added that Connie always suspected that her boyfriend was also dating other women at the time when they were supposed to be together. The doctor added that Connie had given him the impression that she was not in control of her own life but that she was living the life that those around her expected.

The doctor added that he had spoken to Connie's mother, and she informed him that Connie was a shy introverted child from an early age. The overall picture is one of a family life that was not hugely dysfunctional.

JM then asked for clarification of the significance of the death of the nephew's godfather with the onset of psychosis. Was that person a significant person in Connie's life? The doctor clarified that that person did not have a meaningful relationship with Connie, and it was Connie who had changed the temporal association into a causative one. Furthermore, Connie claimed that event caused a resurfacing, a resurgence of earlier, almost psychotic, delusional ideas of being followed. The doctor clarified that he had explored this relationship with Connie, and there did not seem to be a significant emotional connection with that person. Her nephew's godfather was only someone whom she met during large family gatherings.

JM then asked if Connie was overweight. This was confirmed, and Connie was found to have a body mass index (BMI) of 32. Her obesity was attributed to lack of exercise and to the second-generation antipsychotic medication that she was taking.

JM then asked about her reported lack of confidence. More specifically JM asked in what areas of her life did Connie feel she lacked confidence. As this was a difficult area to address, JM clarified that normally people see their confidence in certain areas such as confidence as a spouse, confidence as a woman, confidence as a friend, confidence as a mother, confidence as a child, a daughter of the family, or confidence as a worker. These are some of the areas where one feels that they are confident or inadequate.

JM pointed out that normally we develop the sense of confidence based on the feedback we get from other people. JM gave the example of a doctor relying on feedback from his seniors and his peers (as well as his patients) to develop their own sense of capacity in that function. Did Connie develop the lack of confidence on the basis of such information, or did she carry this vague sense of lack of confidence from her experience as a child?

There is often a healthy association between what people think of us in a certain function and what we think of ourselves. JM pointed out that there are a few people who are so cut off from feedback from others that they continue thinking of themselves as competent despite negative feedback from others. It became clear that Connie had not developed a sense of confidence in any specific way. She continued having this vague sense of not being confident. JM suggested that it would be useful, therapeutically, if this area of competence was explored further with Connie so that she could be helped to develop a realistic view of her self-worth.

JM suggested that Connie's confidence as a woman may have been undermined by the fact that her husband was looking elsewhere for a more satisfying sexual or personal relationship. Her obesity may have been a factor in seeing herself as failing as a woman. JM then asked about the degree to which Connie had insight into her idiosyncratic ideas. For example, did Connie realize that her thoughts of being followed were related to a disturbance in her own mind, or did she feel that this was an actual event happening from outside her mind? It became clear that Connie had virtually no insight into these paranoid ideas.

As Connie seemed to have no insight into her condition, it would be virtually impossible to engage in psychotherapy with her. The situation being such, JM asked, what should the objective of therapy be? The doctor responded that the objective of therapy was to reduce the distress that she felt. JM pointed out that it would be difficult to engage with her in therapy if she did not feel that any of her ideas or feelings were originating from within her mind. JM pointed out that if a person's reality is that of being persecuted, no amount of psychotherapy could reduce this distress. Further discussion clarified that Connie was not coming to therapy with the objective of changing her thoughts and feelings but only with the objective of being made to feel better. JM clarified that a basis for therapy seemed to be absent in Connie's case. The therapist needed to be clear that they are not in a position to make Connie feel better by changing the other people, the people that Connie believes are following or persecuting her.

JM summarized that Connie is seriously dysfunctional in the sense that she does not work and does not fulfill any roles to any satisfactory level. Both she and her boyfriend rely on social security. JM concluded that psychotherapy—in terms of a process of bringing about change in her mind and in her emotions—was not the appropriate process because it was unlikely to bring about a desired change. Connie needed to be helped with support and medication. Any therapeutic attempts would be likely to be counterproductive. Perhaps Connie could be helped by occupational therapy, physiotherapy, and other less dynamic interventions.

In conclusion, this was a case in which dynamic psychotherapy would not only be inappropriate but also a process that would threaten the competence of the therapist and may lead to them becoming disheartened. A therapist treating her would need to be satisfied with limited gains.

For a study of the effect of CBT on early onset psychosis (not in this case), see Jackson et al. (2018)

Reference

Jackson, H., McGorry, P., Edwards, J., Hulbert, C., Henry, L., Francey, S., Maude, D., Cocks, J., Power, P., Harrigan, S., & Dudgeon, P. (2018). Cognitively-oriented psychotherapy for early psychosis (COPE): Preliminary results. *British Journal of Psychiatry*, 172(S33), 93–100.

18
Ideas of Reference; Hallucinations

Susan

Presenting condition

Susan is a 14-year-old female, a Form 2 student, living with her mother in a public housing unit. Susan was admitted 2 weeks prior to this presentation because she was troubled by ideas of being followed and by hearing nonexistent voices; these complaints made her unable to attend school.

History of present complaint

Susan's mental state began deteriorating late in 2017. This was precipitated by increased academic stress related to the high expectations she had of herself. She became increasingly anxious and afraid when her godfather suddenly appeared and reentered their family flat; her godfather still wandered around their building. She heard a nonexistent banging sound from a flat above, heard the doorbell and her mother's voice talking to her (calling her name) in the form of second person; this was not derogatory. She still felt anxious despite repeated reassurance by mother. She also harbored a vague idea of being followed by a stranger; this was based on a stepping sound behind her. She was afraid that she would be abducted or hit by a stranger. She repeatedly looked back and checked for anyone following her. Such symptoms were present at school, at home and on the street. She needed her mother's company continuously (e.g., during a grocery stroll and even when asleep). Susan felt she needed to sleep with her mother. She had no pervasive depressive symptoms. She had no suicidal or violent ideas. Susan had refused school for 1 week prior to the present admission. Her mother and she agreed for admission on the day of follow-up on account of her poor mental state.

Susan was thin-built, tidy, appeared worrisome, and established good contact. She was not suspicious. She was forthcoming and stayed focused during interview. Her mood was not overtly depressed, and her affect was restricted. Her speech was coherent and relevant with normal tempo and soft voice.

Dynamic Consultations with Psychiatrists: Understanding Severely Troubled Patients, First Edition. Jason Maratos.
© 2022 John Wiley & Sons Ltd. Published 2022 by John Wiley & Sons Ltd.

She harbored second-person and elementary auditory hallucinations. She had a referential idea that was not fixed and an idea of being followed. She had no suicidal or violent ideas. Her insight was partial: She was aware that her perceptual disturbances and beliefs were abnormal; she attributed them to mental illness. She was aware of the consequences of mental illness for herself and was willing to receive psychiatric treatment.

Family history

Susan's mother has a history of depression and had defaulted follow-up for at least 1 year.

Personal history

Her mother's pregnancy with Susan was unplanned. Susan was born in the city. Her birth and developmental histories are unremarkable. She is an only child and was cared for by her mother.

Her mother is 39years old and has been a housewife since Susan's birth. Neither Susan nor her mother had contact with Susan's biological father after Susan was born.

Susan's mother was described as "demanding and neurotic," with high expectations on Susan's academic performance. She had an enmeshed relationship with Susan. Her mother's parenting involved corporal punishment, especially around examinations, together with critical comments. Her mother often compared Susan's studying efforts with Susan's classmates. At times, her mother forced Susan to leave home as punishment. As a result, Susan was ambivalent toward her mother.

Susan had good academic results and ranked first across classes (out of more than 100 students) until the last examination in January 2018, in which her ranking dropped to about 20th. This was related to her difficulty in concentrating on her subjects because she was highly anxious and troubled by paranoid ideas.

Susan was introverted and had low self-esteem. She enjoyed reading books and listening to music.

Past psychiatric history

Susan was known to psychiatric services since 2010, when she was 6 years old. She was initially diagnosed with an adjustment disorder. At that time, she was wrongly accused of theft at school, and she attempted to climb out of a window while at school. She defaulted follow-up when she was 7 years old and attending primary class 2. Her case was reactivated when she was 11 years old. She once climbed out of a fourth-floor window at school, allegedly with the intention of ending her life after she learned that her language examination results were poor. She was thought to have a moderate depressive episode and was given fluoxetine.

Susan had one psychiatric admission for 2 weeks, 2 years previously because of impulsive dashing into the road when her mother asked her to go to her maternal grandmother's home and she refused.

After her last discharge, her godfather suffered from an injury on duty at work and started to live with the mother and Susan. Before that, the godfather was caring toward Susan. After the injury, the godfather became more irritable and was repeatedly asking Susan's mother for money. Susan felt that she was being abandoned when she saw that her godfather showed more care toward another girl. She attempted to relieve her distress by banging her head against a wall without major injury. Finally, her mother asked the godfather to leave their home during the last year's summer holiday. Susan enjoyed good past physical health.

The provisional diagnosis was early onset psychosis with the possibility of a strong component of separation anxiety from her mother. Predisposing factors included loss of a paternal figure (both from her biological father and godfather) and her mother's high expressed emotions. Academic stress was considered a precipitating factor. The enmeshed relationship and ambivalence toward her mother plus the limited social support and coping mechanisms were considered perpetuating factors.

Present treatment　Susan is being treated with antipsychotic medication.

Consultation　JM thanked the doctor for the thorough presentation. JM then asked the doctor to clarify the family's relationship with the godfather. The doctor replied this had asked about, and although he was a single man living in a home with a lone woman, they did not have a personal relationship; they were simply good friends. Having clarified that the relationship between the godfather and mother was only friendly, we proceeded to clarify the relationship of godfather to Susan. Susan had grown up to see the godfather as her father. JM asked whether Susan had any affection or love for her godfather and the response was that Susan had treated him as her father. Susan seemed to feel that the godfather was like a father to her from the time that she attended kindergarten up to the previous year (until she reached the age of 13).

JM proceeded to explore further the nature of this "daughter-to-substitute-father" relationship. It seemed that up to the time of the incident at work, there was considerable affection toward him. The godfather was also providing for her and attending to her emotional needs. Her godfather was injured when Susan was about 12 years old. JM inquired about the nature of godfather's accident. It was not clear whether he had a brain injury as part of the accident or if it was only the other systems that were involved in this serious event. It was understood that he needed intensive care and that he had multiple intubations. The object of this line of questioning was exploring any association between the godfather's change of behavior with any possible brain injury. One would expect a lower tolerance of frustration, dysthymia, and greater impulsivity following a serious brain injury. JM also asked if there was any cognitive loss and, in particular, any difficulty in concentrating, focusing, and maintaining attention. From the psychological point of view, the accident meant that the godfather had not been able to return to work and financially he had to depend on Susan's mother. JM pointed out that godfather's status in the family must have changed since the accident. As a result of this change of status, his relationship with Susan would have changed as well since the accident, and instead of a source of support and care, he became a burden to the family. The accident had consequently meant that Susan lost an important source of support.

JM then asked if it was known why her mother remained unmarried after the relationship with Susan's father ended. This was unclear. The doctor explained that Susan's mother was not keen to divulge further information on this subject.

JM then asked if the impression was that Susan was getting warmth from her godfather but only expectations and criticism from mother and that her mother's expectations were harsh and that she was punitive if her expectations were not met. The doctor confirmed this. JM asked if her mother's expectations were proportional to Susan's abilities or was her mother expecting way above what was reasonable. The doctor responded that Susan was a bright girl who ranked first among 100 in her class and she only reduced her ranking to 20th when she became emotionally troubled. In the process of this consultation, it was clarified that mother did not have expectations of the girl that were beyond the girl's ability.

JM then diverted the focus on to Susan's expectations of herself. The doctor stated that Susan also expected to excel to the same level as her mother expected. Susan attributed her reduced performance to increased anxiety. The doctor clarified that the anxiety was about being abducted. JM then suggested that the anxieties were in the psychotic range and were not related in any understandable way to the anxiety that most children have before exams. The same fear of being abducted caused Susan to insist that she be accompanied to school by her mother. Susan did not explain why she felt she would be the target of abduction. She also had some doubts whether these thoughts were real but still insisted that her mother accompany her to school because she found mother's presence as "soothing." It was clarified that during the time of consultation Susan was still an inpatient at the psychiatric unit.

JM then proceeded to agree with the diagnosis of early onset psychosis and advised great caution in making psychoanalytic interpretations of this girl. The doctor clarified that there was no family history of psychiatric illness other than maternal depression. JM pointed out that it would be difficult to explain the onset of psychosis in Susan purely on environmental and psychoanalytical grounds.

Having accepted that there are biological factors contributing to the development of this Susan's psychosis, environmental factors should be examined to gain a fuller picture. Her early life was not optimal because she was brought up by a lone parent, had lost her father (and we know little about his input after the separation from her mother), and had a godfather who played a part as a part-parent without having a relationship with her mother. JM then suggested that it would be helpful for the direction of support to be toward making it possible for her to accept that grades other than the top 1% could be good enough for her. For example, achieving a rating of being in the top 20%, considering all the circumstances, is quite a good outcome. JM pointed out that the top 20% of people can be educated at university and can have a professional career. It is not as if 20% is a disaster, although it does represent a loss if her original expectations were of being placed in the top 1%. JM then suggested that the reason for not accepting a 20% ranking should be sought in mother's criticism, which later became self-criticism. Having adopted her mother's attitude toward herself, Susan needs now to be helped to adopt a more mature and balanced expectation for herself. One form of restoring her self-respect would be for her to believe that achieving a 20% ranking, despite the serious illness that she has, is an achievement that she can be proud of.

JM then suggested that there may be unhelpful dynamics prevalent in the idiosyncratic family relationships with the mother, the godfather, and Susan. JM suggested that further understanding be obtained about the godfather's financial status. The assumption is that if someone is injured at work, then the employer would bear some responsibility for the injury and that the employing company would have a budget to compensate its employees who are injured while at work. Therefore, the godfather relying on the mother's budget remains a puzzle that needs to be solved. The godfather would normally be able to contribute to the family expenses by drawing funds from his compensation.

JM pointed out that the godfather had to cope not only with the physical injury and the reduction of physical ability but also with the loss of status and the loss of a prospect of employment when he is too young to be retired and possibly too old and impaired to find a new job. The godfather's predicament gives a justifiable cause for serious concern. Faced with such a predicament, one can understand why the godfather would be irritable and short-tempered. One would expect that such a change in his psychological makeup would have an impact on Susan who previously had a positive relationship with him.

JM then focused on the possibilities of treatment. He gave a word of caution about using too intrusive or dynamic psychology interpretations. The treatment package should necessarily include medication, a large element of support in the sense of helping Susan regain some self-esteem based on the reality of her abilities and some sense of self-worth (despite the serious difficulties).

Susan needs to be helped to move on in her life despite these difficulties. One example is how she was able to make progress toward attending school by recruiting mother as her escort for the journey to school. Susan may need to be shown that there are ways of overcoming or bypassing the difficulties imposed on her life by her mental state or by her illness.

JM spent a little time explaining the link between performance and arousal. Too low and too high arousal leads to poor performance with the best performance being when a person is appropriately keyed up for the task. Susan ran the risk of being too highly aroused and, as a result, underperforming. Susan can be told that she should not have an expectation of herself to perform in a same way that she would have had she not been troubled by her illness. She should be proud for what she manages to achieve despite it. Susan needs to make some accommodation of her expectations considering her mental illness.

Antipsychotic medication does have an effect on the level of arousal, and for this reason, the level of medication needs to be monitored and regulated closely. It was clarified that Susan is currently on Abilify (aripiprazole). The doctor explained that olanzapine had been tried previously but it made her tired and she had put weight on, so it was changed. JM confirmed that Susan was in the right environment and on the right medication.

JM then focused on the need for such patients to have a sense of continuity of care. As this continuity is unlikely to be provided by individual doctors, who rotate between posts and move on to other parts of their training, Susan and her family need to be reassured that the institution will offer continuity. That means that she should be sure that the hospital will always be there for her and will always accept her as a patient and she will always be able to get the best possible treatment from the hospital even though the individual personnel will change. (For the matter of patients' relationship to a treating institution, see Safirstein [1967]).

A girl who had experienced a father to whom she could not rely on because he disappeared, and a godfather to whom she cannot rely on because he equally disappeared in a different way, she would be particularly vulnerable to fears of being abandoned by the treatment team. Susan needs to be helped to have realistic expectations so that she is not disappointed when she finds that the individual doctors are no longer available for her. JM mentioned that the paranoid fear of being abducted may be related to her fear of being abandoned. Such an explanation may account for why Susan feels more secure in the presence of her mother, particularly on the way to school.

Reference

Safirstein, S. L. (1967). Institutional transference. *The Psychiatric Quarterly*, 41(3), 557–566.

19

Forensic: Shoplifting

Antonia

Presenting condition

Antonia, a single, 27-year-old woman, worked as an executive assistant at a university in the city and lived with her family in a public housing unit. Antonia was first seen in the outpatient clinic for a medical report in relation to a charge of theft.

History of present complaint

Antonia is new to public mental health service. She had been known to a private psychiatric service since 2016.

Regarding the index offense, Antonia reported that the day of theft in 2017 was her last date of contract at work because she was dismissed, having not been able to pass the probation period. She had no work that day because she needed to clear up some annual leave, but that day was her last official date. She was in a poor mental state because of the dismissal, her mood was low, and she had had slept poorly for few days. She suddenly recalled she had a ticket to visit Disneyland, so she decided to go alone. She felt irritable in the crowded area, so she went into a souvenir shop. Throughout this time, she was ruminating about her failures at work and other past unhappy events. She was tearful and walked aimlessly. The next thing she could recall clearly was that she had already been stopped by a security guard around 100 meters outside the souvenir shop. She recalled the guard asked her about the souvenir bag and she did not know what the guard was talking about, and only realized she was carrying the souvenir bag when the guard pointed to the bag she was holding. She reported she could not recall any of the process of putting the cartoon badges inside the bag initially, but after repeated statements she made, she could recall vaguely some of the pieces.

Antonia reported she did not steal the badges intentionally. She denied acting under any influence of a perceptual disturbance, alcohol, or illicit substance during the index offense. She liked going to Disneyland but reported no habit of collecting Disneyland cartoon accessories. The badges were of no use to her.

She had no financial debts and had no history of pathological gambling.

Family history

Antonia reported to have a family history of mental illness; her maternal aunt had been diagnosed with depression, and her mother was suffering from long-term depressive symptoms.

Personal history

Antonia was born in the city and was second of four siblings. Her paternal grandmother was her main carer when she was young. She had a distant relationship with her parents but was close to her siblings and paternal relatives with whom she lived.

Antonia was under a lot of pressure from a young age because her family had high expectations on her academic achievements. Her three other siblings had a smooth academic path, whereas Antonia had considerable difficulty in catching up, despite being hardworking. She needed to repeat a year during primary school one. She gained 12–13 out of 30 marks in the end of secondary education examinations. She then completed 2 years of an associate degree (business) at the city Polytechnic university, and this was followed by a BBA in accounting at a management college. She was currently in year one at the education university of the city (master of education) part-time.

Antonia had worked briefly as an accountant and administrative assistant but could not sustain or pass the probation period because she could not meet the work standard on each occasion. She started her last job in October 2017 as an executive assistant in the education university of the city and was earning US$1,740 a month.

Antonia is single and has been in a stable courtship with her boyfriend for 3 years. They planned to get married in 2020. She is a nonsmoker and nondrinker. She is not religious.

Past psychiatric history

Antonia was known to a private mental health service since 2016. She had presented with low mood and anxiety. However, her mood problem could be dated back to the time she was studying in secondary school. She had developed a habit of pulling her hair when she felt frustrated and anxious; this resulted in baldness, and she had to wear a wig. She had the ongoing habit of hair pulling (trichotillomania). She was also reported to have poor emotional regulation and poor temper control since she was young, and she tended to have temper outbursts at home.

Antonia presented in 2016 with low mood, anxiety, and poor sleep for 2 to 3 years. This was precipitated by work stress because she could barely meet the work requirement and standard. Her mood had become depressed, which was associated with poor sleep, loss of interest, lack of energy level, poor concentration, and a chronic headache. Antonia also had increased anxiety, with hair pulling, and some obsessive features including checking and lining things in an orderly way.

Antonia reported that her first incident of stealing was in 2016. She stole a few bottles of lotion from a department store. That day, she had failed an exam despite putting in a great effort and taking a week of leave from work to study. She felt ashamed and upset because most of her class passed. She walked aimlessly in the streets afterward. She then went into a department store and stole the lotion. She reported that she had not realized that she was stealing and could not recall the process at all.

Antonia started to visit a private psychiatrist in December 2016 after the theft incident. She had been attending monthly follow ups. She had been prescribed an unknown psychiatric medication for anxiety and sleep.

Present Management of Case   Antonia was polite and timid. She was tense and was wriggling with a slip of paper in her hand. Her mood was anxious and depressed. Her affect was congruent. Her speech was relevant and coherent. No formal thought disorder was noted. She was forthcoming with her history. She burst into tears a few times when she talked about her frustration in repeated failures at school and work. She had the negative cognition of uselessness. There were no hallucinations or delusions. She had no ideas of self-harm or harming others. She had preserved insight of her mental illness, and she readily received follow up treatment because she realized the consequences of her poor mental state.

Antonia was diagnosed with mixed anxiety and depressive disorder, as well as trichotillomania.

She had undergone a critical event on day of the offense because she had been dismissed from work. She was depressed and anxious and was preoccupied with negative thoughts. She stressed that she had no intention of stealing during the index offense.

Together with the similar pattern of her past thefts, she was thought to be suffering from episodes of dissociation fugue, which was thought to be a defense against trauma and that this defense helped her to disconnect from extreme psychological distress and to escape an environment that she saw as threatening or intolerable to her.

Her condition was thought to have been based on the following predisposing factors: Insecure attachment, a nonvalidating environment, high expectations from her family, comparison with siblings, poor academic performance, limited academic ability, and low self-esteem. The following perpetuating factors were identified: tendency to set high standards for herself and an excessive effort to study and work. The precipitating factors were the critical events of failing an examination and being dismissed from work.

Antonia had been prescribed an antidepressant and was offered psychological treatment aimed at exploring her inner and interpersonal patterns of handling stressful situations, conflicts, and moods that precipitated the fugue states so to prevent subsequent fugue behaviors, explore core beliefs, and develop healthy coping skills that would help her to manage stress and psychological pain more effectively.

Consultation   At first JM congratulated the doctor for the thoroughness of the presentation. The doctor explained that Antonia decided to accept treatment, including a health service psychologist and to take the advice of the public health psychiatrist to use medication on regularly and not on an as-required basis.

JM then asked if the doctor had identified a trauma or traumata that Antonia had experienced in her childhood. The doctor pointed out that Antonia had been brought up not by her parents but by her paternal relatives and that she has had numerous carers. Regarding her parents, they were absent figures when she was young, but later, their influence was that of expressing high expectations of her. The overall impression was that her attachments were insecure. The doctor felt that Antonia was brought up in an environment that did not validate her. The doctor also felt that Antonia was less intellectually able than her siblings, and despite this, her family expected of her to achieve as well as her more able siblings. The doctor believed that this experience undermined her self-esteem. JM stated how impressed he was with the thoroughness of the formulation and the traumata that this lady experienced when growing up in this family.

JM then summarized the doctor's formulation as follows: Antonia was not brought up in a supportive environment, the environment was not constant, the only influence that she had was that of unrealistically high expectations, these expectations could not be met, and comparing herself with her siblings left her feeling a "lesser person." JM then added that her emotional lability could be understood on the basis that she did not have the internal strength to contain her feelings but neither did she have any external support to do so.

JM then asked what Antonia's treatment plan was. JM explained that the dissociation that Antonia was experiencing and expressing was a manifestation of her difficulty in dealing with trauma because she had neither a solid sense of her own value nor support from her environment. The doctor explained that one of the objectives of therapy would be to build up her self-esteem. The doctor intended on working with her to build her self-esteem on her realistic abilities. JM acknowledged that Antonia needs to develop a positive sense of self based on a realistic self-esteem. To value the abilities of herself and not only to see herself as a person who is lesser than her siblings or other people. If her expectations are adjusted to be near her potential, she stands a reasonable chance of succeeding and, therefore, developing a positive view of herself. JM pointed out that Antonia's performance throughout her school years was problematic or at least lower than that of her siblings. Although a psychological assessment would have been desirable, for pragmatic reasons one can plan her therapy based on studying her academic track record.

JM then pointed out that by simply advising her to set realistic targets for career and performance may not be enough because her emotional basis her core belief is that of her relationships with her parents and her siblings. If she is to develop new core beliefs, these need to arise out of new relationships, which will be emotionally significant to her. Such a new relationship is that which she will develop with her psychiatrist or psychotherapist. Although these professionals need to maintain the professional distance, they are nevertheless human, and their relationship is a human-to-human relationship. Based on such a significant relationship does Antonia stand a chance of basing new views about herself that are in contrast to those that she built on the basis of her relationships with her family.

The new emotional experience is the experience of receiving therapy. JM repeated the point that psychotherapy differs from counseling or advice giving because it is based on a real, professional but, nevertheless, significant relationship between therapist and patient. JM then gave an example how Antonia may be feeling about herself: "I will only be valued if I achieve as much as my siblings." This needs to be changed to: "I will value myself on the basis of what I can realistically achieve and what I can realistically offer to others." This new attitude will help her to overcome the shame that she was feeling at not being as successful as her siblings. JM pointed out that the symptoms of stealing, pulling her hair, and the emotional lability are the result of her being unable to cope with additional traumata (derived from failures or threats of failures) to her already vulnerable self-esteem.

If therapy is successful and she develops realistic expectations for herself, then she is more likely to engage in activities (such as having a job) that are within her capacity and, therefore, she is more likely to succeed. This success will in turn build her self-esteem further. What I described was a virtuous circle that would replace the vicious circle in which she was trapped.

JM then asked if the boyfriend is somebody who really loves Antonia and if he could be recruited to be an ally in the effort to construct a healthy and more positive self-esteem for Antonia, that is, if he is somebody who loves and appreciates her.

For an excellent overview of the problem of shoplifting see the commentary of Professor Gibbens (1981), and for a more focused study of the link with anxiety and depression, see Lamontagne et al. (2000)

References

Gibbens, T. C. N. (1981). Shoplifting. *British Journal of Psychiatry, 138*(4), 346–347.

Lamontagne, Y., Boyer, R., Hétu, C. I. L. L., & Lacerte-Lamontagne, C. (2000). Anxiety, significant losses, depression, and irrational beliefs in first-offence shoplifters. *The Canadian Journal of Psychiatry, 45*(1), 63–66.

Index

Dynamic Consultations with Psychiatrists: Understanding Severely Troubled Patients, First Edition. Jason Maratos.
© 2022 John Wiley & Sons Ltd. Published 2022 by John Wiley & Sons Ltd.